A Clinical Guide for Management of Overweight and Obese Children and Adults

CRC Series in Modern Nutrition Science

Series Editor

Stacey J. Bell

Ideasphere, Inc.
Grand Rapids, Michigan

Phytopharmaceuticals in Cancer Chemoprevention
Edited by Debasis Bagchi and Harry G. Preuss

Handbook of Minerals as Nutritional Supplements
Robert A. DiSilvestro

Intestinal Failure and Rehabilitation: A Clinical Guide
Edited by Laura E. Matarese, Ezra Steiger, and Douglas L. Seidner

Nutrition and Wound Healing
Edited by Joseph A. Molnar

A Clinical Guide for Management of Overweight and Obese Children and Adults
Edited by Caroline M. Apovian and Carine M. Lenders

A Clinical Guide for
Management of Overweight and Obese Children and Adults

EDITED BY
Caroline M. Apovian
Carine M. Lenders

CRC Press
Taylor & Francis Group
Boca Raton London New York

CRC Press is an imprint of the
Taylor & Francis Group, an informa business

Cover design by Sherman Bigornia, MS and Wen Guo, PhD.

CRC Press
Taylor & Francis Group
6000 Broken Sound Parkway NW, Suite 300
Boca Raton, FL 33487-2742

Printed in the United States of America on acid-free paper
10 9 8 7 6 5 4 3 2 1

International Standard Book Number-10: 0-8493-3085-8 (Hardcover)
International Standard Book Number-13: 978-0-8493-3085-8 (Hardcover)

Library of Congress Cataloging-in-Publication Data

Obesity and overweight : a clinical guidebook / editor(s), Caroline M. Apovian, Carine M. Lenders.
p. ; cm. -- (CRC series in modern nutrition science)
Includes bibliographical references and index.
ISBN-13: 978-0-8493-3085-8 (alk. paper)
ISBN-10: 0-8493-3085-8 (alk. paper)
1. Obesity. I. Apovian, Caroline M. II. Lenders, Carine M. III. Series.
[DNLM: 1. Obesity--therapy. 2. Adolescent. 3. Adult. 4. Obesity--surgery. WD 210 O112185 2006]

RC628.O24 2006
616.3'98--dc22 2006018582

Visit the Taylor & Francis Web site at
http://www.taylorandfrancis.com

and the CRC Press Web site at
http://www.crcpress.com

Introduction: Obesity as Realm for the Physician Nutrition Specialist

Caroline M. Apovian and Carine M. Lenders

RATIONALE FOR THIS GUIDEBOOK

Overweight and obesity have approached concerning proportions in both adults and children in the U.S. [1,2] and worldwide [3]. The trend in prevalence is steadily rising each year, with no plateau in sight. While efforts to combat this trend range from targeting the individual to community and public health programs, the clinician has an important role to play in treating the obese patient as provider and coach, for both medical and surgical treatments. Obesity significantly increases the risk of morbidity and mortality from hypertension, dyslipidemia, type 2 diabetes, heart failure, stroke, and coronary artery disease. Excess fat mass is strongly linked to insulin resistance, and 70% of diabetes risk in the U.S. is directly attributed to increased weight. Poor diet and physical inactivity are now second only to smoking as the leading preventable causes of death in the U.S. With an estimated 65% of adults and 31% of children considered overweight and obese, an unprecedented number of individuals are exposed to increased cardiovascular risk.

These statistics highlight the fact that obesity is one of the most common chronic diseases seen by primary care clinicians. It is estimated that 11% of the U.S. population are seen every month in the primary care office and that overweight or obese patients are over-represented in this patient population [4–6]. The U.S. Preventive Services Task Force recommends periodic height and weight measurements for all adult patients in addition to counseling to encourage physical activity and healthy diet practices [7]. While the U.S. Preventive Services Task Force concluded that the evidence was insufficient to recommend routine screening for overweight in children and adolescents [8], the American Academy of Pediatrics and the Expert Committee from the Maternal and Child Health Bureau, Health Resources and Services Administration as well as the Committee on Prevention of Obesity in Children and Youth from the Institute of Medicine [9–11], do recommend using the body mass index to follow the weight status of children and adolescents. Despite these recommendations, less than 45% of adult and pediatric obese patients received any prior advice from a physician to lose weight [12,13].

An analysis of over 55,000 adult physician office visits sampled in the 1995–1996 National Ambulatory Medical Care Survey revealed that physicians reported obesity in only 8.6% of all patient office visits, a rate significantly lower than the 22.7% obesity prevalence rates for the same time period [15]. Likewise, obesity was identified by only half of the clinicians in a study of 2515 pediatric visits (n=244) [16]. The identification of obesity was affected by the age of the patient and the degree of obesity: rates were lowest among preschool children (31%) and highest among adolescents (76%). One study also reported that less than 10% pediatric clinicians followed all recommendations for history and physical examination [17].

The low rate of identification and treatment of obesity by physicians appears to be due to several factors that are commonly noted as barriers to adherence to practice guidelines. These include lack of awareness, lack of familiarity, lack of agreement, lack of self-efficacy, lack of outcome expectancy, inertia of previous practice, and external factors [18]. For example, some physicians may believe that counseling patients to lose weight is futile because long-term studies show a high rate of recidivism in patients who do manage to lose weight. In a study of 444 registered dietitians, 202 pediatricians, and 293 primary care nurse practitioners, pediatric clinicians were concerned about pediatric obesity and associated complications and felt that intervention was important, although several barriers interfered with treatment efforts [18–20]. The barriers identified by these clinicians were lack of parent involvement, lack of patient motivation, lack of support services, and self-reported low proficiency in counseling-related skills needed to manage pediatric obesity effectively. Despite the movement towards including more nutrition education in medical school curricula which led the National Heart, Lung, and Blood Institute (NHLBI) in 1997 to create the Nutrition Academic Award Program (NAA) [21], it is still insufficient, and physicians may still feel inadequately prepared to offer diet and physical activity counseling (especially in pediatrics), and do not feel successful in helping their patients make these changes [18–20,22]. Findings from these studies provide priorities for training, education, and advocacy efforts.

This book is designed to be a guide for the primary care clinician and the specialist who are interested in providing a comprehensive weight management program to their patients in need. We do not feel however, that this guidebook is all that is required to combat the nutritional glut this country seems to be in. Major changes in policy are required to modify the toxic environment we live in and to provide the resources, counseling and reimbursement capacity that physicians, nurse practitioners, psychologists, physical therapists/exercise physiologists, and dieticians need to treat obesity.

Several authors have called for nutrition as a subspecialty in both adult and pediatric medicine [23–26]. There seems to be no more poignant time than now for physician nutrition specialists. There are too few of us currently to make a difference; however the wheels are in motion with the founding of the Intersociety Professional Nutrition Education Consortium and the American Board of Physician Nutrition Specialists [23–27] and the support from societies such as the American Society for Nutrition and NAASO—the Obesity Society. We have observed an increase in physicians taking the Nutrition Boards each year, and what is lacking to continue this momentum is the inclusion of more nutrition fellowship training programs in the U.S., and eventually recognition by the American Board of Medicine. With 65% of adults and 31% of children considered overweight or obese in the U.S., many physicians are interested in learning the tools they need to treat this overwhelming disease. Isn't it time to take another look at a nutrition subspeciality in medicine and pediatrics?

REFERENCES

1. Flegal, K.M., Carroll, M.D., Ogden, C.L., Johnson, C.L., Prevalence and trends in obesity among US adults, 1999–2000, *JAMA* 288, 1723–1727, 2002.
2. Hedley, A.A., Ogden, C.L., Johnson, C.L., Carroll, M.D., Curtin, L.R., Flegal, K.M., Prevalence of overweight and obesity among US children, adolescents, and adults, 1999-2002. *JAMA* 291, 2847–2850, 2004.
3. Kim, S., Popkin, B.M., Commentary: understanding the epidemiology of overweight and obesity — a real global public health concern, *Int. J. Epidemiol.* 35, 60–67, 2006.
4. Green, L.A., Fryer, G.E., Jr, Yawn, B.P., Lanier, D., Dovey, S.M., The ecology of medical care revisited, *N. Engl. J. Med.* 344, 2021–2025, 2001.
5. Noel, M., Hickner, J., Ettenhofer, T., Gauthier, B., The high prevalence of obesity in Michigan primary care practices. An UPRNet study. Upper Peninsula Research Network, *J. Fam. Pract.* 47, 39–43, 1998.
6. Orzano, A.J., Scott, J.G., Diagnosis and treatment of obesity in adults: an applied evidence-based review, *J. Am. Board Fam. Pract.* 17, 359–369, 2004.
7. McTigue, K.M., Harris, R., Hemphill, B., Lux, L., Sutton, S., Bunton, A.J., Lohr, K.N., Screening and interventions for obesity in adults: summary of the evidence for the U.S. Preventive Services Task Force, *Ann. Intern. Med.* 139(11), 933–949, 2003.
8. U.S. Preventive Services Task Force, Screening and interventions for overweight in children and adolescents: recommendation statement, *Pediatrics* 116(1), 205–209, 2005.
9. American Academy of Pediatrics. Overweight and Obesity: AAP recommendations. Elk Grove Village, IL: American Academy of Pediatrics; 2003. Available at www.aap.org/obesity/recommendations.htm. Accessed April 1, 2006.
10. Barlow, S.E., Dietz, W.H., Obesity evaluation and treatment: Expert Committee recommendations, *Pediatrics* 102, 29–40, 1998. Available at: www.pediatrics.org/cgi/content/full/102/3/e29 Accessed April 1, 2006.
11. Koplan, J.P., Liverman, C.T., Kraak, V.I., *Preventing Childhood Obesity: Health in the Balance.* 2005. National Academies Press: Washington, DC. Available at http://www.iom.edu/?id=25048 Accessed April 1, 2006.
12. Galuska, D.A, Will, J.C., Serdula, M.K., Ford, E.S., Are health care professionals advising obese patients to lose weight? *JAMA* 282, 1576–1578, 1999.
13. Sciamanna, C.N., Tate, D.F., Lang, W., Wing, R.R., Who reports receiving advice to lose weight? Results from a multistate survey, *Arch. Intern. Med.* 160, 2334–2339, 2000.
14. Barlow S.E., Trowbridge F.C., Klish W.J., Dietz W.H. Treatment of children and adolescent obesity: reports from pediatricians, pediatric nurse practitioners, and registered dietitians. *Pediatrics*, 110, 229–235, 2002.
15. Stafford, R.S., Farhat, J.H., Misra, B., Schoenfeld, D.A., National patterns of physician activities to obesity management, *Arch. Fam. Med.* 9, 631–638, 2000.
16. O'Brien, S.H., Holubkov, R., Reis, E.C., Identification, evaluation, and management of obesity in an academic primary care center, *Pediatrics* 114(2), e154–e159, 2004.
17. Barlow, S.E., Dietz, W.H., Klish, W.J., Trowbridge, F.L., Medical evaluation of overweight children and adolescents: reports from pediatricians, pediatric nurse practitioners, and registered dietitians, *Pediatrics* 110(1 Pt 2), 222–228, 2002.

18. Story, M.T., Neumark-Stzainer, D.R., Sherwood, N.E., Holt, K., Sofka, D., Trowbridge, F.L., Barlow, S.E., Management of child and adolescent obesity: attitudes, barriers, skills, and training needs among health care professionals, *Pediatrics* 110 (1 Pt 2), 210–214, 2002.
19. Perrin, E.M., Flower, K.B., Garrett, J., Ammerman, A.S., Preventing and treating obesity: pediatricians' self-efficacy, barriers, resources, and advocacy, *Ambul. Pediatr.* 5(3), 150–156, 2005.
20. Kolagotla L., Adams W. Ambulatory management of childhood obesity. *Obes. Res.* 12(2), 275–283, 2004.
21. NAA National Site. http://www.nhlbi.nih.gov/funding/training/naa/index.htm. Accessed April 1, 2006.
22. Ammerman, A.S., DeVellis, R.F., Carey, T.S., Keyserling, T.C., Strogatz, D.S., Haines, P.S., Simpson, R.J., Siscovick, D.S., Physician-based diet counseling for cholesterol reduction: current practices, determinants, and strategies for improvement, *Prev. Med.* 22, 96–109, 1993.
23. Kushner, R.F., Will there be a tipping point in medical nutrition education? *Am. J. Clin. Nutr.* 77, 288–291, 2003.
24. Heimburger, D.C., Physician-nutrition-specialist track: if we build it will they come? Intersociety Professional Nutrition Education Consortium, *Am. J. Clin. Nutr.* 71, 1048–1053, 2000.
25. McLaren, D.S., The need for physician nutrition specialists, *Am. J. Clin. Nutr.* 62, 446–447, 1995.
26. MacLean, W.C., Lucas, A., Pediatric nutrition: a distinct subspecialty. In: Walker W, Watkins J, Duggan C, Eds. *Nutrition in Pediatrics: Basic Science and Clinical Applications*, 3rd ed. B.C. Decker, 2003.
27. Intersociety Professional Nutrition Education Consortium (IPNEC). http://ipnec.org. Accessed April 1 2006.

Preface

A Clinical Guide for Management of Overweight and Obese Children and Adults originated from our perception of a need for a reference that offered a distinction between childhood and adult obesity and addressed both in a practical fashion for the busy health care provider. This guidebook is a collaborative effort edited by adult and pediatric nutrition specialists and reflects our experiences treating obesity in our respective domains.

In this reference, you, the practitioner, will find helpful information on assessment and treatment for simple overweight to complex severe obesity with multiple comorbidities. Treatment modalities range from lifestyle change to bariatric surgery. The core management strategy for any modality of treatment is the weight maintenance phase, and hence much attention has been placed on maintenance strategies and follow-up of the weight management patient.

In keeping with the emergence of a new discipline called "obesity medicine," we start with getting the office ready for the particular needs of this patient population. One of the most important first steps is making sure patients feel comfortable in your office even before seeing you, be it an academic hospital setting or private practice. Your entire staff should be well prepared to ensure that the environment is welcoming to this patient population. Assessment strategies are covered including psychological tools, as is the core prescription of nutrition and physical activity with a focus on behavior change. Pharmacotherapeutic options and surgical options are explored.

We consider *A Clinical Guide for Management of Overweight and Obese Children and Adults* to be a review of state-of-the-art management of this burgeoning disease state. We dedicate this book to the millions of people worldwide who suffer the devastating psychological and physical consequences of obesity, especially the children.

Caroline M. Apovian, M.D.

Carine M. Lenders, M.D., M.S.

Editors

Carine M. Lenders, M.D., M.S. is chief of the Division of Pediatric Nutrition at Boston Medical Center, where she directs two programs: the Nutrition and Fitness for Life program (pediatric weight management program) and Pediatric Nutrition Support Services (2003–present). She is attending physician of the Nutrition Support Team at the Children's Hospital of Boston (1998–present). She is assistant professor at the Boston University School of Medicine since 2004 and is also on faculty at the Harvard School of Medicine (1998–present). She is an active member of multiple national and local obesity and nutrition committees.

Dr. Lenders is the recipient of the *Ninth Physician Nutrition Specialist Award,* a prestigious teaching award (2006, American Society for Nutrition, to advance nutrition education in medical schools and medical practices). Past awards include the *New Investigator Award* (1993, Society of Adolescent Medicine) for her nutrition research in adolescents and *National Research Service awards* (5T32DK007477-14 [PI: Walker] and 5T32DK007703-07 [PI: Willett]) for her training in gastroenterology and in nutrition.

Dr. Lenders has published many articles, abstracts, and book chapters related to the field of nutrition and health conditions associated with insulin resistance. Her chapter "Nutrition Epidemiology" in *Nutrition in Pediatrics: Basic Science and Clinical Applications*, 3rd edition (B.C. Decker; 2003) was described as important and very useful in an article titled "Nutrition in Pediatrics: Basic Science and Clinical Applications" (*JAMA*. 2004; 291(7):885-886).

Her current research interests include the effect of diet and medications on weight gain and conditions associated with obesity. Some of Dr. Lenders' research findings have resulted in press releases, and her work and programs have been featured on the World Wide Web and other media. She serves as a manuscript reviewer of multiple journals and was an external reviewer for the "The Strategic Plan for NIH Obesity Research," National Institute of Health (NIH, 2004) and "Preventing Childhood Obesity: The Health in the Balance," Institute of Medicine (IOM, 2005).

Dr. Lenders is a former family practitioner (1985) with a master's degree in tropical medicine (1986). She graduated with honors from the State University of Liege, Belgium. She spent several months in the Congo with Médecins sans Frontières and three years in Bangladesh at the International Center of Diarrhoeal Diseases and Research, and was a consultant for Project Vietnam, American Academy of Pediatrics California, Chapter 4. She was a fellow in pediatric nutrition from 1991 to 1994 at the Children's Hospital of Philadelphia, a resident in pediatrics at the Massachusetts General Hospital, and a fellow in pediatric gastroenterology (MGH and Children's Hospital of Boston) in a fast-track program from 1994 to 1999. She also served as the codirector of the Optimal Weight for Life program (pediatric weight management program) at the Children's Hospital of Boston from

1998 to 2003. Dr. Lenders is board certified by the American Board of Pediatrics (2000) and the American Board of Physician Nutrition Specialists (2001).

Caroline M. Apovian, M.D., F.A.C.P. is the director of the Nutrition and Weight Management Center and co-director of Nutrition and Metabolic Support Service at Boston University Medical Center. She also serves as Director of Clinical Research at the Obesity Research Center of Boston University Medical Center, and is an associate professor of medicine at Boston University School of Medicine. Dr. Apovian is also a principal investigator for the Centers for Obesity Research and Education in New England. She has been an active member of the Boston Obesity Research Nutrition Center since 2000. She is codirector of a BONRC Core (Human Metabolic and Genetic Core) and serves on its executive committee.

Dr. Apovian was awarded the Physician Nutrition Specialist Award given by the American Society of Clinical Nutrition to advance nutrition education to doctors and medical students

She served as medical director of the Program for Weight Management, Division of Metabolic Support Service, at Brigham and Women's Hospital/Harvard Medical School from 1998 to 2000, and was the Director of Weight Management and Nutritional Medicine at Spence Centers for Women's Health from 1996 to 2000. Prior to moving to Boston, she was the director of the High Risk Obesity Clinic and the director of Nutrition Support Fellowship at the Geisinger Medical Center in Danville, Pennsylvania.

Dr. Apovian has published numerous original papers, abstracts, reviews, and book chapters on nutrition, obesity, and nutrition support in hospitalized patients. Her ongoing research interests include novel medical treatments for obesity, monitoring type 2 diabetes, endothelial cell dysfunction and obesity, and cytokine expression of adipose cells after weight loss treatment in humans. Dr. Apovian serves as manuscript reviewer for several journals including the *New England Journal of Medicine,* the *American Journal of Clinical Nutrition,* and the *Journal of Parenteral and Enteral Nutrition,* as well as serving on the editorial board of *Obesity Research.*

Dr. Apovian serves as nutrition consultant to NASA at the Lyndon B. Johnson Space Center in Houston, Texas. She has been selected to participate in clinical status evaluation workshops to develop the nutrition program for astronauts on future long-term space missions. She is currently serving on the Betsy Lehman Center for Patient Safety and Medical Error Reduction Expert Panel on Weight Loss Surgery for the Massachusetts Department of Public Health.

Dr. Apovian earned her M.D. from the University of Medicine and Dentistry of New Jersey in 1985. She completed her residency in internal medicine at New England Deaconess Hospital from 1985 to 1988, where she was also a fellow in nutrition support from 1989 to 1990.

Contributors

Louis J. Aronne, M.D.
Weill Medical College of Cornell University

Diana Cullum-Dugan, R.D., L.D.
Boston Medical Center
Boston, Massachusetts

Francis A. Farraye, M.D., M.Sc.
Boston University School of Medicine
Boston, Massachusetts

R. Armour Forse, M.D., Ph.D., F.A.C.S.
Creighton University School of Medicine
Omaha, Nebraska

Christopher S. Huang, M.D.
Boston University School of Medicine
Boston, Massachusetts

Nawfal Istfan, M.D.
Boston University School of Medicine
Boston, Massachusetts

John M. Jakicic, Ph.D.
University of Pittsburgh Medical School
Pittsburgh, Pennsylvania

Cheryl Jesuit, H.S., R.D., L.D.N.
Boston Medical Center
Boston, Massachusetts

Robert F. Kushner, M.D.
Feinberg Medical School of Northwestern University
Chicago, Illinois

Shaheen U. Lakhani, Psy.D.
Boston University School of Medicine
Boston, Massachusetts

Stephen Luippold, A.P.R.N.
Boston University School of Pediatrics
Boston, Massachusetts

Angela Marinilli Pinto, Ph.D.
Brown Medical School
Providence, Rhode Island

Margaret Marino, Ph.D.
Boston University School of Medicine
Boston, Massachusetts

Alan F. Meyers, M.D., M.P.H.
Boston University School of Medicine
Boston, Massachusetts

Vivien Morris, M.S., R.D., M.P.H., L.D.N.
Boston University School of Medicine
Boston, Massachusetts

Valerie H. Myers, Ph.D.
Louisiana State University
Baton Rouge, Louisiana

Heather Niemeier, Ph.D.
Brown Medical School
Providence, Rhode Island

Holly Oh, M.D.
Boston University School of Medicine
Boston, Massachusetts

Amy D. Otto, Ph.D., R.D., L.D.N.
University of Pittsburgh School of Medicine
Pittsburgh, Pennsylvania

Judy C.C. Phillips, M.S., R.D.
South End Community Health Center
Boston, Massachusetts

Kristen Polzien, Ph.D.
University of Pittsburgh School of Medicine
Pittsburgh, Pennsylvania

Gita Rao, B.A.
Boston University School of Medicine
Boston, Massachusetts

Timothy M. Rivinus, M.D.
Boston University School of Medicine
Boston, Massachusetts

Gary S. Rose, Ph.D.
Tufts University School of Medicine
Boston, Massachusetts

Donna H. Ryan, M.D.
Louisiana State University
Baton Rouge, Louisiana

Ranjan Sudan, M.D., F.A.C.S.
Creighton University Medical Center
Omaha, Nebraska

Marie Thearle, M.D.
Columbia University Medical Center
New York, New York

Garry Welch, Ph.D.
Bay State Medical Center
Springfield, Massachusetts

Rena R. Wing, Ph.D.
Brown Medical School
Providence, Rhode Island

Alene J. Wright, M.D.
Creighton University Medical Center
Omaha, Nebraska

Table of Contents

1 Getting the Office Ready for the Patient

Robert F. Kushner

CONTENTS

1.1 INTRODUCTION

Obesity is one of the most common chronic medical problems in primary care; over 60% of U.S. adults and 30% of children and adolescents are currently categorized as overweight or obese [1]. Since obesity is associated with an increased risk of multiple health problems, these patients are also more likely to present with silent diseases (e.g., hypertension, type 2 diabetes, or dyslipidemia) or with a variety of complaints requiring further medical attention. Thus, it is important for physicians to routinely identify, evaluate, and treat patients for obesity. However, a review of the medical literature shows that obesity is under-recognized and undertreated in the primary care setting. Studies conducted among patients [2–9] and physicians [10–12] uniformly demonstrate that physicians fail to adequately identify the overweight and mildly obese patient at a stage when early prevention and treatment could be implemented; however, there is greater recognition of the moderately to severely obese patient, particularly when comorbid conditions are present. In general, less than 50% of obese adults are advised to lose weight by health care professionals [2–6]. In a study of over 400 adult patients attending two primary care practices, Potter et al. [5] found that the most common weight loss approach physicians used was to not mention the subject at all — a "don't ask, don't tell" strategy was reported by 61% of the patients.

The failure of health care providers to initiate or intensify therapy when indicated was recently termed *clinical inertia* by Phillips et al. [13]. The low rate of identification and treatment of obesity is likely due to several factors, including lack of training in obesity care, low confidence in the ability to treat and change behaviors, limited time during office visits, competing demands, and inadequate reimbursement [14,15]. In large part, these barriers are representative of the global problem of trying to care for chronically ill patients within an acute care setting. Rather than emphasizing short appointments, brief patient education, rendering a rapid diagnosis, and dispensing a prescription, the chronic care model focuses on relationship-centered communication to create informed, active patients with improved self-management skills [16]. Although the implementation of obesity care at some level can be initiated within any office setting, physicians should not rely on intuition, convenience, and habit to address this problem. Successful treatment will depend on two factors: systematic organization of office-based processes and functions, and physician training in obesity care. The focus of the system comes from organizational theories that promote change by altering the system of care. The emphasis is not on the "bad apple" (i.e., the doctor who does not practice obesity care) but on the "bad system" (i.e., the practice environment that does not facilitate provision of obesity care) [17]. Physicians can be trained through seminars, conferences, workshops, primers, Web sites, and journal articles.

1.2 PERFORMING AN OFFICE-BASED SELF-AUDIT

1.2.1 Retooling the Office for Chronic Care

Several tools are available to assist physicians in evaluating their office practice and systems with regard to preventive and chronic care services. One such tool is Put Prevention Into Practice (PPIP), a national campaign by the Agency for Health Care Policy and Research (AHCPR) to improve the delivery of clinical preventive services such as counseling for health behavior change [18]. The office audit, adapted from PPIP, can be used for assessing current obesity care (Table 1.1). This will help highlight current strengths and deficiencies in the office and focus on targeted information needed to improve obesity care. PPIP identifies key components that can expedite or hinder the care of patients in the office. These include organizational commitment, clinicians' attitudes, staff support, establishing policies and protocols (using simple office tools), and delegating tasks.

Another useful tool is Improving Chronic Illness Care (ICIC), a national program of the Robert Wood Johnson Foundation [19]. Perhaps not surprisingly, the essential elements for improving the care of people with chronic illnesses overlap with the components described by PPIP; these include assistance with self-management, decision support based on guidelines, development of clinical information systems, use of well-designed delivery systems that meet the needs of patients, adoption of a unified organizational philosophy of health care, and involvement of community resources. ICIC provides several useful tools, including a step-by-step manual for improving one's practice, a care model checklist, and a self-assessment of chronic illness care. These tools are excellent resources for initiating and conducting ongoing quality improvement initiatives in obesity care.

TABLE 1.1
Office Audit for Delivery of Office-Based Obesity Care

Do you routinely assess and evaluate patients for overweight and obesity?

What kinds of services or programs do you routinely provide to your overweight patients, e.g., dietary and exercise counseling, group support, referral to a registered dietitian, and use of antiobesity medications?

Are the services or programs recorded in the patient's chart?

What policies and procedures do you have in place for providing obesity care; e.g., all patients have their height, weight, and BMI measured and recorded in their chart, patient readiness is assessed before initiating treatment, and weight loss goals are established and tracked in the progress notes?

What forms, patient handouts, and educational materials are you using?

How does your office environment support or inhibit delivery of obesity care; e.g., sturdy armless chairs, large arm and thigh blood pressure cuffs, large gowns, measuring of body weight in a private setting, and a sensitive and informed office staff?

What functions do staff currently perform in the provision of obesity care; e.g., office nurse obtains weight, height, and BMI; physician's assistant reviews food and activity diaries and medication side effects; and receptionist schedules referral appointments with dietitian and clinical psychologist?

What can you do differently?

Source: Adapted from: *10 Steps: Implementation Guide. Put Prevention into Practice*. Agency for Healthcare Research and Quality, 1998.

Although currently there are few evidence-based interventions that have been shown to specifically improve health professionals' management of obesity [20–22], this chapter reviews the office-based systems that should be considered when caring for the obese patient (Table 1.2). While some practices may need only a small adjustment in their current systems, others may require a deliberate redesign of the entire patient care process. In either case, the ICIC recommends that the system undergo a "PDSA" cycle of evaluation — Plan, Do, Study, Act. By planning, trying,

TABLE 1.2
Office-Based Obesity Care

The physical environment	Accessibility and comfort: stairs, doorways, hallways, restrooms, waiting room chairs and space; magazines and pictures
Equipment	Large adult arm and thigh blood pressure cuffs, large gowns, step stools, weight and height scales, and tape measure
Materials	Educational and behavioral: promoting brochures, pamphlets, and handouts on BMI, obesity-associated diseases, diet, exercise, medications, and surgery
Tools	Previsit questionnaires, BMI chart stamps, body weight flow sheets, food and activity diaries, and pedometers
Protocols	Patient care treatment protocols for return visit schedule, medications, referrals to dietitians, exercise specialists, and psychologists, and commercial programs
Staffing	Team approach to include office nurse, physician assistant, nurse practitioner, health advocate, or educator

observing the results, and acting on what is learned, a systematic method is used for improving the care of the overweight and obese patient population. For practices that choose to adopt a more rigorous and comprehensive approach, a curriculum modeled on that of the National Standards of Diabetes Self-Management Education (DSME) could be developed [23]. The DSME curriculum mandates the development of ten content areas ranging from nutritional and physical activity management, medications, and monitoring, to goal setting, problem solving, and psychological adjustment. However, no national standards of care specifically aimed for obesity management currently exist.

1.3 THE PRACTICE ENVIRONMENT

1.3.1 Tools, Protocols, and Procedures

A significant portion of the time spent in evaluation and treatment of the obese patient can be reduced by the use of tools, protocols, and procedures. Tools assist in patient risk assessment, prompting and tracking of counseling and referral, and education [24]. Perhaps the most commonly used is the questionnaire. A self-administered medical history questionnaire can be mailed to the patient before the initial visit, posted on the Internet for downloading, or completed in the waiting room. Attention to literacy level is important [25]. In addition to standard questions, sections of the form could inquire about past obesity treatment programs, a graphical body weight history (i.e., patients are asked to graph their weight with concurrent life events), current diet and physical activity levels, social support, and goals and expectations. The review-of-systems section can include medical prompts that are more commonly seen among the obese, such as snoring, morning headaches and daytime sleepiness (obstructive sleep apnea), menstrual irregularities, hirsutism and acne (polycystic ovarian syndrome), urinary incontinence, skin fold infections, sexual dysfunction, and symptoms of binge eating disorder. An example of a patient history questionnaire can be obtained from the American Medical Association's Assessment and Management of Adult Obesity: A Primer for Physicians [26]. Adding a question such as, "Are you concerned about your weight?" may help broach the subject with reluctant patients. Additional questions should address readiness to change, to allow a more targeted approach to the multiple facets of obesity care [27].

Obesity is one of the easiest diseases to diagnose since it is based on height and weight measurements [28]. These measurements and determination of body mass index (BMI) are endorsed by multiple societies and organizations for routine screening [29–35]. However, despite the uniformity of these recommendations, the single best strategy to ensure ongoing performance of these measurements is not certain. One approach is to have a laminated BMI table adjacent to the height and weight scale for easy determination and documentation in the patient's chart. BMI tables are available for free from several Internet sites and pharmaceutical companies. Identifying BMI as a fifth vital sign may also increase physician awareness and prompt counseling. This method was successfully used in a recent study on smoking: a smoking status stamp was placed on the patient's chart, alongside blood pressure, pulse, temperature, and respiratory rate data [36]. Use of such prompts, alerts, or other reminders has been shown to significantly increase physician performance in other health maintenance activities as well [37,38]. Once the patient is identified as overweight or obese, printed education tools, such as brochures and pamphlets, can be provided. Food and activity diaries and patient information sheets on a variety of topics such as the U.S. Department of Agriculture (USDA) food guide, deciphering food labels, healthy snacking, dietary fiber, aerobic exercise and resistance training, and dealing with stress can be used to support behavior change and facilitate patient education. Ready-to-copy materials can be obtained from a variety of sources free of charge, such as those found in the USDHHS's Practical Guide [29], or for a minimal fee from other public sites and commercial companies. Additional resources are listed in the section entitled "Selected Internet Resources for Patients" at the end of the chapter. It is useful to have these materials readily available in the examination room at the time of counseling.

Health promotion literature recommends the use of written materials and counseling protocols for more effective and efficient obesity care. In a study of community-based family medicine physicians, Kreuter at el. [39] showed that patients are more likely to reduce smoking, increase physical activity, and limit dairy fat consumption when physician advice is supported by health education materials. In another randomized intervention study by Swinburn et al. [40], a written, goal-oriented exercise prescription in addition to verbal advice was more effective than verbal advice alone in increasing the physical activity level of sedentary individuals over a six-week period. Several exercise assessment and counseling protocols that can be easily incorporated into obesity care have been developed. These include Project PACE (Provider-based Assessment and Counseling for Exercise) [41], ACT (Activity Counseling Trial) [42], and STEP (Step Test Exercise Prescription) [43]. Finally, protocols for various treatment pathways can be established for obtaining periodic laboratory monitoring and referral to allied health professionals, such as registered dietitians, exercise specialists, and clinical psychologists. The USDHHS's Practical Guide provides a treatment algorithm, "A Quick Reference Tool to ACT" (an acronym for Assessment, Classification, and Treatment). The American Medical Association (AMA) [34] and the American Pharmaceutical Association (APA) [44] have also developed treatment algorithms. The treatment algorithm from the National Heart, Lung, and Blood Institute (NHLBI) Clinical Guidelines on the Identification, Evaluation, and Treatment of Overweight and Obesity in Adults [45] is shown in Figure 1.1. Helpful as these and other guidelines are, information on how to apply them in practice is usually missing. This is where physicians need to assess their practice environment and identify tools and protocols to facilitate care.

1.3.2 Accessibility and the Waiting Room

Accessibility to the office is critical for the obese patient. Facility limitations include difficult access from the parking lot or stairs, narrow doors and hallways, and cramped restrooms. These are similar to the problems that patients with other disabilities face

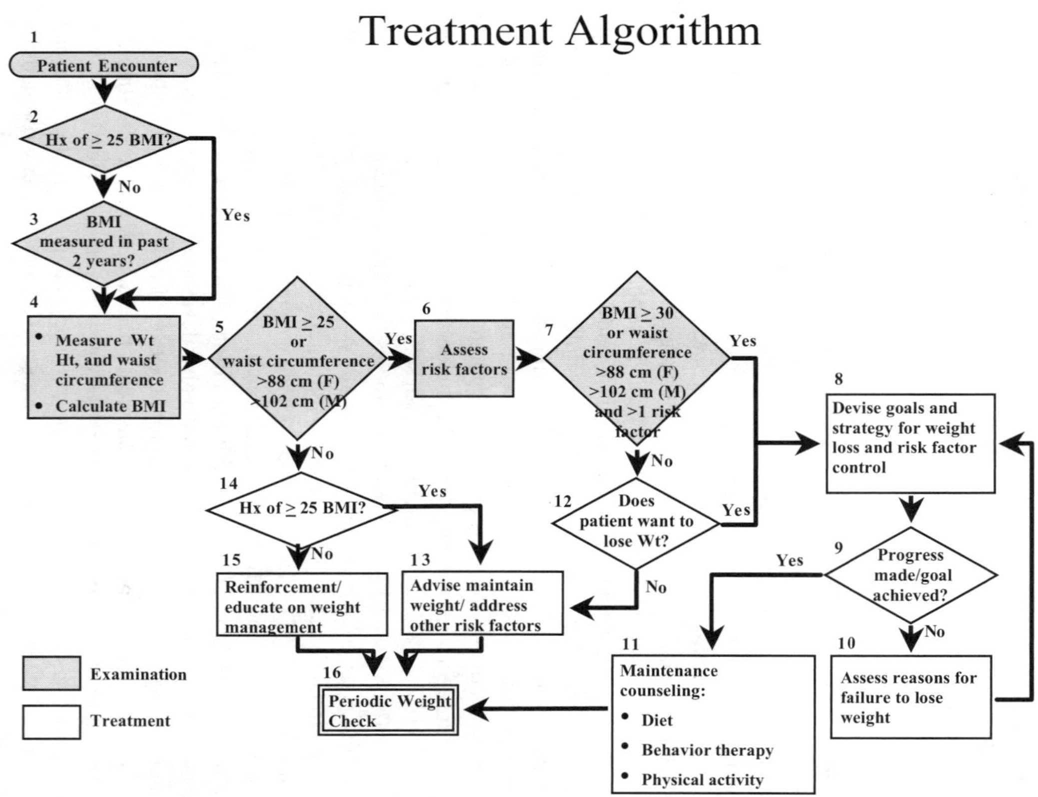

FIGURE 1.1 Treatment algorithm for obesity. (Clinical Guidelines on the Identification, Evaluation, and Treatment of Overweight and Obesity in Adults. National Heart, Lung, and Blood Institute [45].)

and are covered under the regulations of the Americans with Disabilities Act of 1990. The National Association to Advance Fat Acceptance (NAAFA [46]), an advocate group for overweight persons, provides guidelines for health care providers in dealing with obese patients. Recommendations for the waiting room include having several sturdy, armless chairs, with at least 6 to 8 inches of space between them, and firm high sofas if possible. Although often considered insignificant, hanging art, magazines, newspapers, television programs, movies, and billboards that celebrate society's beauty ideals should not find any place in the waiting and examination rooms, as these can convey wrong messages to patients. Magazines, newsletters, and artwork can be chosen that do not contribute to these unattainable images.

1.3.3 Equipment

Accurate measurement of height and weight is vital to treating patients with obesity. All too often, the scale in the physician's office does not measure above 350 lb, or the **foot platform is too narrow to securely balance the overweight individual**. Although a wall-mounted sliding statiometer is best, a firm height meter attached to the scale will suffice. The weight scale should preferably have a wide base with a nearby handle bar for support if necessary. Depending on the patient population, it is reasonable to select a scale that measures in excess of 350 lb. The scale should be placed in such a location **to protect the privacy of the patient and avoid causing embarrassment**.

Examination rooms should be equipped with large-sized gowns as well as a sturdy step stool to mount the examination tables. In addition, adult and large adult thigh blood-pressure cuffs must be available. A bladder cuff inappropriate to the patient's arm circumference will cause a systematic error in blood pressure measurement. The tighter the cuff, the bigger the error — a situation commonly encountered among the obese. It has been demonstrated that the most frequent error in measuring blood pressure is "miscuffing," with undercuffing accounting for 84% of the "miscuffings" [47]. According to an updated American Heart Association (AHA) Scientific Statement on blood pressure measurement, the "ideal" cuff should have a bladder length that is 80% and a width that is at least 40% of arm circumference (a length-to-width ratio of 2:1) [48]. Therefore, a large adult cuff (16 × 36 cm) should be chosen for patients with mild to moderate obesity (or arm circumference 14–17 in) while **an adult thigh cuff** (16 × 42 cm) will need to be used for patients whose arm circumferences are **greater than 17 inches**. In patients whose arm circumferences are very large and upper arms are short, blood pressure can be measured by placing the cuff on the forearm and listening for sounds over the radial artery (although this may overestimate systolic blood pressure). Lastly, a cloth or metal tape should be available for the measurement of waist circumference, as per the NHLBI Practical Guide for Obesity Classification [29].

1.4 USING AN INTEGRATED TEAM APPROACH

How practices operate on a day-to-day basis is extremely important for the provision of chronic disease management. Establishing an integrative team approach is one such strategy [49–50]. Teamwork entails coordination and delegation of tasks between providers and staff [24]. Starfield defines a patient care team as "a group of diverse clinicians who communicate with each other regularly about the care of a defined group of patients and participate in that care" [51]. However, the team should be considered more than the clinical staff — nonclinical staff (customer service, business, managerial) play a role as well. This is addressed in the ICIC component of delivery system redesign that outlines the creation of multidisciplinary teams to create both cooperation and division of labor because no physician alone can improve the care of patients with chronic diseases [19]. Such teams ensure that key elements of care that doctors may not have the training in or time to do well are competently performed [52]. Such team members are often better qualified than the physician to provide the self-management aspects of care — dietary, physical activity, and behavioral counseling, along with scheduling and arranging follow-up. Accordingly, there is an opportunity for other office staff to play a greater role in the care of obese patients. A sense of "groupness," defined as the degree to which the group practice identifies itself and functions as a team, will enhance the quality and efficiency of care [53].

The optimal team composition and management structure will vary between practices. However, as an example of an integrative model, receptionists can provide useful information about the program, including general philosophy, staffing, fee schedules, and other written materials; registered nurses can obtain vital measurements including height and weight (for BMI) and waist circumference, instruction on and review of food and activity journals and other educational materials. Similarly, physician assistants can monitor the progress of treatment and assume many of the other responsibilities of care. Customer service staff could be responsible for flagging charts and inserting prompts, and for patient education materials and reminder calls. A new position of health advocate, whose role is to serve as a resource to the physician and to patients by providing additional information and assisting in arranging recommended follow-up, may be particularly useful [54]. Regardless of how the workload is delegated, the power of the physician's voice should not be underestimated. The physician should be perceived as the team leader and the source of common philosophy of care [32]. According to Crabtree et al. [53], the keys to success include physician commitment and a supportive organizational structure.

1.5 SUMMARY

Effective obesity care will not be accomplished without the implementation of a well-planned, office-based organizational system designed to assess, evaluate, and treat the overweight and obese patient. An office audit (as in Table 1.1) should be useful in triggering quality improvement opportunities in obesity care. Similarly, the chart audit in Table 1.3 can be used to assess current and future practice behavior.

This chapter has reviewed the key office-based components for the delivery of obesity care. Although most of this work focuses on adult obesity, many recommendations may be used for the pediatric office. The strategies and techniques for treatment are addressed in the remaining chapters.

TABLE 1.3
Chart Audit for Obesity Care

	Yes	No	D/N/A
Weight noted in medical record			
Height noted in medical record			
BMI documented in medical record			
Patient weighed on follow-up office visits			
Obesity included on the patient's problem list			
	Yes	**No**	**D/N/A**
Weight loss addressed with overweight/obese patient without existing comorbid medical conditions			
Dietary counseling provided to overweight/obese patient			
Exercise counseling provided to overweight/obese patient			
Weight management provided to patient with a diagnosis of diabetes, hypertension, and/or hyperlipidemia			
Weight loss goal set for overweight/obese patient			
Weight loss counseling provided to overweight/obese patient			
Referral to ancillary staff (dietitians, psychologists, exercise specialists) for obese patient			

Source: Adapted from the Centers for Obesity and Research and Education (CORE).

SELECTED INTERNET RESOURCES FOR PATIENTS

www.collagevideo.com Collage Video sells exercise videos and includes detailed information and reviews to assist in selecting videos based on preferences and physical limitations.

www.eatright.org The American Dietetic Association offers information on nutrition, healthy lifestyle, and how to find a registered dietitian.

www.fitday.com FitDay.com gives nutrition analysis of calories, fat, protein, carbohydrates, and fiber in table and graph form as well as offering journals, and goal-setting and activity-tracking tools.

www.healthetech.com Healthetech offers information on its Palm or Windows software program for personalized weight management.

www.nal.usda.gov/about/oei/index.htm National Heart, Lung, and Blood Institute Obesity Education Initiative offers information on selecting a weight loss program, menu planning, food label reading, and BMI calculation and interpretation.

www.niddk.nih.gov/health/nutrit/win.htm Weight Control Information Network has weight loss articles from the National Institutes of Health.

www.diet.com Subscription-based online program based on personal identification of eating, exercise, and coping lifestyle patterns. Coaching is available by a physician and registered dietitian. Includes interactive boards, chat rooms, recipes, and trackers.

www.eDiets.com Subscription-based online diet, fitness, and counseling network providing a personal profile. Management team consists of licensed dietitians and psychologists.

www.Cyberdiet.com Provides free planning for meals and exercise profile designed by a registered dietitian.

www.Calorieking.com Searchable database of over 40,000 foods. Diet and food tracker.

www.efit.com A free e-newsletter on nutrition tips. Also offers weight loss counseling services by a registered dietitian.

www.WebMD.com Eating plan based on small changes to current reported eating behaviors, food preferences, and lifestyle. Staff includes a registered dietitian and exercise physiologists.

www.obesityhelp.com Information for and by gastric bypass patients, and individuals considering weight loss surgery. All aspects of the surgical process are discussed, including insurance issues, as well as chat rooms and message boards.

REFERENCES

1. Ogden C.L., Carroll, M.D., Curtin L.R., McDowell M.A., Taback, C.J., Flegal, K.M. Prevalence of overweight and obesity in the United States, 1999–2004. *JAMA*, 295, 1549–1555, 2006.
2. Galuska, D.A., Will, J.C., Serdula, M.K., Ford, E.S., Are health care professionals advising obese patients to lose weight?, *JAMA*, 282, 1576, 1999.
3. Nawaz, H., Adams, M.L., Katz, D.L., Weight loss counseling by health care providers, *Am. J. Public Health*, 89, 764–767, 1999.
4. Sciamanna, C.N., Tate, D.F., Lang, W., Wing, R.R., Who reports receiving advice to lose weight? Results from a multistate survey, *Arch. Intern. Med.*, 160, 2334–2339, 2000.
5. Potter, M.B., Vu, J.D., Groughan-Minhane, M., Weight management: what patients want from their primary care physicians, *J. Fam. Prac.*, 50, 513, 2001.
6. Mehrotra, C., Naimi, T.S., Serdula, M., Bolen, J., et al., Arthritis, body mass index, and professional advice to lose weight. Implications for clinical medicine and public health, *Am. J. Prev. Med.*, 27, 16, 2004.
7. Huang, J., Yu, H., Marin, E., Brock, S., et al., Physicians' weight loss counseling in two public hospital primary care clinics, *Acad. Med.*, 79, 156, 2004.
8. Wittchen, B.P., Kirch, P.D., Krause, P., Lehnert, H., et al., Recognition and management of overweight and obesity in primary care in Germany, *Int. J. Obes. Relat. Metab. Disord.*, 28, 1299, 2004.
9. Simin-Silverman, L.R., Gleason, K.A., King, W.C., Weissfeld, L.A., et al., Predictors of weight control advice in primary care practices: patient health and psychosocial characteristics, *Prev. Med.*, 40, 71, 2005.
10. Kristeller, J.L., Hoerr, R.A., Physician attitudes toward managing obesity: differences among six specialty groups, *Prev. Med.*, 26, 542, 1997.
11. Stafford, R.S., Farhat, J.H., Misra, B., Schoenfeld, D.A., National patterns of physician activities to obesity management, *Arch. Fam. Med.*, 9, 631–638, 2000.
12. Block, J.P., DeSalvo, K.B., Fisher, W.P., Are physicians equipped to address the obesity epidemic? Knowledge and attitudes of internal medicine residents, *Prev. Med.*, 36, 669, 2003.

13. Phillips, L.S., Branch, W.T., Cook, C.B., Doyle, J.P., El-Kebbi, I.M., Gallina, D.L., et al., Clinical inertia, *Ann. Intern. Med.*, 135, 825–834, 2001.
14. Hiddink, A., Nutrition guidance by primary care physicians: perceived barriers and low involvement, *Eur. J. Clin. Nutr.*, 49, 842, 1995.
15. Kushner, R.F., Barriers to providing nutrition counseling by physicians. A survey of primary care practitioners, *Prev. Med.*, 24, 546, 1995.
16. Casalino, L.P., Disease management and the organization of physician practice, *JAMA*, 293, 485, 2005.
17. Gross, P.A., Greenfield, S., Cretin, S., Ferguson, J., et al., Optimal methods for guideline implementation. Conclusions from Leeds Castle meeting, *Med. Care*, 8, IIs–855, 2001.
18. 10 Steps: Implementation Guide. Put Prevention into Practice, Adapted from *The Clinicians' Handbook of Preventive Services*, 2nd ed, Publication No. 98-0025, Agency for Healthcare Research and Quality, Rockville, MD, 1998 http://www.ahrq.gov/ppip/ Available at: impsteps.htm.
19. Bodenheimer, T., Wagner, E.H., Grumbach, K., Improving primary care for patients with chronic illness, *JAMA*, 288, 1775, 2002.
20. Harvey, E.L., Glenny, A.M., Kirk, S.F.L., Summerbelt, C.D., A systematic review of interventions to improve health professionals' management of obesity, *Int. J. Obes.*, 23, 1213–1222, 1999.
21. Harvey, E.L., Glenny, A.M., Kirk, S.F.L., Summerbelt, C.D., Improving health professionals' management and the organization of care for overweight and obese people. The Cochrane database of systematic reviews. The Cochrane Library, 2002.
22. The Counterweight Project Team, A new evidence-based model for weight management in primary care: the counterweight programme, *J. Hum. Nutr. Diet.*, 17, 191, 2004.
23. Mensing, C., Boucher, J., Cypress, M., Weinger, K., et al., National standards for diabetes self-management education, *Diabetes Care*, 28, S72, 2005.
24. Dickey, L.L., Gemson, D.H., Carney, P., Office system interventions supporting primary care-based health behavior change counseling, *Am. J. Prev. Med.*, 17(4), 299–308, 1999.
25. Kennen, E.M., Davis, T.C., Huang, J., Yu, H., et al., Tipping the scales: the effect of literacy on obese patients' knowledge and readiness to lose weight, *South. Med. J.*, 98, 15, 2005.
26. Kushner, R.F., Roadmaps for Clinical Practice: Case Studies in Disease Prevention and Health Promotion. American Medical Association, Chicago, IL, 2003. Available at: www.ama-assn.org/ama/pub/category/10931.html.
27. Logue, E., Sutton, K., Jarjoura, D., Smucker, W., Obesity management in primary care: assessment of readiness to change among 284 family practice patients, *J. Am. Board Fam. Pract.*, 13, 164, 2000.
28. Wolf, C., Tanner, M., Obesity, *West. J. Med.*, 176, 23, 2002.
29. The Practical Guide Identification, Evaluation, and Treatment of Overweight and Obesity in Adults. NIH Publication No. 00-4084, U.S. Department of Health and Human Services, Public Health Service, National Institutes of Health, National Heart, Lung, and Blood Institute, 2000.
30. McTigue, K.M., Harris, R., Hemphill, B., Lux, L., Sutton, D., Bunton, A.J., Lohr, K.N., Screening and interventions for obesity in adults. Summary of the evidence for the US Preventive Services Task Force, *Ann. Intern. Med.*, 139, 933–949, 2003.
31. Pearson, T.A., Blair, S.N., Daniels, S.R., Eckel, R.H., Fair, J.M., Fortmann, S.P., et al., AHA guidelines for primary prevention of cardiovascular disease and stroke: 2002 update. Consensus panel guide to comprehensive risk reduction for adult patients

without coronary or other atherosclerotic vascular diseases, *Circulation*, 106, 388–391, 2002.
32. Guzman SE and the American Academy of Family Physicians Panel on Obesity. Practical Advice for Family Physicians to Help Overweight Patients. An American Family Physician Monograph, AAFP, Leawood, KS, 2003. Available at: www.aafp.org/ obesitymonograph.xml. Accessed March 21, 2005.
33. Nawaz, H., Katz, D.L., American College of Preventive Medicine practice policy statement. Weight management counseling of overweight adults, *Am. J. Prev. Med.*, 21(1), 73–78, 2001.
34. Lyznicki, J.M., Young, D.C., Riggs, J.A., Davis, R.M., Obesity: assessment and management in primary care, *Am. Fam. Physician*, 63(11), 2185–2196, 2001.
35. Cummings, G.P., Coulston, A.M., Dalton, S., Hayes, D., Ikeda, J.P., Manore, M., Position of the American Dietetic Association: weight management, *J. Am. Diet. Assoc.*, 102(8), 1145–1155, 2002.
36. Ahluwalia, J.S., Gibson, C.A., Kenney, E., Wallace, D.D., Resnicow, K., Smoking status as a vital sign, *J. Gen. Intern. Med.*, 14, 402–408, 1999.
37. Yano, E.M., Fink, A., Hirsch, S.H., Robbins, A.S., Rubenstein, L.V., Helping practices reach primary care goals. Lessons from the literature, *Arch. Intern. Med.*, 155, 1146–1156, 1995.
38. Balas, E.A., Weingarten, S., Garb, C.T., Blumenthal, D., Boren, S.A., Brown, G.D., Improving preventive care by prompting physicians, *Arch. Intern. Med.*, 160, 301–308, 2000.
39. Kreuter, M.W., Chheda, S.G., Bull, F.C., How does physician advice influence patient behavior? Evidence for a priming effect, *Arch. Fam. Med.*, 9, 426–433, 2000.
40. Swinburn, B.A., Walter, L.G., Arroll, B., Tilyard, M.W., Russell, D.G., The green prescription study: a randomized controlled trial of written advice provided by general practitioners, *Am. J. Pub. Health*, 88, 288–291, 1998.
41. Calfas, K.J., Long, B.J., Sallis, J.F., Wooten, W.J., Fratt, M., Patrick, K., A controlled trial of physician counseling to promote the adoption of physical activity, *Prev. Med.*, 25, 225–233, 1996.
42. Albright, C.L., Cohen, S., Gibbons, L., Miller, S., Marcus, B., Sallis, J., et al., Incorporating physical activity advice into primary care. Physician-delivered advice within the activity counseling trial, *Am. J. Prev. Med.*, 18, 225–234, 2000.
43. Petrella, R.J., Wight, D., An office-based instrument for exercise counseling and prescription in primary care. The step test exercise prescription (STEP), *Arch. Fam. Pract.*, 9, 339–344, 2000.
44. Albrant, D.H., Fernstrom, M.H., Foster, G.D., Jorgensen, A., Kushner, R.F., AphA drug treatment protocols: comprehensive weight management in adults, *J. Am. Pharm. Assoc.*, 41(1), 25–31, 2001.
45. Expert Panel Clinical guidelines on the identification, evaluation, and treatment of overweight and obesity in adults. The evidence report. National, Heart, Lung, and Blood Institute, Public Health Service, U.S. Department of Health and Human Services, 1998.
46. NAAFA: National Association to Advance Fat Acceptance. http://www.naafa.org.
47. Manning, D.M., Kuchirka, C., Kaminski, J., Miscuffing: inappropriate blood pressure cuff application, *Circulation*, 68, 763, 1983.
48. Pickering, T.G., Hall, J.E., Appel, L.J., Falkner, B.E., et al., Recommendations for blood pressure measurement in humans and experimental animals. Part 1: blood pressure measurement in humans. A statement for professionals from the subcommittee of professional and public education of the American Heart Association Council on high blood pressure research, *Circulation*, 111, 697, 2005.

49. Kushner, R.F., Pendarvis, L., An integrated approach to obesity care, *Nutr. Clin. Care*, 2, 285–291, 1999.
50. Frank, A., A multidisciplinary approach to obesity management: the physician's role and team care alternatives, *J. Am. Diet. Assoc.*, 98 (Suppl. 2), S44–S48, 1998.
51. Starfield, B., *Primary Care Concepts, Evaluation, and Policy*, Oxford University Press, New York, 1992.
52. Wagner, E.H., The role of patient care teams in chronic disease management, *BMJ*, 320, 569–572, 2000.
53. Crabtree, B.F., Miller, W.L., Aita, V.A., Flocke, S.A., Stange, K.C., Primary care practice organization and preventive services delivery: a qualitative analysis, *J. Fam. Pract.*, 46(5), 404–409, 1998.
54. Scholle, S.H., Agatisa, P.K., Krohn, M.A., Johnson, J., McLaughlin, M.K., Locating a health advocate in a private obstetrics/gynecology office increases patient's receipt of preventive recommendations, *J. Womens Health Gend. Based Med.*, 9(2), 161–165, 2000.

2 Steps for the Medical Evaluation of the Obese Patient

Nawfal W. Istfan and Wendy A. Anderson

CONTENTS

2.1 INTRODUCTION

The medical evaluation of an obese patient centers on understanding the factors that contribute to the patient's condition and the impact of excessive body fat accumulation on his or her health. These factors can then be taken into consideration when discussing therapeutic options. Effective evaluation includes a physical examination and detailed medical and social histories. Objectives are to identify pertinent etiologies, assess the severity and medical complications of obesity-related conditions, and determine the patient's readiness to address his or her obesity. This chapter is intended as a guide for clinicians. Our approach to the evaluation of obese patients is summarized in Table 2.1 [1,2].

TABLE 2.1
Steps for the Medical Evaluation of the Obese Patient

Etiologies of abnormal energy balance
Thyroid and endocrine
Genetic syndromes
Eating disorders
History of weight gain
Temporal characteristics
History of weight loss and weight regain cycles
Quantitative assessment and classification
BMI classification
Body fat
Metabolic
Medical assessment
Is the patient ready to implement a weight management plan?

2.2 ETIOLOGIC CONSIDERATIONS

We evaluate etiologies of obesity mainly to identify patients with treatable causes. Obesity is a common phenotype, but its behavioral and metabolic manifestations are not readily apparent. Despite recent advances in the molecular biology of adipose tissue, current understanding of the genetics of obesity limits our ability to classify etiologies in the majority of patients. However, obesity is a secondary manifestation of primary diseases that can be identified and treated. In that many patients might benefit from such treatment, it is essential that every effort be made to identify syndromes associated with obesity.

2.3 THYROID AND ADRENAL SYNDROMES

In most instances, a routine medical history and physical examination will be sufficient to identify a primary endocrine etiology. However, further evaluation may be necessary. Blood-screening tests for thyroid disease, e.g. TSH levels, are routinely obtained in patients with obesity. Such diagnostic work can help identify patients at an early stage of the disease process.

Patients with obesity who present with cushinoid features require further evaluation on the use of corticosteroid medications; this is important in the management of obesity, especially when considering weight loss surgery. Decisions about the appropriate treatment modalities — including eligibility for weight loss surgery — depend upon the etiology of Cushing's syndrome. For example, patients with a long history of steroid-dependent asthma may be appropriate candidates for bariatric surgery because withdrawal of steroid medications is unlikely to reverse their obesity. On the other hand, patients with hypersecreting adrenal tumors often improve significantly with treatment of the primary disease.

Presence of cushinoid facial features with classic findings on physical examination (e,g., abnormal body fat distribution, signs of skin fragility, and masculinization in women) may be further assessed by measuring morning serum cortisol levels and 24-hour urinary excretion of free cortisol, and testing cortisol suppression. The latter is typically sufficient to exclude adrenal hypersecretion (tumors and adrenal hyperplasia) in the majority of patients with morbid obesity. However, further evaluation by an endocrinologist may be needed.

2.4 GENETIC SYNDROMES

Genetic obesity syndromes are almost always associated with extreme obesity, and those who suffer from them require special care. Although underlying metabolic mechanisms of these syndromes are unclear, patients at risk can be identified at an early age based on a constellation of features, including mental retardation and abnormal physical findings. Such individuals often pose serious medical and surgical treatment challenges. However, it is important to note that a diagnosis of genetic obesity does not necessarily preclude weight loss surgery if there is sufficient evidence that weight loss is medically necessary and that post-surgical treatment will not cause harm. Signs and symptoms of syndromic obesity require appropriate referrals by primary care clinicians and weight management teams for further genetic assessment and counseling. In general, symptoms of a genetic obesity syndrome include short stature, hypotonia, hypogonadism, movement disorders, and structural abnormalities (e.g., bradydactyly [short fingers], structural cardiac defects, renal anomalies, retinal degeneration, and peculiar facial features). Table 2.2 presents a summary of autosomal and x-linked obesity syndromes (also see Chapter 11).

2.5 EATING DISORDERS

Eating disorders among obese patients remain ill-defined [3]. However, identification of eating behaviors that contribute to obesity is an important part of overall medical assessment (see Chapter 13). The prevalence of eating disorders among obese adults is approximately twice that of the non-obese population (21 vs. 9%) [4]. It is well recognized that obese individuals with a diagnosis of binge eating have clinically

TABLE 2.2
Genetic Syndromes in which Morbid Obesity is a Main Feature

Syndrome	Stature	Features
Prader-Willi	Short	Hypogonadism; short extremities
Angleman's	Normal	Movement disorder; happy affect
Albright's osteodystrophy	Normal/Short	Bradydactyly; subcutaneous ossification
Bardet-Biedl	Normal/Short	Rod-cone dystrophy; polydactyly; renal structural defects
Alstrom	Normal/Short	Deafness; cardiomyopathy; cone-rod dystrophy
Carpenter's	Short	Acrocephaly; polydactyly; hypogonadism
Cohen	Normal/Short	Facial features; retinochondrial dystrophy; granulocytopenia
Down	Short	Typical facial features; cardiac malformations; hypotonia

significant emotional distress associated with the disorder as well as obesity-related physical complications [5,6]. Therefore, it is important to seek psychiatric help in establishing the diagnosis and planning treatment of an eating disorder [7]. There are concerns about possible adverse effects of dieting when patients with eating disorders join weight loss programs. However, results from a recent randomized trial suggest that the benefits of weight loss in a multidisciplinary setting outweigh the risks [8].

2.6 HISTORY OF BODY WEIGHT CHANGES

A history of body weight changes will provide information about the patient's understanding of his or her own eating behavior as well as environmental factors that trigger weight gain. The sequential account of body weight changes can help establish potential for the success of weight control efforts. For example, a patient with a BMI >40 kg/m^2 (also referred to as Class III obesity; see Table 2.3) may not have had previous medical and behavioral treatments, may have failed weight loss attempts, or may have a history of weight cycling. The latter is especially important as it could impact future behavior. While the presence of weight-cycling behavior may indicate an eating disorder, it might also be a sign of significant metabolic risks. Weight cycling often involves periods of positive energy balance and rapid weight gain. Although rapid weight gain is often ignored, there is mounting evidence of its harmful effects [9–12].

Weight gain is an important contributor to cardiovascular and metabolic pathophysiology in obese individuals [13–15]. Its risk may be modified by weight loss but not by liposuction [16–18]. After exhausting possible weight loss strategies, bariatric surgery may be an option for these patients. Weight cycling is associated

TABLE 2.3
Metabolic Assessment of Obesity

Parameter	Measurement	Critical Value
Obesity	Body mass index (BMI): $\frac{Weight(kg)}{[Height(m)]2}$	Up to 24.9: Normal 25–29.9: Overweight 30–34.9: Class I obesity 35–39.9: Class II obesity ≥40: Class III obesity
Body fat distribution	Waist circumference	Men: >40 Women: >35
Fasting lipid profile	HDL Triglycerides	HDL Men: <40 HDL Women: <50 TG: >150
Insulin resistance	Fasting blood glucose (mM) Fasting insulin (μU/ml)	HOMA-IR ≥5
Hypertension	Blood pressure	Systolic >130 Diastolic >85

with greater weight gain over time [9–12,14]. Although weight cycling has been linked to mortality [19,20], there is no accepted definition that calls for immediate medical intervention. Thus, potential negative effects of weight cycling must be considered on a patient-by-patient basis. For example, weight cycling in a patient with congestive heart failure (CHF) could be detrimental in view of possible fluid retention during weight gain. In that further liver lipid deposition can lead to fibrosis and cirrhosis, similar arguments can be made for patients with fatty liver disease.

2.7 CLASSIFICATION

Assessing the degree of obesity is an essential component of the medical evaluation. Obesity is classified according to level of BMI, extent to which excess body fat contributes to pathophysiology, and the existence of medical conditions directly related to obesity.

2.7.1 Body Mass Index

Body mass index (BMI) is widely used to assess the degree of a patient's obesity according to current criteria (summarized in Table 2.3). BMI is calculated using the patient's weight and height according to the following equation:

$$\text{BMI} = \text{Weight (kg)}/\text{Height (m)}^2$$

This classification of obesity, which has been validated, shows that overweight and obesity are associated with increased risk for cardiovascular [21,22] and other chronic diseases [23,24]. An individual with a BMI of ≥30 kg/m^2 is considered obese. Further classification of obesity as Classes I through III (Table 2.3) is based on BMI, and is useful in the management of obesity. For example, at a BMI ≥40 kg/m^2, bariatric surgical options become reasonable treatment choices.

2.7.2 Body Fat Distribution and Metabolic Assessment

Several criteria have been proposed to define the metabolic syndrome (or insulin resistance syndrome). Those from the Adult Treatment Panel III of the National Cholesterol Education Program (ATP III) provide a practical tool for identifying patients at increased risk of cardiovascular disease (CVD), which is considered the primary outcome of the metabolic syndrome (Table 2.3) [25–27]. Central body fat, measured by waist size and waist-to-hip ratio, is associated with insulin resistance, hypertension (HTN), and diabetes [1]. It is therefore recommended that clinicians measure waist circumference and waist/hip ratio, and perform a routine metabolic assessment of patients with BMI >25 kg/m^2. In adults, this assessment includes fasting lipid profile and insulin and glucose levels. The latter can also be used to determine the degree of insulin resistance according to the homeostatic model assessment-insulin resistance (HOMA-IR) [28]. This index is calculated from fasting glucose and insulin levels according to the following equation:

$$[\text{Fasting insulin } (\mu\text{U/ml}) \times \text{Fasting glucose (mM/L)}]/22.5$$

Values of HOMA-IR ≥5 are indicative of significant insulin resistance. Although HOMA-IR is still considered a research tool, clinicans may gain additional knowledge of a patient's metabolic status from its use. In addition to HOMA-IR and blood lipid profiles, measurement of homocysteine and high sensitivity C-reactive protein (hsCRP) levels may help assess risk and determine whether a patient is in need of immediate weight loss management. Routine measurement of nontraditional parameters, such as homocysteine and hsCRP, is still controversial [29]. If traditional parameters are normal in the obese individual, nontraditional parameters can be considered.

2.8 COMPLICATIONS ASSOCIATED WITH OBESITY

The identification of one or several serious conditions associated with obesity may influence the clinician's approach to weight management. As comorbidities worsen, the need to to discuss more aggressive means of weight reduction, including bariatric surgery, become apparent to both physician and patient. Type 2 diabetes mellitus, severe hypertension, severe degenerative joint disease, hypoventilation syndrome, sleep apnea, and coronary atherosclerotic heart disease are common comorbid conditions that influence clinical decision making. Weight loss surgery can lead to dramatic and permanent weight loss, with improvement or reversal of obesity-related comorbidities. Even moderate weight loss of 5 to 10% can improve metabolic status (e.g., improve glycemic control in diabetic patients and control of blood pressure in diabetic or non-diabetic patients) [30,33]. Obesity-related medical conditions in the patient with morbid obesity (Class III) should alert the clinician to an immediate need for weight loss of at least 20% of initial body weight. Bariatric surgery is the most likely means to that end. A list of common comorbid conditions and evaluations is presented in Table 2.4.

2.8.1 Cardiovascular Disease

Hypertension is very prevalent in obese patients. In fact, obesity is now recognized as an etiologic factor in hypertension. The pathophysiologic contribution of obesity to blood pressure control has been reviewed elsewhere [34–36]. Briefly, hyperinsulinemia and insulin resistance are major contributors to endothelial cell dysfunction [37,38]. It is not unusual for obese patients presenting for medical weight management to be taking antihypertensive medications. Special attention to the obese hypertensive patient is indicated if appetite suppressants are considered. Over-the-counter and prescription appetite suppressants have potent sympathomimetic activity that renders their use in hypertensive patients risky. Therefore, it is essential that blood pressure is thoroughly assessed in all obese patients to ensure adequate control prior to adding additional pharmacologic agents intended to improve compliance with dietary restriction. Blood pressure in obese hypertensive patients may change significantly during weight loss. While these changes often lead to better blood pressure control, antihypertensive medications may also result in symptomatic low blood pressure during rapid weight loss. Therefore, clinicians caring for obese patients need to frequently assess blood pressure and adjust the number and doses of medications in relationship to weight loss and obesity treatment.

TABLE 2.4
Medical Assessment of Comorbidities Associated with Obesity

System	Condition	Evaluations
Cardiovascular	CAD CHF	**Minimal:** PE, ECG, CXR **Additional:** cardiac echo, stress testing, cardiology consult
Metabolic	Diabetes Hypercholesterolemia	**Minimal:** fasting glucose and insulin; lipid profile; hemoglobin A1C **Additional:** HOMA-IR calculation
Pulmonary	Obesity Hypoventilation Sleep Apnea Asthma COPD	**Minimal:** PE, CXR, PFT's **Additional:** sleep study
Gastrointestinal	Fatty liver Gallstones GERD	**Minimal:** PE; abdominal ultrasound **Additional:** endoscopy
Musculoskeletal	DJD	**Minimal:** PE **Additional:** radiology; MRI; orthopedic consultation

Obese patients with congestive heart failure also pose significant challenges during weight loss and need to be thoroughly evaluated by the clinician. Since these patients are often treated with pharmacologic diuretics, the additional diuretic effect of calorie restriction could induce clinical dehydration and electrolyte imbalances. Patients with cardiomyopathy as the etiologic basis of heart failure are especially at high risk of developing arrhythmias. Additionally, obese patients with a history of congestive heart failure are at a high risk of sustaining dangerous fluid retention during the early phases of positive energy balance and weight gain. This situation is frequently encountered in patients who initially undergo rapid weight reduction and reduce their usual medications but subsequently fail to maintain their weight loss. Therefore, obese patients with a history of congestive heart failure should have an assessment of renal function and blood electrolyte levels at the beginning of weight loss treatment and periodically during weight loss. We also recommend that these patients have an echocardiogram for assessment of cardiac function at the beginning of their weight reduction effort.

2.8.2 Pulmonary Disease

Obesity is an independent risk factor for deep vein thrombosis (DVT) and pulmonary embolism (PE) [39–42]. Patients with DVT are more likely to be heavy [43] and have abdominal fat distribution. They are also more likely to smoke [44], be older [45], have venous insufficiency [39,43] and venous stasis due to immobilization [43], have obesity hypoventilation syndrome or severe sleep apnea as well as CHF [39], use oral contraceptives and hormone replacements containing estrogen [40,45], and have inborn or acquired hypercoagulable states [41].

Assessment of the risks of VTE and PE are especially important in obese patients being considered for surgical procedures. Retrospective reviews of case series in which patients with clinically suspected VTE were assessed after weight loss surgery suggest that both DVT and PE occur in <1% of patients; however, incidence rates as high as 8% for DVT and 4% for PE have been described in patients with other risk factors, such as severe venous stasis [46–48]. A more recent review found respective average rates of DVT and PE of 0.05 and 0.21% in patients with Roux-en-Y gastric bypass (RYGB); those with laparoscopic adjustable gastric banding (LAGB) had DVT and PE rates of 0.05 and 0.01%, respectively [49]. Findings from a nationwide survey in 1997 showed a decline of PE rates to 0.07% [50]. Although the incidence of PE after obesity surgery appears to be low, PE accounts for 25 to 66% of postoperative mortality [51,52], and thus is important to identify.

2.8.3 Obstructive Sleep Apnea

Obstructive sleep apnea (OSA) is considered a serious and potentially life-threatening pulmonary disorder that may be caused by repeated cessation of breathing, either from collapse of the upper airway during sleep or lack of respiratory effort. OSA pathophysiology associated with obesity involves anatomic and functional aspects of the pharyngeal airway, the central nervous system, central obesity, and possibly hormonal regulators, such as leptin and ghrelin. OSA has been associated with the initiation and progression of cardiovascular diseases. Some data also implicate OSA in the development of HTN, cardiac ischemia, CHF, arrhythmias, and possibly cerebrovascular accidents [54].

It is well established that there is a high prevalence (12 to 40%) of OSA in adult patients with obesity [55] and a high prevalence of obesity in patients with OSA [56]. OSA is among the most underdiagnosed weight-related comorbidities. It is estimated that up to 93% of middle-aged women and 82% of men of the same age are undiagnosed [57]. In studies where patients were evaluated with polysomnography, 35 to 71% were diagnosed with OSA [57–59]. One study indicates that BMI does not correlate with, nor is it a predictor of, OSA [54]. In a study of 170 patients presenting for weight loss surgery, the prevalence of sleep apnea was 77% independent of BMI. The data from this study and others [55] support the use of routine-screening polysomnography in patients with symptoms of OSA. Another study on incidence of OSA involved polysomnography in all patients, regardless of symptoms; it found that patients with obesity had an 88% incidence of obstructive breathing-related disorders, and 71% of those patients had OSA [60].

Based on a physiologic rationale, the presence of OSA is thought to be a predisposing factor for perioperative cardiovascular and pulmonary complications [61,62], especially in obese patients with other comorbidities who are being considered for bariatric surgery. However, data from multivariate statistical models do not consistently support OSA as an independent risk factor in perioperative morbidity [63]. Currently there is no support for the routine use of CPAP in the immediate postoperative period of weight loss surgery. Rather, postoperative decisions about use of positive pressure ventilation should be individualized.

2.8.4 Liver Disease

Nonalcoholic fatty liver disease (NALFD) represents a spectrum of liver disease associated with obesity. Microscopic analysis of fatty liver disease reveals either accumulation of fat alone (statuses) or fat accompanied by inflammation and fibrosis (hepatitis); the latter is generally defined as non-alcoholic steatohepatitis (NASH). The prevalence of NAFLD is estimated at 10 to 24% of the general population and 30 to 100% of adults with obesity [64]. Up to 25% of cases of patients with NAFLD may progress to cirrhosis [65]. In studies of patients undergoing bariatric surgery, intraoperative liver biopsies revealed hepatic steatosis in 65 to 89% of patients, NASH in 10 to 56%, fibrosis in 1 to 51%, and cirrhosis in 0 to 6% [66–69].

NAFLD is commonly associated with type 2 diabetes mellitus, insulin resistance or hyperinsulinemia, older age, male gender, BMI. The association with other components of the metabolic syndrome, such as abdominal obesity measured by anthropometry or imaging, is less consistent [70,71]. Data indicate that the best predictor of the histological severity of NAFLD is the presence of type 2 diabetes, glucose tolerance, insulin resistance, HTN, and older age [66–68]. Although hepatic transaminase concentrations are unreliable predictors of histological severity, alanine aminotransferase (ALT) is a very sensitive biomarker of steatosis, and is therefore recommended as part of the evaluation of liver steatosis. Concentration of aspartate aminotransferase (AST) or a ratio of AST to ALT >1 have been associated with more advanced inflammation or fibrosis; these measures, however, should not be used to guide clinical management at this time [72]. In some studies, hyperferritinemia and CRP have also been associated with NAFLD histology [73,74].

2.9 EVALUATING THE PATIENT'S MOTIVATION FOR BEHAVIOR CHANGE

Successful treatment of obesity involves a behavioral approach targeted to patient readiness and motivation. For many clinicians, discussing body weight and related behaviors can be sensitive topics for the patient. Therefore it is important for the clinician to determine if and when the patient is ready to implement a weight reduction plan. Identification of a patient's state of readiness to adopt health behaviors that may lead to a healthier weight is an important step in the evaluation of the obese patient and should be considered during the discussion of treatment options (See Chapter 13). Counseling strategies that combine motivational interviewing and the stages of change approach can be found in Chapter 3 and Chapter 13.

2.10 CONCLUSION

The clinical evaluation of the obese patient prior to medical or surgical weight loss treatment involves a determination of the etiology and history of weight change. Obesity-related comorbidities, including a psychological profile for eating disorders, should be assessed. The physical examination should include laboratory tests and the measurement of height, weight, BMI, and waist circumference. Lastly, a determination of the patient's motivation and readiness to change is crucial in gauging the patient's chance for a successful treatment outcome.

REFERENCES

1. National Institutes of Health, National Heart, Lung, and Blood Institute, and North American Association for the Study of Obesity. *The practical guide to the identification, evaluation, and treatment of overweight and obesity in adults.* Available from http://www.nhlbi.nih.gov/guidelines/obesity/prctgd_c.pdf . Accessed April 1, 2006.
2. National Institutes of Health, National Heart, Lung, and Blood Institute. and the National Institute of Diabetes and Digestive and Kidney Diseases. *Clinical guidelines on the identification, evaluation, and treatment of overweight and obesity in adults.* NIH Publication No. 98-4083 Available from http://www.nhlbi.nih.gov/guidelines/obesity/ob_gdlns.pdf. Accessed April 1, 2006.
3. American Psychiatric Association. *Diagnostic and Statistical Manual of Mental Disorders,* 4th ed. American Psychiatric Association. Washington, DC, 1994.
4. French SA, Jeffery RW, Sherwood NE, Neumark-Sztainer D. Prevalence and correlates of binge eating in a nonclinical sample of women enrolled in a weight gain prevention program. *Int J Obes Relat Metab Disord* 1999; 23:576–585.
5. Grilo CM. Binge eating disorder. In *Comprehensive Textbook of Obesity and Eating Disorders,* 2nd ed., CG Fairburn and KD Brownell (Eds.), New York: Guilford Press, pp. 178–182, 2002.
6. Dunkley DM and Grilo CM. Self-criticism, low self-esteem, depressive symptoms, and over-evaluation of shape and weight in binge eating disorder patients. *Behav Res Ther* 2006; Epub ahead of print.
7. Brody ML, Masheb RM, Grilo CM. Treatment preferences of patients with binge eating disorder. *Int J Eat Disord* 2005; 37:352–356.
8. Wadden TA, Foster GD, Sarwer DB, Anderson DA, Gladis M, Sanderson RS, Letchak RV, Berkowitz RI, Phelan S. Dieting and the development of eating disorders in obese women: results of a randomized controlled trial. *Am J Clin Nutr* 2004; 80(3):560–568.
9. National Task Force on the Prevention and Treatment of Obesity. Weight Cycling. *JAMA* 1994; 272:1196–1202.
10. Folsom AR, French SA, Zheng W, Baxter JE, Jeffrey RW. Weight variability and mortality: the Iowa Women's Health Study. *Int J Obes Relat Metab Disord* 1996; 20:704–709.
11. Blair SN, Shaten J, Brownell K, Collins G, Lissner L. Body weight change, all-cause mortality, and cause-specific mortality in the Multiple Risk Factor Intervention Trial. *Ann Intern Med* 1993; 119(7 Pt 2):749–757.
12. Jeffrey RW, Wing RR, French SA. Weight cycling and cardiovascular risk factors in obese men and women. *Am J Clin Nutr* 1992; 55:641–644.
13. Wannanethee SG, Sharper AG, Walkere M. Overweight and obesity and weight changes in middle-aged men: impact on cardiovascular disease and diabetes. *J Epidemiol Community Health* 2005; 59:134–139.

14. Field AE, Manson JE, Laird N, Williamson DF, Willettt WC, Colditz GA. Weight cycling and the risk of developing type 2 diabetes among adult women in the United States. *Obes Res* 2004; 12:267–274.
15. Field AE, Coakley EH, Must A, Spadano JL, Laird N, Dietz WH, Rimm E, Colditz GA. Impact of overweight on the risk of developing common chronic diseases during a 10-year period. *Arch Intern Me*d 2001; 161:1581–1586.
16. Kelley DE. Thermodynamics, liposuction, and metabolism. *N Engl J Med* 2004; 350:2542–2544.
17. Kelley DE, Wing R, Buonocure C, Sturis J, Plolonsky K, Fitzsimmons M. Relative effects of calorie restriction and weight loss in noninsulin-dependent diabetes mellitus. *J Clin Endocrinol Metab* 1993; 1287–1293.
18. Klein S, Fontana L, Young VL, Coggan AR, Kilo C, Patterson BW, Mohammed BS. Absence of an effect of liposuction on insulin action and risk factors for coronary heart disease. *N Engl J Med* 2004; 350:2549–2557.
19. Wannamethee SG, Shaper AG, Walker M. Weight change, weight fluctuation, and mortality. *Arch Intern Med* 2002; 162:2575–2580.
20. Wannamethee SG, Shaper AG, Lennon L. Reasons for intentional weight loss, unintentional weight loss, and mortality in older men. *Arch Intern Med* 2005; 165:1035–1040.
21. Rexrode KM, Carey VJ, Hennekens CH, Walters EE, Colditz GA, Stampfer MJ, Willett WC, Manson JE. Abdominal adiposity and coronary heart disease in women. *JAMA* 1998; 280:1843–1848.
22. Flaherty KT, Fuchs CS, Colditz GA, Stampfer MJ, Speizer FE, Willett WC and Curhan GC. A prospective study of body mass index, hypertension, and smoking and the risk of renal cell carcinoma (United States). *Cancer Causes Control* 2005; 16:1099–1106.
23. Carey VJ, Walters EE, Colditz GA, Solomon CG, Willett WC, Rosner BA, Speizer FE, Manson JE. Body fat distribution and risk of non-insulin-dependent diabetes mellitus in women. The Nurses' Health Study. *Am J Epidemio*l 1997; 145:614–619.
24. Colditz GA, Feskanich D, Chen WY, Hunter DJ, and Willett WC. Physical activity and risk of breast cancer in premenopausal women. *Br J Cancer* 2003; 89:847–851.
25. Grundy SM, Brewer HB Jr, Cleeman JI, Smith SC Jr, Lenfant C; American Heart Association; National Heart, Lung, and Blood Institute. Definition of metabolic syndrome: Report of the National Heart, Lung, and Blood Institute/American Heart Association conference on scientific issues related to definition. *Circulation* 2004; 109:433–438.
26. Third Report of the National Cholesterol Education Program (NCEP) expert panel on detection, evaluation, and treatment of high blood cholesterol in adults (Adult Treatment Panel III). Final report. *Circulation* 2002; 106: 3143–3421.
27. Klein S, Burke LE, Bray GA, Blair S, Allison DB, Pi-Sunyer X, Hong Y, Eckel RH. Clinical implications of obesity with specific focus on cardiovascular disease: a statement for professionals from the American Heart Association Council on Nutrition, Physical Activity and Metabolism. *Circulation* 2004; 110:2952–2967.
28. Abbasi F, Reaven GM. Evaluation of the quantitative insulin sensitivity check index as an estimate of insulin sensitivity in humans. *Metabolism* 2002; 51:235–237.

29. Ridker PM, Wilson PW, Grundy SM. Should C-reactive protein be added to metabolic syndrome and to assessment of global cardiovascular risk? *Circulation* 2004; 109:2818–2825.
30. Bosello O, Armellini F, Zamboni M, Fitchet M. The benefits of modest weight loss in type II diabetes. *Int J Obes Related Metab Disord* 1997; 21(Suppl 1):S10–13.
31. Wedick NM, Mayer-Davis EJ, Wingard DL, Addy CL, Barret-Connor E. Insulin resistance precedes weight loss in adults without diabetes: the Rancho Barnardo Study. *Am J Epidemiol* 2001; 153:1199–1205.
32. Muscelli E, Camastra S, Catalano C, Galvan AQ, Ciociaro D, Baldi S Ferrannini E. Metabolic and cardiovascular assessment in moderate obesity: effect of weight loss. *J Clin Endocrinol Metab* 1997; 82:2937–2943.
33. Mavri A, Alessi MC, Bastelica D, Geel-Georgelin O, Fina F, Sentocnik JT, Stegnar M, Juhan-Vague I. Subcutaneous abdominal, but not femoral fat expression of plasminogen activator inhibitor-1 (PAI-1) is related to plasma PAI-1 levels and insulin resistance and decreases after weight loss. *Diabetologia* 2001; 44:2025–2031.
34. Frontoni S, Bracaglia D, Gigli F. Relationship between autonomic dysfunction, insulin resistance and hypertension, in diabetes. *Nutr Metab Cardiovasc Dis* 2005; 15:441–449.
35. Walcher D, Marx N. Insulin resistance and cardiovascular disease: the role of PPAR-gamma activators beyond their anti-diabetic action. *Diab Vasc Dis Res* 2004; 1:76–81.
36. Biddinger SB, Kahn CR. From mice to men: insights into the insulin resistance syndromes. *Annu Rev Physiol* 2006; 68:123–158.
37. Desideri G, De Simone M, Iughetti L, Rosato T, Iezzi ML, Marinucci MC, Cofini V, Croce G, Passacquale G, Necozione S, Ferri C. Early activation of vascular endothelial cells and platelets in obese children. *J Clin Endocrinol Metab* 2005; 90:3145–3152.
38. Sjöholm Å, Nyström T. Endothelial inflammation in insulin resistance. *Lancet* 2005; 365: 610–612.
39. Samama MM. An epidemiologic study of risk factors for deep vein thrombosis in medical outpatients: the Sirius study. *Arch Int Med* 2000; 160(22):3415–3420.
40. Goldhaber S, Grodstein F, Stampfer M, et al. A prospective study of risk factors for pulmonary embolism in women. *JAMA* 1997; 277:642–645.
41. Blaszyk H, Bjornsson J. Factor V leiden and morbid obesity in fatal postoperative pulmonary embolism. *Arch Surg* 2000; 135:1410–1413.
42. Blaszyk H, Wollan PC, Witkiewicz AK, Bjornsson J. Death from pulmonary thromboembolism in severe obesity: lack of association with established genetic and clinical risk factors. *Virchows Arch* 1999; 434:529–532.
43. Sugerman HJ, Sugerman EL, Wolfe L, Kellum JM, Jr., Schweitzer MA, DeMaria EJ. Risks and benefits of gastric bypass in morbidly obese patients with severe venous stasis disease. *Ann Surg* 2001; 234:41–46.
44. Hansson PO, Eriksson H, Welin L, Svardsudd K, Wilhelmsen L. Smoking and abdominal obesity: risk factors for venous thromboembolism among middle-aged men: "the study of men born in 1913". *Arch Int Med* 1999; 159:1886–1890.
45. Lowe GD, Haverkate F, Thompson SG, et al. Prediction of deep vein thrombosis after elective hip replacement surgery by preoperative clinical and haemostatic variables: the ECAT DVT Study. European Concerted Action on Thrombosis. *Thromb Haemost* 1999; 81:879–886.

46. Westling A, Bergqvist D, Bostrom A, Karacagil S, Gustavsson S. Incidence of deep venous thrombosis in patients undergoing obesity surgery. *World J Surg* 2002; 26:470–473.
47. Eriksson S, Backman L, Ljungstrom KG. The incidence of clinical postoperative thrombosis after gastric surgery for obesity during 16 years. *Obes Surg* 1997; 7:332–335; discussion 336.
48. Printen KJ, Miller EV, Mason EE, Barnes RW. Venous thromboembolism in the morbidly obese. *Surg Gynecol Obstet* 1978; 147:63–64.
49. Chapman AE, Kiroff G, Game P, et al. Laparoscopic adjustable gastric banding in the treatment of obesity: a systematic literature review. *Surgery* 2004; 135:326–351.
50. Pope GD, Birkmeyer JD, Finlayson SR. National trends in utilization and in-hospital outcomes of bariatric surgery. *J Gastrointest Surg* 2002; 6:855–860.
51. Livingston EH, Huerta S, Arthur D, Lee S, De Shields S, Heber D. Male gender is a predictor of morbidity and age a predictor of mortality for patients undergoing gastric bypass surgery. *Ann Surg* 2002; 236:576–582.
52. Peltier G, Hermreck AS, Moffat RE, Hardin CA, Jewell WR. Complications following gastric bypass procedures for morbid obesity. *Surgery* 1979; 86:648–654.
53. Shamsuzzaman ASM, Gersh BJ, Somers VK. Obstructive sleep apnea. Implications for cardiac and vascular disease. *JAMA* 2003; 290:1906–1914.
54. O'Keeffe T, Patterson EJ. Evidence supporting routine polysomnography before bariatric surgery. *Obes Surg* 2004; 14:23–26.
55. Young T, Shahar E, Nieto FJ, et al. Predictors of sleep-disordered breathing in community-dwelling adults: the Sleep Heart Health Study. *Arch Int Med* 2002; 162:893–900.
56. Young T, Evans L, Finn L, Palta M. Estimation of the clinically diagnosed proportion of sleep apnea syndrome middle-aged men and women. *Sleep* 1997; 20:705–706.
57. Frey WC, Pilcher J. Obstructive sleep-related breathing disorders in patients evaluated for bariatric surgery. *Obes Surg* 2003; 13:676–683
58. Serafini FM, MacDowell Anderson W, Rosemurgy AS, Strait T, Murr MM. Clinical predictors of sleep apnea in patients undergoing bariatric surgery. *Obes Surg* 2001; 11:28–31.
59. van Kralingen KW, de Kanter W, de Groot GH, et al. Assessment of sleep complaints and sleep-disordered breathing in a consecutive series of obese patients. *Respiration* 1999; 66:312–316.
60. Guardiano SA, Scott JA, Ware JC, Schechner SA. The long-term results of gastric bypass on indexes of sleep apnea. *Chest* 2003; 124:1615–1619.
61. Benumoff JL. Obstructive sleep apnea in adult obese patient; implications for airway management. *J Clin Anesth* 2001; 13:144–156.
62. Peiser J, Ovnat A, Uwyyed K, Lavie P, Charuzi I. Cardiac arrhythmias during sleep in morbidly obese sleep-apneic patients before and after gastric bypass surgery. *Clin Cardiol* 1985; 8:519–521.
63. Fernandez AZ Jr, Demaria EJ, Tichansky DS, Kellum JM, Wolfe LG, Meador J, Sugerman HJ. Multivariate analysis of risk factors for death following gastric bypass for treatment of morbid obesity. *Ann Surg* 2004; 239:698–702; discussion 702–703.
64. Angulo P, Lindor KD. Treatment of non-alcoholic steatohepatitis. *Best Pract Res Clin Gastroenterol* 2002; 16:797–810.

65. Scheen AJ, Luyckx FH. Obesity and liver disease. *Best Pract Res Clin Endocrin Metab* 2002; 16:703–716.
66. Luyckx FH, Desaive C, Thiry A, Dewe W, Scheen AJ, Gielen JE, Lefebvre PJ. Liver abnormalities in severely obese subjects: effect of drastic weight loss after gastroplasty. *Int J Obes Relat Metab Disord* 1998; 22:222–226.
67. Gholam PM, Kotler DP, Flancbaum LJ. Liver pathology in morbidly obese patients undergoing Roux-en-Y gastric bypass surgery. *Obes Surg* 2002; 12(1):49–51.
68. Beymer C, Kowdley KV, Larson A, Edmonson P, Dellinger EP, Flum DR. Prevalence and predictors of asymptomatic liver disease in patients undergoing gastric bypass surgery. *Arch Surg* 2003; 138:1240–1244.
69. Spaulding L, Trainer T, Janiec D. Prevalence of non-alcoholic steatohepatitis in morbidly obese subjects undergoing gastric bypass. *Obes Surg* 2003; 13:347–349.
70. Marchesini G, Bugianesi E, Forlani G, et al. Nonalcoholic fatty liver, steatohepatitis, and the metabolic syndrome. *Hepatology* 2003; 37:917–923.
71. Dixon JB, Bhathal PS, O'Brien PE. Nonalcoholic fatty liver disease: predictors of nonalcoholic steatohepatitis and liver fibrosis in the severely obese. *Gastroenterology* 2001; 121:91–100.
72. Angulo P, Keach JC, Batts KP, Lindor KD. Independent predictors of liver fibrosis in patients with nonalcoholic steatohepatitis. *Hepatology* 1999; 30:1356–1362.
73. Hsiao TJ, Chen JC, Wang JD. Insulin resistance and ferritin as major determinants of nonalcoholic fatty liver disease in apparently healthy obese patients. *Int J Obes* 2004; 28:167–17.
74. Park SH, Kim BI, Yun JW, Kim JW, Park DI, Cho YK, Sung IK, Park CY, Sohn CI, Jeon WK, Kim H, Rhee EJ, Lee WY, Kim SW. Insulin resistance and C-reactive protein as independent risk factors for non-alcoholic fatty liver disease in non-obese Asian men. *J Gastroenterol Hepatol* 2004; 19:694–698.

3 Motivational Interviewing and Health Behavior Change Counseling

Gary S. Rose, Judy C.C. Phillips, and Garry Welch

CONTENTS

3.1 INTRODUCTION

The purpose of this chapter is to introduce Motivational Interviewing (MI), an evidence-based style of health behavior change consultation, and to discuss the implications of MI for the challenges faced in treating the obese patient. Our goal is to provide readers with a set of ideas to stimulate creative thought about health behavior change and a toolkit of techniques that may be readily integrated into professional practice.

3.2 SETTING THE STAGE

We are at the beginning of a new era with respect to the assessment and treatment of obesity. Training in obesity treatment is finally available for generalist and specialist practitioners through many venues, and as body mass index (BMI) becomes a basic vital sign, screening for overweight will quickly become standard practice. Overweight or obese patients will be identified with greater frequency, as will the correlated risks associated with increased weight; but how will the subject of obesity and lifestyle change be effectively addressed by the clinician?

Obesity and weight are inherently difficult topics to discuss. Patients are often reluctant to broach the subject because of previous failures of weight management, misinformation, fear, guilt, embarrassment, or concern about the costs of treatment [1]. Practitioners are equally reluctant to raise the topic. Less than half of obese adults report being advised to lose weight by health care professionals [2]. Primary care practitioners report confusion regarding clinical guidelines and treatment tools. Few receive training in behavior change counseling strategies, and many report an acute lack of consultation time [3]. Practitioners are also reluctant to raise the topic without being able to offer a quick solution or a simple prescriptive approach to weight loss. Unlike smoking cessation or seatbelt use, where the messages are simple, with obesity, the means (lifestyle changes) to achieving the desired outcome (weight loss) are complex.

Even when obesity and weight are addressed, the communication is often problematic. The usual practice of asking questions and providing directives regarding change leaves patients passive, confused, and disengaged. Furthermore, according to a recent report from the Institute of Medicine, "90 million adult Americans have difficulty understanding the health information they get from their doctors" [4]. Attempts to increase motivation through exhortation, explanation, and coercion generally fail. All too often, the outcome of these consultations is frustration and demoralization for both patient and practitioner.

There is a clear need for increased competence **in communication skills**. Practitioners need to learn how to communicate more effectively to foster change. Only through skillful communication will they be able to effectively raise concern and direct patients on a reasonable course of treatment. The Accreditation Council for Graduate Medical Education has acknowledged this need and now recommends that physicians demonstrate competence in five key communication skills: listening effectively; eliciting information through questioning skills; providing information via explanatory skills; counseling and educating patients; and making informed decisions on the basis of patient information and preference [5].

MI holds promise as a means to meet the need for increased effectiveness of practitioner–patient communication. With demonstrated effectiveness in the treatment of addictive disorders [6], there is a growing body of evidence that supports the efficacy of MI in consultations addressing weight management and dietary modification and obesity-related diseases such as diabetes [7,8].

3.3 HISTORY AND DEFINITION

Evolving from the earlier work of William R. Miller [9] and Stephen Rollnick [10], the 1991 seminal volume, *Motivational Interviewing: Helping Clients Change Addictive Behavior* [11] introduced MI to an international audience as a "client centered yet directive" interviewing style that promoted behavior change through the "analysis and resolution of ambivalence." With the 2002 publication of the 2nd edition of the MI text [12], we saw a broadening of the application of MI to behavior change in general including preventative medicine and chronic medical illnesses. These then are the two key features of MI: directed listening and the resolution of patient ambivalence to change. A central premise of MI is that, prior to the initiation of change, the practitioner must understand and appreciate the idiosyncrasies of the patient's often conflicting ideas, attitudes, and feelings about the targeted health behaviors. Through a process of directed or strategic listening, the practitioner promotes the resolution of the ambivalence in a manner that increases the patient's commitment to changing his/her behaviors toward healthier options.

Four key elements of MI address both what one discusses with the patient and how one discusses this: express empathy, roll with resistance, develop discrepancy, and support self-efficacy. The first two elements, *express empathy* and *roll with resistance*, pertain to the practitioner–patient relationship. Empathic listening (accurately understanding the patient's story) is fundamental to MI as it provides the vehicle for both understanding the patient's unique connection to the targeted health behavior and is the venue through which rapport is developed and maintained. *Roll with resistance* is a particular manifestation of empathy, wherein argumentation is avoided and attempts are made to thoroughly understand the patient's reluctance to change. Furthermore, unsolicited advice-giving is avoided in an attempt to maintain the collaborative spirit of MI.

Develop a discrepancy refers to the engine of change. MI is a self-advocacy model of behavior change. The focus is on increasing intrinsic motivation, changing "because I want to," by helping patients become aware of the discrepancy between current behavior and highly cherished personal values and goals.

The fourth element, *support self-efficacy*, simply asserts that wanting to change is only half of the behavior change battle. Patients need to also believe that change is possible, that there is a way to succeed, to persist with health behavior change. Empowerment and offering choice are critical to the development of patient self-efficacy.

MI, then, is an approach to health behavior change consultation that employs high-quality listening to discuss the "whys" and "hows" of change, with goal of increasing patients' readiness for, and commitment to, the adoption of a healthier lifestyle.

3.4 THREE STYLES: TOWARD INTEGRATION

Before further pursuing the discussion of MI, let us look at where this consultation fits into the world of the health care practitioner. Rose et al. [13] have proposed that practitioners adopt one of three styles in their patient consultations: *Instruct, Guide,* and *Listen*. They further propose that each of these styles is critical to communication,

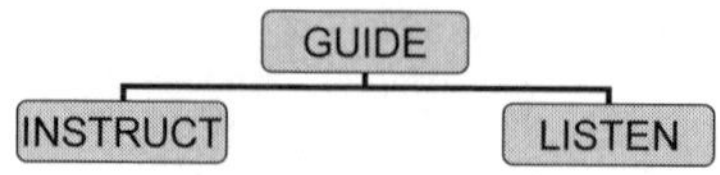

FIGURE 3.1 The three styles of motivational interviewing.

and that to be effective, the practitioner needs to be flexible, adaptable, and competent in the delivery of all three styles (Figure 3.1).

The three styles are defined as follows:

1. Instruct: *Give information or advice*. Other activities associated with this style include directing, informing, leading, educating, telling and using one's expertise. These are used when there is specific information that one wants to provide, hopefully which the person wants to receive.
2. Listen: *Understand the person's experience.* Other activities used include gathering information, following, eliciting, attending and empathizing. These are used when one wishes to understand how the person feels or what has happened to him or her.
3. Guide: *Encourage person to set his/her own goals and find ways of achieving them.* Other activities associated with this style include coaching, negotiating, mobilizing and motivating. These are used when the person is facing change, having to make decisions and to act upon them.

The guiding style is best understood as a higher-order style of communication that integrates elements of both instruction and listening, but differs fundamentally from these other two styles. Critical to effective guiding are activities such as collaboration, empowerment, affirmation, and the entertaining of alternatives.

Our model does not suggest that any one style is *a priori* more effective. Rather, we propose that each style has a place in the armamentarium of the health care practitioner, and the challenge is one of matching the consultation style to a specific clinical context and the expectations of the patient. **The guiding style is particularly effective when addressing health behavior change**. This is due to the nature of the desired change, which is almost completely under the control of the patient and entails the patient learning to integrate changes with day-to-day habitual activities in the face of competing nonhealth interests.

MI is essentially a sophisticated, evidence-based example of the guiding style of consultation. To the extent that guiding is appropriate, MI serves as a model of effective practice.

As we shall see later, however, MI is not just a form of guiding. Rather, the style also includes elements of collaborative instruction and purposeful listening.

3.5 LEARNING MI

The representation of the MI learning process as a pyramid (see Figure 3.2) has proven to be an effective heuristic vehicle. MI as a style of health behavior change consultation is built upon a theoretical/attitudinal foundation called the *Spirit of MI* [14].

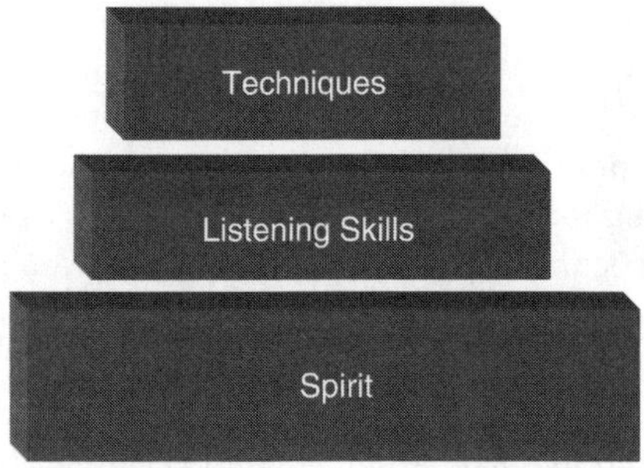

FIGURE 3.2 MI learning pyramid.

Sophisticated listening skills serve to operationalize the spirit, and structured techniques offer opportunities for productive behavior change conversations between practitioner and patient. We will discuss each of these levels of the MI pyramid in turn (Figure 3.2).

3.5.1 Spirit of MI: The Principles of Guiding

There is strong anecdotal evidence that the attitudes comprising the spirit of MI are critical variables in the effective implementation of this consultation style. Embracing the spirit of MI often yields significant changes in the manner that practitioners engage their patients. Conversely, implementation of the techniques without the context of these attitudes generally misses the mark and results in ineffectual MI at best. The Spirit of MI can be described as follows: collaborate and empower, appreciate ambivalence, and elicit intrinsic motivation — a desire to change grounded in personal goals and values.

3.5.1.1 Collaboration

Consistent with the patient-centered method in medicine [15], MI promotes practitioner–patient collaboration and the sharing of power [14]. Traditional health care consultation is "top-down," with a power differential in the favor of the "expert practitioner." Consider the following depiction of traditional health education:

Collect data, to…
Assess health status, to…
Make decisions, to…
Deliver information, to…
Improve health!

The active practitioner–passive patient relationship is a wonderful example of the "instructional" style and is perfectly adapted to the demands of acute and emergency medicine and surgery. One cannot imagine, for example, that while being wheeled into the surgical ward, the surgeon offers his patient choices regarding procedures to repair a cranial injury. However, there are serious limitations with this "expert" consultation style when the goal is to encourage the lifestyle change that often is needed for preventative medicine and chronic illness management. It is important to consider the nature of the requested change and the factors associated with enduring health behavior change. When we ask patients to modify health behavior, we are invariably asking them to both initiate and persist with change. Initiation of change may not be particularly difficult, especially if reward strategies are in place. It is the nonpersistence of new behaviors that can cause problems. Ask any smoker how many times he or she has initiated smoking cessation or any dieter how many "successful" diets he or she has experienced. The challenge with regard to persistence of change has to do with the need to integrate the healthier behavior into everyday life and competing nonhealth-related priorities. Factors that result in successful integration include a sense of empowerment or personal self-efficacy [16] and compatibility between the new behavior and daily life. From an MI perspective, the collaborative relationship provides access to both of these factors. Shared decision making empowers the patient and allows selection of a change plan consistent with the patient's style of initiating and maintaining change. Rather than a "*practitioner knows best*" relationship, in the spirit of MI, we suggest entertaining the concept of "*dual expertise*" [17]. The practitioner is an expert in medical science and health; the patient provides expertise in self-change [18] and in the whys and hows of health behavior change. Only the patient has the depth of understanding as to what might work and what might not, given his or her lifestyle and priorities; therefore, it is critical that the patient's own life is understood and integrated into the treatment plan.

One perceived barrier to the adoption of a dual expertise relationship is time. The busy, time-constrained practitioner often fears that collaboration and empowerment just takes too much time. The top-down expert relationship may not always work, but there is a comfort in the perceived ability to "get things done quickly." Furthermore, there is a pervasive fear among health care practitioners that to ask an open-ended question is to initiate a runaway conversation or a "Pandora's box" of problems. However, the typical patient only needs 3 to 4 minutes of good active listening to thoroughly inform the practitioner, and this information correlates with effectiveness and efficiency of health care [19].

To anticipate our discussion of listening, we would suggest that an attitude of empowerment accompanied by a few key words and phrases will set the stage for shared decision making. For example, the phrases "Let's put our heads together and review the options," and "I can offer an opinion but you'll need to tell me what will work best in your daily life," clearly elicit dual expertise in a timely manner.

3.5.1.2 Appreciate Ambivalence

Ask any health care practitioner what proportion of patients have mixed feelings toward change and they will say the majority. Ambivalence is thus a normal aspect of the behavior change quandary. From the MI perspective, the goal is to understand and use ambivalence in the service of change rather than in the service of staying the same. We will now elaborate on this goal.

The decisional matrix [20] provides a visual tool for understanding the concept of ambivalence as it pertains to health behavior change. One might assert that the

	Eat Whatever I Desire	Healthier Eating Habits
BENEFITS	I like the taste It's cheaper and more convenient I feel fine At least I don't smoke I'm not that bad	Stay healthy Less medications Control sugars Good role model In control of my life I don't want to die!
COSTS	My Doc lectures me I've gained another 20 Out of control sugars I don't want insulin I feel guilty	Too expensive No recipes We hate veggies!! Dining out? No time!

FIGURE 3.3 A decisional matrix.

matrix presents both sides of the change–no change argument in the debate about health behavior change. With respect to the argument for the status quo, the decisional matrix illustrates common losses and barriers associated with adopting a healthier lifestyle. Figure 3.3 presents data regarding the adoption of healthier eating habits. The upper left quadrant (benefits of current behavior) describes, from the patient's point of view, positive attributes of the current "unhealthy" eating style. Included here are attributes associated with taste, convenience, sociability, culture, and psychological coping strategies, to name a few. The lower right quadrant (*costs of change*) likewise describes perceived barriers to adopting healthier eating behavior. Here we observe attributes including cost, inconvenience, fear of failure, disruption of daily habits, and cultural discordance. These factors comprise what we call the *Status Quo* side of ambivalence, which perhaps can be referred to as, "I like my life/your plan won't work for me!" The remaining two cells of the matrix present the arguments in favor of change, otherwise known as *Change Talk*; Concerns about current behavior and benefits anticipated from change can be referred to as, "I've got problems /Life could be better."

A moment's reflection yields the observation that both sides of the ambivalence have credibility. Patient-identified barriers and anticipated losses associated with change have credibility in at least the short term, as do mitigations of risk associated with likely health deterioration. It is our contention that traditional approaches to health behavior change have generally ignored these aspects of ambivalence, in favor of the items listed in the remaining two quadrants of the matrix: the problems, costs, and risk factors associated with current behavior, and the potential or predictable benefits that accrue upon implementation of change. This bias causes problems for the conscientious health care practitioner in a number of ways. First, consider how ambivalence operates in normal daily social interactions. If one is ambivalent about a certain matter, such as work, personal relationships, etc., and one is conversing with somebody who strongly supports one side of the ambivalence, there is a strong tendency to defend the other side, e.g. "Why don't you quit that job! You work long hours for short pay. There's no chance for promotion, and your boss is always breathing down your neck!" "But I like the people I work with; I've been there long enough to get a nice corner office, and I feel good about the work we do here!" This wrestling match in the form of point–counterpoint is all too familiar to parents of teenagers, spouses, etc. When it occurs in the heath care setting, it is what we call the *Righting Reflex* [12]. The harder the practitioner argues for change, the harder the patient talks about, and thinks about, the benefits of staying the same. "You need to lose weight" — "I feel fine" "You can do it" — "I've tried before and I always fail." "You're going to have a heart attack at this rate!!" — "Everybody is fat in my family. This is just how we are built, and, besides, we all live to be 90!"

Not only does the wrestling match of the righting reflex result in apathy and a loss of rapport between practitioner and patient, but it leads to a second, equally enduring problem. Social psychology informs us that **people are more likely to remember what they say aloud (or say with their internal voice)** than that which is simply told to them by others. Every parent and teacher who asks the demure child, "Repeat what I said so I know that you heard it correctly," implicitly understands this principle. Furthermore, self-perception theory [21] suggests that what people hear themselves say influences what they believe. Accordingly, this righting reflex generates a double whammy. Ambivalent patients verbalize their reasons for wanting to maintain the status quo and their concerns about our change plans; these words that they hear themselves utter actually reinforce their commitment to *staying the same!* Simply put, when we are dealing with highly ambivalent patients, the righting reflex becomes a powerful means for demotivating patients. The harder the practitioner tries to persuade the patient to change by differentially asserting current health risks and future gains, the more committed the patient becomes to maintaining the status quo. In the practice of MI, we try to reverse the righting reflex. Using the guiding style, we provide patients with opportunities to verbalize change talk. For it is through the verbalization of change talk in all its variations that people increase their readiness for change [12].

In MI, the goal is to appreciate ambivalence regarding change, to allow the patient to give voice to the status quo, to roll with any resistance. Listening then substitutes for arguing, guiding for debate. Key questions are used strategically to demonstrate an openness to understand both sides of the change–status quo debate, such as this dialog between general practitioner and patient, "I can smell a bit of smoke about you, so I'll shortly have to give you advice and some options for quitting. But, before I do, I'd like to ask, what do you still like about smoking? What will make it difficult to quit?" Rather than fall into a confrontation–denial trap, the MI practitioner rolls with resistance [11].

Curiosity about status quo yields at least three positive products: first, one identifies often personal and highly idiosyncratic positive reinforcers and barriers to change; second, the patient is delivered a message loud and clear, that, "I am not simply going to tell you what to do. Instead, I would like to discuss your mixed feelings here." Thirdly, by avoiding falling into the righting reflex, the practitioner allows the patient freedom to safely discuss concerns about the present and hopes for the future. These utterances then subtly shift the motivation toward, rather than away from, change.

3.5.1.3 Elicit Intrinsic Motivation

"I do everything I can to motivate my patients. They seem ready to do what I tell them when they leave the clinic, but when they come back they are even heavier. They just don't listen!" Sounds familiar? We have heard it thousands of times across all fields of health care. From the perspective of the spirit of MI, we assert that health care practitioners operate under a misassumption that health is naturally a high-priority goal. A bit of self-reflection reveals that **health is generally not a high-priority goal for most people** unless there is some sense of immediacy regarding change. Otherwise, the more immediate demands of daily home and work life take precedence, "I'd love to exercise before work, but I just don't have the time." "I'm happy if I can just pick up a take-out meal of hamburgers and french fries for dinner. That's the best I can do." It is no wonder that patients' ears are not open when it comes to conversations about healthiness.

From the perspective of MI, the challenge is one of increasing intrinsic motivation, the desire to change because *I* think it is a good idea. We must help the patient identify healthiness, holding onto it or getting it back, as a means to a personally valued goal. Take, for example, the obese teenaged boy who is only willing to change his diet and exercise routine when he sees its connection to his becoming a better wrestler; the renal dialysis patient who is willing to modify fluid intake so that she might have the energy posttreatment to walk her grandchild home from school; the smoker who will discuss quitting not because she wants to live to be 90, but because personal discipline is a core spiritual value. These are all people who have identified a connection between healthiness and something they want. It is this discrepancy between current behavior and personal goals, values, and desires that pushes healthiness further up the list of daily priorities. Help a patient develop a discrepancy and watch his ears open up regarding a conversation about change. Discrepancies are discovered through careful listening and strengthened by the reinforcement of patient change talk [12].

Summarizing, at its foundation, MI embraces a core set of attitudes: collaborate and empower, avoid the righting reflex, and develop intrinsic motivation by discovering the discrepancy between current lifestyle and personal goals and values. These attitudes facilitate the *guiding* style that is intrinsic to MI. In the next section, we will address the manner in which listening — what you say and how you say it — brings these attitudes into the consultation room.

3.5.2 Listening: The Implementation of MI

MI is a client-centered, yet directive, interviewing style. Miller and Rollnick [12] refer to the basic listening skills with the acronym OARS: Ask open-ended questions, affirm, listen reflectively, and summarize. These listening skills serve at least two functions within MI. First, the skills operationalize the concept of empathy that is central to MI, the practitioner's goal of understanding all sides of the issue regarding behavior change. In the context of discovery, a few well-conceived open questions followed by small summaries of what the patient says and means are critical to the development of a comprehensive understanding of the patient's beliefs pro/con change.

Second, careful listening is an effective alternative to instruction and confrontation in the face of patient resistance to change. From an MI perspective, the first line of intervention in dealing with a resistant patient is to listen well. Confrontation alternately breeds more confrontation and the overuse of direct persuasion may be considered a principal source of conflict in a practitioner–patient relationship [13].

Summarization is a deceptively simple listening skill that is critical to the directive side of MI. Summarization allows the practitioner to present a comprehensive yet pithy overview of the behavior change dilemma to the patient in a fashion that allows for gentle prods in the direction of increased commitment to change. For example:

Practitioner: So, you used to be somebody who could eat whatever you wanted, just eat things that tasted good, not worry about the amount you ate, and you were big into exercise.

Patient: Yes, and now that you mention taste I don't find food tastes that good; I don't feel like I taste it. I just eat it, but before, I remember "Oh that tasted so good" or I have memories of the past, "Oh, I always liked that" and now I eat it and it's like ugh, but I eat it anyway.

Practitioner: Things used to taste good and now when you eat the same things…

Patient: They have no taste to them. They are just a means for me to fill my stomach.

Practitioner: Kind of lost some of the fun and pleasure of eating. And back in the old days, not only did you enjoy the tastes, but exercise was a big part of your life and there may have been some connection between the exercise and being able to eat and maintain the weight you wanted.

The fourth listening skill, affirmation, serves two distinct functions: first, the patient's participation in the health behavior change discussion is clearly reinforced; second, affirmation leads to empowerment. For example, consider these statements of affirmation: "I can see that you're very invested in becoming healthier." "You're making some difficult choices regarding your diet. It's very important to you to control your blood sugars without insulin." Affirm and empower patients and they are more likely to persist with health behavior change.

3.5.3 Instructing Well

MI is, at its core, an example of the guiding style of consultation — a style of great utility when working with patients regarding the initiation and maintenance of lifestyle change. There are, however, within MI, and within the world of health care, times when effective instruction is critically important. From an MI perspective, the goals of effective health education are twofold: 1) provide relevant information, and 2) maintain rapport. The best dose of education is ineffective when it falls upon closed ears. Maintain the balance of power, keep the information relevant, and patient interest will be sustained.

Instruction is "top-down" by its very nature and, as such, creates a challenge with respect to collaboration. To counter this natural noncollaborative tendency, the MI clinician can employ a very simple but effective technique — Ask permission first: "Do you mind if I ask you a few personal questions?" "With your permission, I'd like to propose a plan." "If you don't mind, may I share a bit of information…?" *Ask Permission First* is similar to the now ubiquitous knock on the door of health care practitioners just prior to entering the examination room — a very simple, inexpensive tool for communicating respect and empowerment. MI practitioners have found that the simple asking of permission frequently allows them to provide expert information and advice without falling into the "expert trap," wherein the patient stops listening not as much out of disinterest but rather because of the experience of being infantilized or talked down to. Maintain rapport by balancing interpersonal power and patients will become more amenable to instruction.

A second challenge regarding effective instruction is the need to keep information relevant and succinct. Consistent with the spirit of MI, we follow the formula, *Elicit-Provide-Elicit*, to effectively exchange information. Rather than delivering a chunk of information based upon our *a priori* assumptions of what the patient needs to know, we begin by simply eliciting, from the patient, questions and concerns, followed by careful listening. Here is an example:

Practitioner: I'd be interested in just getting a sense from you what you know about nutrition and healthy diet and maybe what questions you have. And you've done some reading and thinking about this. Would this be OK?

Patient: Well, I know that that you shouldn't skip meals, and that people think if they haven't had breakfast, it's good because they haven't consumed those calories, then they feel that they can eat lunch and even dinner. But if I do that, if I don't eat breakfast, most of the time by lunchtime I will eat anything, stuff I wouldn't even touch normally. I'm not a big French fry person but where I work, right next door, there's a lunch counter with french fries.

Practitioner: French fries coming out of the woodwork.

Patient: Yes, you order a sandwich and you get 20 lbs of French fries. And I know that for lunch, almost every day, I eat that. I know that's not good. Then I'm stuffed 'til like about seven o'clock. By the time I get home, I'm hungry again and I need to *do something quick*. I don't have anything to prepare, so I open up a can of something, usually something cheesy or fat. And I know it's fat and I don't add any vegetables or anything and that's what I eat.

Practitioner: So you know that skipping meals is a problem, that it is healthier to eat three meals a day. And you've experienced that if you do skip a meal at lunchtime, you're just so ravenous that you go ahead and eat for dinner the things you wouldn't normally eat because you don't particularly like their taste. You have this sense about yourself that if you don't kind of pace out your eating, you start to make the wrong choices. Perhaps we could put our heads together and discuss some options regarding pacing, healthy choices, and how to manage that stressful evening meal."

Having elicited a short list of patient concerns, the practitioner is now challenged with the task of providing information in a manner that maintains rapport and patient involvement; in other words, to instruct in the spirit of MI. Three keys to success are: 1) use neutral conditional language; 2) offer a menu of choices; and 3) take "reflection breaks," small bits of listening interspersed in with the instruction.

Affectionately called "wiggle words," the use of neutral and conditional language is fundamental to MI-spirited information exchange. Substitute "I think" and "you should" with phrases that empower the patient by allowing for personal choice, "one option you might consider…; perhaps you could start with…" Deliver information in the third person tense. Rather than, "I recommend," try, "Experts suggest." For "You should," substitute "Some of my patients have found…" Words that allow choice empower patients and maintain their interest.

The concept of a menu of choices is also critical to maintaining the spirit of MI while providing instruction and negotiating treatment goals. Offer patients a short list of choices and you will find that they feel more empowered. The act of decision-making by patients when working with a menu of choices also facilitates their commitment; people are more likely to persist with goals they have self-selected. Furthermore, the menu provides hope in the face of failure, as there is always another plan of action to try if the first plan fails.

Reflection breaks are the third key to successful MI-spirited instruction. A reflection break is merely an opportunity to maintain rapport and avoid information overdose through the use of small summaries of the patient's utterances. Consider this example: deep into a period of education about the importance of eating more vegetables, the patient interjects, "Well, I guess I could start eating a bit of broccoli and asparagus for lunch." The nutritionist might respond in one of two ways to this utterance: 1) continued instruction: "Yes, you're absolutely right, and I'd also recommend some carrots and lettuce..." or 2) provide a reflection break, "So you're thinking of adding some broccoli and asparagus to your lunch," to which the patient might respond, "Yes, and maybe there are some other veggies I could try like carrots and celery."

What are the benefits of the reflection break? Patient interest is maintained through active participation, the practitioner gains direction, and collaborative problem solving is encouraged. Whatever the task, effective listening is key to maintaining the spirit of MI.

3.5.4 Techniques: Reaching into the MI Toolkit

Following the impetus of Rollnick [22] and others, a variety of techniques that are helpful adjuncts to the more open-ended conversational style of MI have been developed. These techniques provide a means of structuring MI-spirited conversations that often integrate easily into the everyday world of the health care practitioner. Three particularly helpful techniques are: Agenda Setting, Good - Not So Good, and Importance–Confidence.

3.5.4.1 Opening the Door: Agenda Setting

"I've got so much to cover and there is so little time; how can I possibly get the job done!" What health care practitioner has not uttered these words now and again?

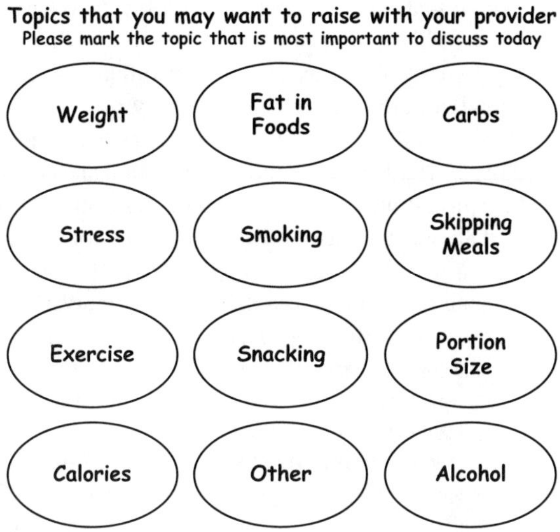

FIGURE 3.4 An agenda-setting chart.

As an MI technique, agenda setting [17] provides a means to both actively engage the patient and increase the effectiveness of the health care consultation. Using a simple chart to elucidate a menu of choices (Figure 3.4), the practitioner elicits from the patient preferences regarding topics to address during their office visit. The chart may be geared toward topics that are often major concerns for patients, such as smoking, stress management, domestic violence, shelter anxiety, weight loss, alcohol use, and sexual concerns. The chart could also be modified to address the needs of a more focused consultation, for example a patient with diabetes: blood sugar monitoring, diet, exercise, medications, foot care, and self-care barriers. The goal of the agenda-setting technique is to provide the patient with the opportunity to discuss that which they are most ready to change and the practitioner with the opportunity to deliver a dose of tailored education to an interested individual. Consider this dialog:

Practitioner: Thanks for coming in today, Mr. Smith. I'd like to spend about 15 minutes talking to you about your eating and weight as factors in your blood sugar control. Would that be all right?

Patient: Well, it's not my favorite subject, but I guess we can give it a go.

Practitioner: Yes, many of my patients feel that way. They have many concerns about their diets, some of which I have on this chart. Would you like to see if any of them relate to you? For some of them, it is not knowing what to eat, whether they are getting too many carbohydrates or fat; others are not sure when they should eat, or worry about how stress affects their eating; sometimes the concern has to do with smoking or alcohol use. And often it is something else altogether, which is why we leave some blank circles. Where would you like to start?

Patient: Well, I know that I need to cut back on the steak and cheese but I just don't fancy myself eating tofu and tuna fish all day long.

Practitioner: So you think you may be eating too much saturated or "bad" fat, but the alternatives are not too appealing to you.

Patient: I used to eat really healthy foods and kept my weight down. But since I started my new job, I seem to crave steaks and fatty food.

Practitioner: So, stress could be a factor in what you eat.

Patient: Yeah. That's what I should work on.

Perhaps there is a pressing clinical concern that must be addressed or another issue of importance to the practitioner. How can these situations be integrated into agenda setting? Try negotiating a primary and a secondary agenda, as follows:

Practitioner: So, let's put our heads together regarding ways to manage stress. I'd also like to reserve a few minutes to discuss blood sugar monitoring. I know from our previous discussions that this has been a challenge and I think it's important to keep our eyes on that. Would that be OK, too?

In the service of patient empowerment and the minimization of resistance, if feasible, address the patient's concerns first, followed by the concerns of the practitioner. Agenda setting is easily adapted to briefer interventions by limiting the choice to a fixed list of two or three topics. Critical, however, is the offering of choice.

Practitioner: When it comes to managing weight some people prefer to focus on changing what they eat; others prefer to look at activity and exercise. What would you prefer to discuss today?

3.5.4.2 Listening to Learn: Good–Not So Good

Faced with the reluctant patient, how does one achieve a productive consultation? Jumping ahead of the patient's readiness often results in the mutual frustration of a one-sided lecture falling upon deaf ears. One option is to reach into the MI toolkit and pull out the Good–Not So Good technique.

Good–Not So Good is simply a structured conversation addressing the content of the leftmost column of the decisional matrix (Figure 3.3), organized in a manner consistent with the spirit of MI: appreciate ambivalence and avoid the righting reflex. Using the listening style, the practitioner first queries the patient about the enjoyable, pleasurable, and hard-to-give-up aspects of the target behavior (status quo talk). This is then followed by a query about the other side of the ambivalence — that which is less good (change talk). Words are chosen carefully so as to avoid an argument. For example, "What is not-so-good" is chosen over "What don't you like about…" or "What's a problem with…." The goal is to provide the opportunity for a brief but balanced conversation about the target behavior in a manner that leaves the patient, not the practitioner, articulating the concerns. Again, people are more effectively influenced by what they say than by what they hear.

Practitioner: I gather that you're not all that excited about discussing cutting down on the carbohydrates and fats. So, I wonder if it might be helpful to take a step back and look at what we're asking you to give up, if you do make some of these changes. How's that sound?

Patient: OK.

Practitioner: Well, what do you like about your current eating? What would you miss if you did change?

Patient: Gosh, No one has ever asked me that! The stuff just tastes good. I guess the worse it is for you, the better it tastes going down. I go crazy over chocolate and I just can't seem to get through the day without some chips.

Practitioner: So, you like the taste of the sweets and crave the salty snacks, too. What else about what you are eating makes you feel good?

Patient: Things at home have been rough lately, with my three teenagers and the little one; the only time we have a bit of peace is when we're sitting down to a family dinner. I know I eat too much then, but I really look forward to that time together.

Practitioner: Big portions seem to be an essential part of the family dinner.

(*Query continues*)

Practitioner: Now, how about the other side. What is not so good about your current eating? What do you like a bit less?

Patient: I hear all the lectures and the threats. If I don't change, I'm headed for insulin, I guess. And it's getting to where even the stretch pants don't fit.

Practitioner: People are really on you about your health and you've also noticed the effects of the weight gain on your body size.

Patient: Yeah, and the breathing is worse. I can hardly get up the two flights of stairs in my house. When the little one cries, it takes me a good 5 minutes to get to her.

Practitioner: Sounds like that really concerns you; not being able to be there for your child.

Patient: Yeah. Can you imagine if there was a fire or something?

The goal of Good–Not So Good is to structure a helpful conversation with the patient not yet ready for health education or treatment planning. Resistance is reduced by first eliciting status quo talk. The more confrontational change talk query follows next, with the patient in the position to articulate concerns, often revealing a particularly personal concern tied to a core value, such as being a good parent who can protect a child. Having articulated concern, interest tends to pique regarding a conversation about steps toward healthiness.

3.5.4.3 Guiding toward Readiness: Importance–Confidence

The Importance–Confidence scaling technique is a wonderful technique developed by Rollnick [22]; incorporated into this simple technique are all the basic elements of MI: listen carefully, appreciate ambivalence, elicit change talk, empower and collaborate. The scaling exercise yields for the practitioner a clear sense of how ready the patient is for change and how to be most helpful.

Importance and confidence reflect two conceptually independent dimensions that underlie patient readiness to change: *Why should I?* (Importance) and *How can I?* (Confidence). Simplifying, a 2 × 2 table of high–low importance vs. high–low confidence yields the following four situations, exemplified by these typical statements:

High Importance/High Confidence: "I really want to lose weight so that I can get off insulin. I know that with a dietitian's guidance, I can do it and keep it off."

High Importance/Low Confidence: "I really want to lose weight so that I can get off insulin, but I have tried a million diets and they just don't work for me."

Low Importance/High Confidence: "I have lost weight before so I know I can do it, but what's the point? My whole family has diabetes so losing weight won't stop me from getting it."

Low Importance/Low Confidence: "There is no point in me trying to lose weight; I have always been fat and couldn't lose it if I tried."

Imagine the possibilities of mismatching professional advice to patient readiness, as follows:

Practitioner: For patients who have already had a heart attack, eating a lot of saturated fat is the worst thing for their health; it's even worse than for people in general. I need to strongly encourage you to cut back!

Patient (High Importance/Low Confidence): With all due respect, Doctor, you're preaching to the choir. I know that ice cream, clam chowder, steak, and cheese are all heart attack foods. I'm scared to death of another heart attack, but I've tried everything and nothing seems to work. I think I'll be eating this stuff 'til my dying day!

Practitioner: All you have to do is go on a diet. I will refer you to a dietitian immediately. We can deal with cravings with some medication. And a little exercise will help, too. We've got plenty of tools at our disposal to make the process simple and easy.

Patient (Low Importance): "I'm sorry Doctor, but what I eat makes me happy, it's a comfort to me since the kids have left home. Since I quit smoking, I don't get much enjoyment from anything else in life. It's my last vice. It's just not that big of a deal!"

In the first case, the practitioner has mistakenly assumed that the barrier to change falls in the "*why should I*" arena and passionately delivers a dose of instruction that at best is redundant with the patient's current knowledge-base and, at worst, is perceived by the patient as evidence that the practitioner just has not listened well. The second case is a fine example of the righting reflex, where, by assuming that the barrier is in the arena of "*how can I*," the practitioner jumps way ahead of the patient's readiness to take action, resulting in a consultation marked by discord and conflict.

Importance–Confidence provides a means of avoiding these rapport-breakers by facilitating an MI-spirited conversation about change that both informs the practitioner about how best to help the patient and also allows the patient to verbalize change talk. This is implemented with six simple questions:

How important is it for you right now to change? On a scale from 0 (not at all important) to 10 (extremely important), what score would you give yourself?
a. Why are you at (*X*) and not at 0?
b. What would need to happen for you to get from (*X*) to (*X* + 2)?

If you did decide to change, how confident are you (0, not at all confident; 10, extremely confident) that you could do it?
a. Why are you at (*X*) and not at 0?
b. What would need to happen for you to get from (*X*) to (*X* + 2)?

Notice that the "*downward*" question precedes the "*upward*" question, with regard to both Importance and Confidence. Often called the "Colombo question" after the 1980s television detective known for his subtle questioning, the downward question is critically important to this MI tool. "*Why is it an 8 and not a 0?*" both demonstrates an attitude of acceptance and also invites the patient to verbalize change talk, expressed as concerns regarding current behavior. The exceptionally important and more confrontational question, "*What would it take to raise your score,*" then follows.

Using Importance–Confidence, a practitioner can, in a matter of minutes, obtain a good idea of how ready a patient is to change the target behavior, and whether to proceed by initially exploring importance or building confidence.

3.5.5 Briefer Interventions

"*But how can we do this in just a few minutes?*" This is the most frequent and most legitimate question posed to MI trainers. The answer is at once both simple and a bit complex. The deceptively simple answer is, try to sandwich as much MI as possible into your conversation. The somewhat more complex answer is, "Think about the three styles and try to flexibly move between them in a manner that meets the needs of your patient."

The MI sandwich refers to the integration of the fundamentals of the MI spirit and listening style into everyday practice [23] For example, the spirit of collaboration is easily established within the first few minutes of a consultation by employing some of these simple strategies: 1) communicate clearly about the purpose of the visit and how this consultation will address the patient's expressed concerns; 2) ask permission before proceeding; emphasize that you will be sharing ideas back and forth, and remember to offer a menu of options at the appropriate moments; 3) set an agenda together when appropriate; and 4) thank the patient and affirm his or her efforts. These strategies are among the options that will promote the spirit of collaboration and empowerment.

As with the longer versions of MI, effective listening is critical to brief implementations. Listen with small summaries. Carefully choose your words. Offer some wiggle words and avoid the use of first person directives. When you instruct, elicit first, and then educate. Look for opportunities for reflection breaks.

Finally, the practitioner who becomes *3 Styles-Savvy* — aware of the communication style being used and purposeful about matching style to situation — will find the integration of MI into briefer conversations quite straightforward. Listen in response to resistance. Guide with the MI toolkit to stimulate interest and to open ears. Instruct with options and then listen some more.

These basic principles will guide the integration of MI into everyday health care practice, whether we are talking about specialist mental health, health behavior change consultations, or of the more frequent corridor conversations that so impact the patient's experience of the health care system.

3.6 WHAT THE RESEARCH SHOWS

There have been several reviews of the clinical usefulness of MI [6,8,24–27]. Over 400 published papers on MI have been published to date, including around 70 outcome trials [27]. Given space constraints, we will discuss these outcome findings only briefly here. However, the reader is encouraged to seek out the reviews mentioned above for a deeper understanding of the findings as well as the complexities of research in this area. It is notable that there are numerous ongoing studies both in the U.S. and overseas, applying much more stringent MI training and intervention standards than were used even 5 years ago, that will come to fruition soon and help further clarify the role of MI in health promotion generally, and obesity in particular [26]. Generally, the findings to date have provided encouragement and support for our clinical methods and have prompted further refinement of MI interventions to fit specific patient groups and settings.

Of particular relevance to the management of obesity are five studies focusing on diet and physical activity that will be outlined below. Overall, it should be noted that the MI clinical approach itself has evolved since the mid-1990s and critical MI counseling elements have been refined. For example, research has clarified the importance of empathy and adherence to the core MI spirit of collaboration, autonomy support, and eliciting change talk. Recent intriguing findings reported by Amrhein et al. [28] have also suggested that fostering strong commitment language from the patient may be one of the most important mediators of behavior change; that is, the best predictor of change is the patient's verbalization of a concrete plan of action. Generally, in MI intervention studies, we have seen dramatic improvements in the standards of interventionist training and treatment fidelity, including routine analysis of audio tapes of interventionist-patient interactions using standardized coding tools to measure, empirically, the presence of important MI counseling attitudes and behaviors [29].

What have MI review studies reported to date on the clinical usefulness of MI? Zweben and Zuckoff [24], in their review of the impact of MI on treatment adherence, identified 21 studies from 1988 to 2001, including interventions targeting alcohol and drug abuse, dual psychiatric diagnoses, diabetes, weight control, exercise, HIV prevention, and eating disorders. Despite problems with internal validity seen in many of these studies (i.e., small samples, lack of control group, limited description of interventionist training or the intervention, insufficient precautions to ensure treatment fidelity across conditions), the adding of an MI component has produced significant adherence effects and helped patients move from one level of treatment adherence to a higher one. For example, Borsari and Carey [30] in a randomized, controlled trial found that MI reduced binge drinking among college students in the MI intervention group (using a single MI session) by 35% compared to 15% for controls. Scales [31] observed that motivational enhancement therapy, a brief MI protocol, produced lower scores for patients in cardiovascular rehabilitation on a linear score combining perceived stress, physical activity, and dietary fat. Treasure et al. [32] found a similar impact when MI was combined with a behavior intervention in the treatment of bulimia. Hodgins, Currie, and el-Guebaly [33] concluded that a single session of MI reduced days gambling and amount of money lost by problem gamblers; this effect was much more robust than that obtained with a self-help book.

More relevant to obesity, Resnicow et al. [34] reviewed five outcome studies evaluating the impact of MI counseling on diet and physical activity change [26,35–40]. Berg-Smith et al. [35] report that children receiving two sessions of MI for diet reported significant improvement in fat and calorie intake. Mhurchu et al. [36] observed no differences in main outcomes between hypertensive patients receiving an MI condition involving three MI sessions and those receiving a standard dietary intervention.

In a pilot study, Smith et al. [37] found older, obese women with type 2 diabetes, receiving an MI intervention to have greater group attendance, more frequent blood glucose monitoring, and improved blood glucose control (i.e., 1% HbA1c drop) compared to a behavior therapy intervention. In a subsequent randomized, controlled trial designed to evaluate the incremental benefit of MI to improve outcomes in behavioral obesity treatment [37], 217 overweight (average BMI = 37) women (38% African-American) with type 2 diabetes received either a group-based behavioral weight control program with supplemental individual MI sessions or the same weight control program with health education sessions (attention placebo control). Women in the MI group lost significantly more weight than those in the control group at 6 months (–4.7 vs. −3.1 kg, $p < 0.02$). This superior weight loss was mirrored by enhanced adherence to the treatment program on all process variables examined over the initial 6 months: session attendance (19 vs. 17, $p < 0.006$); number of weekly self-monitoring diaries submitted (17 vs. 14, $p < 0.002$); average diary rating (1.4 vs. 1.2, $p = 0.002$); and changes in caloric expenditure in moderate to vigorous exercise (+955 vs. +742 kcal, $p < 0.04$). Weight losses were strongly associated with attendance, diary submission, and diary ratings ($r = 0.45$ to 0.52, $p < 0.001$) and modestly associated with increased caloric expenditure ($r = 0.21$, $p < 0.03$), suggesting that enhanced engagement in the treatment program accounted for superior weight losses in the MI condition at 6 months. The pattern remained consistent in the 12 months of follow-up. Thus, MI appears to facilitate adherence to weight loss maintenance efforts, as well as weight loss induction and as such merits consideration for inclusion in standard behavioral weight control programs.

Harland and colleagues [39] obtained data indicating that MI enhanced exercise behaviors among sedentary but healthy general practice patients at 39 months compared to controls; but this difference disappeared at 1 year follow-up. Woollard et al. [40] found significant improvements in systolic blood pressure of 6 to 8 mm Hg as well as reduced alcohol and salt intake for hypertensive patients receiving one of two levels of MI counseling compared to a usual care condition. Resnicow et al.

[26] increased fruit and vegetable consumption among African-American adults by one serving per day following an MI intervention delivered by trained dietitians relative to comparison and control conditions, although analysis of tape-recorded phone intervention sessions, however, suggested only moderate treatment fidelity to the spirit and techniques of MI.

Overall, the data regarding the impact of MI generally, and on obesity and related problem areas specifically, have been promising, particularly the randomized clinical trial (RCT) conducted recently by Smith-West et al. [38] on obese diabetic patients, which is part of a new wave of MI intervention studies with high MI training and treatment fidelity standards. We will continue to be informed by these more sophisticated methodological papers conducted using the behavior change consortium (BCC) guidelines [29] and specifically with use of interview coding strategies such as that provided by the MI Treatment Integrity (MITI) tool [41]. We will see an improved focus on measuring MI-related mediators such as importance of change and self-efficacy as well as the amount and quality of patient change talk that new research is showing to be important. These enhancements, as part of an overall strengthening of the evaluation research in MI studies, will likely lead to a clearer picture regarding what type and dose of MI is required for what patients and in which clinical contexts to produce the maximal health benefits.

3.7 CONCLUSIONS

MI and its derivative, Health Behavior Change Counseling, instructs us to appreciate the limits of a direct-persuasion model of interpersonal influence, guides toward an understanding of ambivalence and the value of eliciting patient change- and confidence-talk, and models the use of effective listening skills to build, engage, understand, and facilitate behavior change. Whether one has the luxury of extended patient contact or must work within the parameters of a brief scheduled or opportunistic exchange, there are opportunities to integrate elements of the MI guiding style into everyday practice. Start at the foundation of the MI learning pyramid, using what you say, and what you avoid saying, to communicate respect, empowerment, and a willingness to hang in there with patients as they struggle with the decision to change. Try to answer the questions, "Why would this particular patient want to modify his or her eating and activity behavior at this particular moment in time?" "What would the patient gain and what would he or she has to give up?" Bring the spirit of MI into the consultation through effective listening: Ask a few open questions to elicit your patient's concerns and ideas regarding change. Follow this with reflective listening, small summaries of what you just heard. Listen, rather than argue when you hear resistance from the patient. As the decisional matrix informs, there are always compelling reasons in the short term not to be eager to change health behavior.

Avoid instructing if patients' ears are not open. Give them some *wiggle room* by couching advice in neutral and conditional language. Reach into the MI toolkit and use a technique to guide toward readiness for health education. Finally, when you start to hear change talk, offer the patient options as you negotiate a plan of action.

RESOURCES

Motivational Interview Network of Trainers, an international organization of MI trainers and researchers all of whom have completed the Training New Trainers workshop under W.R. Miller, Ph.D. and/or S. Rollnick, Ph.D., www.motivationalinterview.org.

Institute for Motivation and Change, an M.I. training institute, www.miinstitute.com.

REFERENCES

1. Olsen, C.L., Schumaker, H.D., and Yawn, B.P., Overweight women delay medical care, *Arch. Fam. Med.*, 3, 888–892, 1994.
2. Galuska, D.A., Will, J.C., Serdula, M.K., and Ford, E.S., Are health care professionals advising obese patients to lose weight? *JAMA*, 282, 1576–1578, 1999.
3. Manson, J.E., Skerrett, P.J., Greenland, P., and VanItallie, T.B., The escalating pandemics of obesity and sedentary lifestyle: a call to action for clinicians, *Arch. Intern. Med.*, 164, 249–258, 2004.
4. Nielsen-Bohlman, L., Panzer, A.M., and Kindig, D.A., Eds., *Health Literacy: A Prescription to End Confusion*, Institute of Medicine, Washington, D.C., 2004.
5. Travaline, M., Ruschinskas, R., and D'Alonzo, G.E., Patient-physician communication: why and how, *J. Am. Osteopath. Assoc.*, 105, 13–18, 2005.
6. Burke, B.T., Arkowitz, H., and Dunn, C., The efficacy of motivational interviewing and its adaptations: what we know so far. In *Motivational Interviewing: Helping People Change,* 2nd ed., Miller, W.R., and Rollnick, S., Eds., Guilford Press, New York, 2002.
7. DiLillo, V., Siegfried, N.J., and Smith-West, D., Incorporating motivational interviewing into behavioral obesity treatment, *Cogn. Behav. Prac.,* 10, 120–130, 2003.
8. VanWormer, J.J. and Boucher, J.L., Motivational interviewing and diet modification: a review of the evidence, *Diabetes Educ.*, 30, 404–419, 2004.
9. Miller, W.R., Motivational interviewing with problem drinkers, *Behav. Psychother.,* 1, 147–172, 1983.
10. Rollnick, S., The value of a cognitive-behavioral approach in the treatment of problem drinkers. In *The Misuse of Alcohol: Clinical Issues in Dependency Treatment and Prevention,* Heather, N., Robertson, I., and Davies, P., Eds., New York University Press, New York, 1985.
11. Miller, W.R. and Rollnick, S., *Motivational Interviewing: Helping People Change Addictive Behavior*, Guilford Press, New York, 1991.
12. Miller, W.R. and Rollnick, S., *Motivational Interviewing: Helping People Change,* 2nd ed., Guilford Press, New York, 2002.
13. Rose, G.S., Rollnick, S.R., and Lane, C., What's Your Style? A model for helping practitioners to learn about communication and motivational interviewing, *MINUET,* 11, 2–4, 2004.
14. Rollnick, S. and Miller, W.R., What is motivational interviewing? *Behav. Cogn. Psychother.*, 23, 325–334, 1995.
15. Stewart, M., Brown, J.B., Weston, W.W., McWhinney, I.R., McWilliam, C.L., and Freeman, T.R., *Patient-Centered Medicine: Transforming the Clinical Method,* Sage Publications, London, 1995.
16. Deci, E.L., *Intrinsic Motivation and Self-Determination in Human Behavior*, Springer Publications, New York, 1985.
17. Rollnick, S., Mason, P., and Butler, C. *Health Behavior Change: A Guide for Practitioners*, Churchill Livingstone, London, 1999.

18. Sobell, M.B. and Sobell, L.C., *Problem Drinkers: Guided Self-Change Treatment*, Guilford Press, New York, 1993.
19. Langewitz, W., Denz, M., Keller, A., Kiss, A., Ruttimann, S., and Wossmer, B., Spontaneous talking time at start of consultation in outpatient clinic: a cohort study, *BMJ*, 325, 682–683, 2002.
20. Janis, I.L. and Mann, L., *Decision-Making: A Psychological Analysis of Conflict, Choice, and Commitment*, Free Press, New York, 1977.
21. Bem, D.J., Self-perception theory. In *Advances in Experimental Social Psychology,* Berkowitz, L., Ed., Academic Press, New York, 1972.
22. Rollnick, S., Readiness, importance, and confidence: critical conditions of change in treatment. In *Treating Addictive Behaviors,* 2nd ed., Miller, W.R. and Heather, N., Eds., Plenum Press, New York, 1998.
23. Wagner, C., personal communication, 2004.
24. Zweben, A. and Zuckoff, A., Motivational interviewing and treatment adherence, In *Motivational Interviewing: Preparing People for Change,* 2nd ed., Miller, W.R. and Rollnick, S., Eds., Guilford Press, New York, pp. 229–319, 2002.
25. Welch, G., Rose, G., and Ernst, D. Motivational interviewing and diabetes: what is it, how is it done, and does it work? *Diabetes Symposium* 19, 5–11, 2006.
26. Resnicow, K., Jackson, A., Wang, T., McCarty, F., Dudley, W.N., and Baranowski, T., A motivational interviewing intervention to increase fruit and vegetable intake through black churches: results of the Eat for Life trial, *Am. J. Public Health*, 91, 1686–1693, 2001.
27. Hettema, J.E., Miller, W.R., and Steele, J.M., A meta-analysis of motivational interviewing techniques in the treatment of alcohol use disorders, *Alcohol Clin. Exp. Res.*, 28, 74A, 2004.
28. Amrhein, P.C., Miller, W.R., Yahne, C.E., Palmer, M., and Fulcher, L., Client commitment language during motivational interviewing predicts drug use outcomes, *J. Consult. Clin. Psychol.,* 71, 862–878, 2003.
29. Belig, A.J., Borrell, B., Resnick, B., Hecht, J., Minicucci, D.S., Ory, M., Ogededbe, G., Orwig, D., Ernst, D., and Czajkowski, S., Enhancing treatment fidelity in health behavior change studies: best practices and recommendations from the NIH Behavior Change Consortium, *Health Psychol.,* 23, 443–451, 2004.
30. Borsari, B. and Carey, K.B., Effects of a brief motivational intervention with college student drinkers, *J. Consult. Clin. Psychol.*, 68, 728–733, 2000.
31. Scales, R., Motivational interviewing and skills-based counseling in cardiac rehabilitation: the Cardiovascular Health Initiative and Lifestyle Education (CHILE) Study, Doctoral dissertation, The University of New Mexico. *Dissertation Abstracts International,* 59-03A, 0741, 1998.
32. Treasure, J.L., Katzman, M., Schmidt, U., Troop, N., Todd, G., and de Silva, P., Engagement and outcome in the treatment of bulimia nervosa: first phase of a sequential design comparing motivation enhancement therapy and cognitive behavioural therapy, *Behav. Res. Ther.,* 37, 405–418, 1999.
33. Hodgins, D.C., Currie, S.R., and el-Guebaly, N., Motivational enhancement and self-help treatments for problem gambling, *J. Consult. Clin. Psychol.,* 69, 50–57, 2001.
34. Resnicow, K., DiIorio, C., Soet, J.E., Borrelli, B., Ernst, D., Hecht, J., and Thevos, A.K., Motivational interviewing in medical and public health settings, In *Motivational Interviewing: Preparing People for Change,* 2nd ed., Miller, W.R. and Rollnick, S., Eds., Guilford Press, New York, pp. 251–269, 2002.
35. Berg-Smith, S.M., Stevens, V.J., Brown, K.M., Van Horn, L., Gernhofer, N., Peters, E., Greenberg, R., Snetselaar, L., Ahrens, L., and Smith, K. (for the Dietary Inter-

vention Study in Children [DISC Research Group]), A brief motivational intervention to improve dietary adherence in adolescents, *Health Educ. Res.,* 14, 399–410, 1999.
36. Mhurchu, C.N., Margetts, B.M., and Speller, V., Randomized clinical trial comparing the effectiveness of two dietary interventions for patients with hyperlipidaemia, *Clin. Sci.*, 95, 479–448, 1998.
37. Smith, D.E., Heckemeyer, C.M., Kratt, P.P., and Mason, D.A., Motivational interviewing to improve adherence to a behavioral weight-control program for older obese women with NIDDM: a pilot study, *Diabetes Care*, 20, 53–54, 1999.
38. Smith-West, D., DiLillo, V., Greene, P., Bursac, Z., and Phillips, M., Motivational interviewing increases adherence to a behavioral weight control program. Paper presented at the Annual Meeting of the Society of Behavioral Medicine, Baltimore, MD, April 21, 2004.
39. Harland, J., White, M., Drinkwater, C., Chinn, D., Farr, L., and Howel, D., The Newcastle exercise project: a randomized controlled trial of methods to promote physical activity in primary care, *BMJ,* 319, 828–832, 1999.
40. Woollard, J., Beilin, L., Lord, T., Puddey, I., MacAdam, D., and Rouse, I., A controlled trial of nurse counseling on lifestyle change for hypertensives treated in general practice: preliminary results, *Clin. Exp. Pharmacol. Physiol.,* 22, 466–468, 1995.
41. Moyers, T., Martin, T., Manuel, J., Miller, W.R., *The Motivational Interviewing Treatment Integrity (MITI) Code (v 2.0)*, CASAA, University of New Mexico, Albuquerque, NM, 2004.

4 Dietary Therapy

Diana Cullum-Dugan and Cheryl Jesuit

CONTENTS

4.1 THE PROBLEM WITH DIETING IN THE OBESE POPULATION — AN OVERVIEW

4.1.1 Bias toward the Obese

Regardless of our belief system and perceived ability to abide by social mores, many of us have garnered internalized prejudices against people of size — the overweight or obese people in our population. Negative attitudes toward the obese in our culture could be a possible contributor to the hesitancy of health care providers to treat the disease. Physicians often hold negative views and stereotype this population as lazy or lacking motivation or willpower to make the lifestyle changes necessary for weight loss; the negativity on the part of the physician and shame on the part of the patient increases as the weight of the patient increases [1]. Nurses agree that obesity could be prevented by self-control and registered dietitians exhibit ambivalent and negative attitudes toward obesity [2], again demonstrating the pervasiveness of a negative outlook toward working with obese patients. Even overweight individuals themselves, unlike other minority group members, do not appear to hold more favorable attitudes toward each other [3], and professionals whose careers emphasize research or the clinical management of obesity show very strong weight bias, indicating pervasive and powerful stigma [4].

In this time of epidemic proportions of obesity [5], it is critical that we take the time to assess our own feelings and potential prejudices about people who are obese, remove a patient's personal responsibility out of the equation of treatment, and turn our attention toward treating obesity as a disease, consistent with its genetic, behavioral, and environmental influences.

4.1.2 Adherence and Compliance to Dieting

In the U.S. at any given time, 45% of women and 30% of men are actively dieting [6], along with as many as 25% of American girls and 13.8% of American boys under the age of 14 [7]. Yet adults often do not follow the recommended guidelines to lower their calorie intake and become physically active [8], and, in fact, most defer to the so-called fad or popular diets published without scientific evidence and hyped by the media and personal testimonials, such as Sugar Busters! [9], Protein Power [10], and the Atkins Diet [11] (Table 4.1). Adolescents who use restrictive dieting to lose weight actually show an increased risk of developing obesity later in life, suggesting that early dieting predicts weight gain in adulthood [12].

Despite a teachable spirit and strong commitment to begin making lifestyle changes through diet, patient compliance is less than adequate in most cases, possibly due to the length of time required for goal-oriented weight loss and maintenance; lack of knowledge in nutrition, meal planning, and making appropriate food choices; previous weight loss failures and yo-yo dieting; inability or lack of desire to maintain an adequate level of physical activity; and living in an unsupportive environment. Even with professional guidance such as that of a health care provider or commercial or medically supervised weight loss program, compliance is low and attrition high in most weight management programs. The burden of weight loss is further complicated by the stringent methods and requirements needed for weight maintenance,

TABLE 4.1
Nutrient Intake in Various Diets

Diet	Total Fat (% kcals)	Protein (% kcals)	CHO (% kcals)
Low Carbohydrate High Fat Diets *(Dr. Atkin's New Diet Revolution)*	55–65	25–30	<20%
Moderate-Fat *(DASH, Weight Watcher's, Food Guide Pyramid)*	20–30	15–20	55–60
Very Low Fat, High Carbohydrate *(Dean Ornish's Program)*	<10–19	10–20	>65
ATP III	25–35	15	50–60
Glycemic Index	30–35	15–25	45–50

Adapted in part from Freedman M.R., *Obes. Res.* 9(1), 2001; Ebberling C., *Am. J. Clin. Nutr.* 2005;81: 976–982; http://www.nhlbi.nih.gov/guidelines/cholesterol/atp3full.pdf

and long-term data indicate most persons regain lost weight within 5 yrs [13], with approximately half returning to their baseline weight [14]. With this in mind, obesity should be considered a disease that requires lifelong treatment.

4.1.3 Diets for a "Quick Fix"

Typically, a low- to moderate-fat, high-carbohydrate diet such as the U.S. Department of Agriculture (USDA) Food Guide Pyramid [15], American Diabetes Association Exchange List [16], and USDA and National Institutes of Health (NIH)-recommended DASH diet [17] that recommend adequate selections of fruit, vegetables, whole grains, low- and nonfat dairy, lean meats, poultry and seafood, and a focus on monounsaturated fats is consensually recommended and prescribed for weight loss. Yet the intrigue of a popular diet offering no calorie counting, measuring, or portioning and palatable, satiating foods lures even wary dieters. Some of the more popular diets can be categorized by macronutrient content:

Low-carbohydrate, high-fat diets (such as Dr. Atkins' New Diet Revolution, Protein Power, Sugar Busters!, and the Zone)
Very-low-fat, high-carbohydrate diets (Eat More, Weigh Less – Dr. Dean Ornish's Life Choices Program, and The New Pritikin Program)

Data published on the short-term effects of the low-carbohydrate, high-fat diets indicate greater weight loss as compared to conventional diets at 6 months, but at 1 yr weight loss is equivalent [6]. There still remain many unanswered questions concerning the adequacy of nutrients in these diets.

4.1.4 Herbal Supplements

"Magic bullet" supplements also intrigued 7% of adults who reported using over-the-counter weight loss supplements in 1998 (28% were young, obese women) [18]. These herbals, botanicals, and other remedies that promise fat burning without caloric restriction or additional exercise continue to reel in a large portion of U.S. dollars each year — most with no scientific evidence of conclusive, positive results. Some of the botanicals and herbal supplements that have offered appeal are Ma Huang or ephedra (since removed from the market due to a ban by the Food and Drug Administration [FDA]), bitter orange, guarana, caffeine, chromium, chitosan, L-carnitine, conjugated linoleic acid, and apple cider vinegar (Table 4.2). The appeal of these sometimes dangerous preparations reflects the increased desperation of many to be thin. Many continue to seek the fast, no-fuss weight loss pill or plan. It is our responsibility as health care providers to educate patients on the inappropriateness of quick fixes and to applaud and encourage their tenacious efforts along the most fruitful, albeit more lengthy, pathways.

4.1.5 Medically Supervised Weight Loss Programs

Health care providers trained in the treatment of obesity often have their own personal preferences for weight loss recommendations, ranging from the more aggressive approaches using pharmacotherapy, full liquid diets, and protein-sparing modified fasts to variations of a balanced calorie deficit diet and partial meal replacement programs. Professional opinion, research, and meta-analyses of diets with varying nutrient composition continuously conclude that not one diet fits all [19]. Weight management is a delicate equilibrium between energy intake and expenditure. The bottom line for successful weight management is to combine a reduction in total calorie intake, while increasing physical output, with a strong focus on behavioral modification, especially in light of our "toxic food environment" [20]. Various modalities of treatment for adult obesity and behavioral modification are based on body mass index (BMI) guidelines (Table 4.3). This chapter's emphasis is on nutrition, while information on physical activity can be found in Chapter 5.

4.2 NUTRITIONAL ASSESSMENT — ADULTS

4.2.1 Determining Caloric Needs Using Energy Expenditure

The number of kilocalories required for maintenance of life over a 24-hr period (total energy expenditure [TEE]) is the total of the kilocalories needed to support respiration, circulation, regulation of body temperature, and support of other vital organs (basal metabolic rate [BMR]) plus the kilocalories required for the digestion, absorption, and metabolism of energy (thermal effect of food [TEF]). Also added to the equation are calories expended in activities of daily living (ADLs) and purposeful physical activity. It is complicated, cumbersome, and inconvenient to obtain a BMR for each patient. The measurement of indirect calorimetry is performed accurately only in the fasted state in a tightly controlled environment. A resting metabolic rate (RMR) is used far more often than BMR; yet this measurement is

TABLE 4.2
Outline of Dietary Supplements

Dietary Supplement	Other Names	Mechanism	Effectiveness	Safety
Ephedra alkaloids	Ma Huang, norepinephrine, ephedrine alkaloids, epitonin	Thermogenic; CNS/CVS stimulant	Yes, with and without caffeine	Unsafe (hypertension, palpitation, tachycardia, stroke, seizures, death); banned from market by FDA 4/04
Caffeine	Guarana (*Paullinia cupana*), Yerba Maté (*Ilex paraguayansis*)	Thermogenic; CNS stimulant	No, when used alone	High doses or combinations may be unsafe (hypertension, tachycardia, nausea, dizziness)
Chromium	Chromium picolinate	↑ insulin sensitivity	Uncertain	Uncertain
Ginseng	Korean ginseng (*Panax ginseng*), American ginseng (*Panax quinquefolux*), Siberian ginseng (*Eleutherococcus senticosus*)	↑ insulin sensitivity; thermogenic; ↑ lipolysis	Uncertain	Uncertain; lowering of INR with warfarin
Fiber	Guar gum, psyllium, flaxseed, glucomannan	Malabsorption; ↑ insulin sensitivity	Unlikely	Generally safe, but some forms may have risk of GI obstruction
Hydroxycitric acid	Malabar tamarind (*Garcinia cambogia*)	↑ de novo fatty acid synthesis	Unlikely	Uncertain
Dehydro-epiandrosterone (DHEA)	Adrenal steroid hormone	↓ fat synthesis	Uncertain	Uncertain; metabolites may stimulate breast and prostate tissue
Chitosan	Chitin (crustacean shells)	Blocks dietary fat absorption	Uncertain	Uncertain
Horsetail	Equisetum sp.	Diuretic	Uncertain	Unsafe (may be K+-wasting)
Senna, Cascara	Cassia sp., *Rhamnus pushiana*	Laxatives	Uncertain	Unsafe for treatment of obesity

(continued)

TABLE 4.2 (Continued)
Outline of Dietary Supplements

Dietary Supplement	Other Names	Mechanism	Effectiveness	Safety
St. John's Wort	SJW "herbal phen-fen" (*Hypericum perforatum*)	Antidepressant	Unlikely	Uncertain; phototoxicity; drug interactions with many psychoactive and HIV drugs
Aristolochic acid	Aristolochia, Bragantia, Asarum	Increases metabolism	Uncertain	Causes nephropathy; 2001-FDA consumer advisory; urged industry to remove from products
Tiratrichol	Trioodothyroacetic acid, Triax Metabolic Accelerator	Potent thyroid hormone	Uncertain	1999-FDA consumer advisory
Phenylpropanola-mine	PPA, norephedrine, Lipokinetix (PPA, caffeine, yohimbine, diiodothyronine, sodium usnate)	CNS stimulant	Yes, short-term	2000-FDA consumer advisory; urged industry to remove from products; 2001-FDA consumer advisory about Lipokinetix-liver toxicity
Phen-fen	Phentermine and fenfluramine	Works on CNS hypothalamus to decrease appetite	Yes, short-term	Mitral valve prolapse, mitral regurgitation, primary pulmonary hypertension; 1997-FDA banned combination and fenfluramine from market

Source: Adapted from Lenders, C., Hoppin, A. Management and treatment of obesity. In *Nutrition in Pediatrics: Basic Science and Clinical Applications*, 3rd ed., Walker, W.W., Watkins, Y., Duggan, C., Eds., B.C. Decker, Ch. 54, pp. 917–934, 2003. With permission.
Note: SJW, St John's Wort; FDA, Food and Drug Administration; HIV, human immunodeficiency virus; CNS, central nervous system.

TABLE 4.3
Body Mass Index (BMI)

	<24.9	25–26.9	27–29.9	30–34.9	35–39.9	>40
Low calorie diet	√	√	√	√	√	√
Physical activity	√	√	√	√	√	√
Behavior modification		√	√	√	√	√
Pharmacotherapy			√*	√	√	√
Surgery				√*	√	

*with co-morbidities

Source: Adapted from NHLBI Guidelines.

also not easily rendered in a clinical versus research setting because of the difficulties of ensuring that a patient has not participated in strenuous physical activity, is fasted, and has lived under low-stress conditions for the preceding several days.

Predictive equations for BMR or RMR (Figure 4.2) prove to be reasonable alternatives to these; yet there are concerns they may over- or underpredict RMR, and they do not provide accurate predictive power for the obese population. For the obese population, predictive equations do not consider excess body fat; therefore, it is suggested that an adjusted body weight (ABW) be obtained and used in the calculations.

Essentially, decreasing the daily total energy intake by 500 to 800 kcal will help achieve a weight loss of approximately 1 to 2 lb/week. Weight loss studies among obese subjects suggest to lower goals for weight loss to 10% body weight rather than ideal body weight because 10% weight loss is typically associated with decreased morbidity [21].

4.3 MEDICALLY SUPERVISED DIETS

4.3.1 Aggressive, Short-Term Diets

In an effort to lose more weight in a shorter time period than a typical low-calorie diet can allow, especially for those suffering from severe obesity-related comorbid diseases, full liquid diets and the protein-sparing modified fast (PSMF) were developed. These diets are classified as very-low-calorie-diets (VLCDs) (>400 kcal and <800 kcal), and it is well documented that a VLCD for weight loss results in a significant loss of lean body weight as well as body fat and a decrease in RMR. Adding an intensive, high-volume resistance training program can preserve lean muscle and RMR during weight loss with a VLCD [22]. These VLCD options should be reserved for those patients whose BMI is ≥30 (or ≥27 with one or more comorbidities). As there is a potential of gallstone formation, dehydration, and electrolyte abnormalities in those on VLCDs, medical monitoring is essential. If a patient has a history of gallstones or sludge, it may be advisable to prescribe ursodiol as prophylaxis. For the prevention of gallstones during rapid weight loss during a

TABLE 4.4
Predictive Equations for Metabolic Rate

Harris-Benedict Equation	Men	RMR[a] = 66 + (13.75 $\times$ weight, kg) + (5.0 $\times$ height, cm) - (6.76 $\times$ age, y)
	Women	RMR = 655 + (9.56 $\times$ weight, kg) + (1.85 $\times$ height, cm) - (4.68 $\times$ age, y)
Mifflin Equation	Men	RMR = (9.99 $\times$ weight, kg) + (6.25 $\times$ height, cm) - (4.92 $\times$ age, y) + 5
	Women	RMR = (9.99 $\times$ weight, kg) + (6.25 $\times$ height, cm) - (4.92 $\times$ age, y) -161
Dietary Reference Intakes[c]	Men	TEE[b] = 864 - (9.72 $\times$ age, y) + PA[(14.2 $\times$ weight, kg) + (503 x height, m)]
	Women	TEE = 387 - (7.31 $\times$ age, y) + PA[(10.9 $\times$ weight, kg) + (660.7 $\times$ height, m)]

Quick Methods Based on Harris-Benedict Equation

For weight gain:	35 kcal/kg ABW
For weight loss:	20-25 kcal/kg ABW
For weight maintenance:	30 kcal/kg ABW

Physical Activity Factors (PAFs):	**Men**	**Women**
Sedentary	1.00	1.00
Low active	1.12	1.14
Active	1.27	1.27
Very active	1.54	1.45

Adjusted Body Weight:	ABW = present weight - ideal body weight (.25) + ideal body weight
Ideal Body Weight for Males:	106 lbs for the 1st 5 ft of height + 6 lbs for every inch over 5 feet
Ideal Body Weight for Females:	100 lbs for the 1st 5 ft of height + 5 lbs for every inch over 5 ft

[a]Resting Metabolic Rate
[b]Total Energy Expenditure
[c]Institute of Medicine, Food & Nutrition Board

Source: Keim, N.L., Blanton, C.A., Kretsch, M.J. America's obesity epidemic: measuring physical activity to promote an active lifestyle. JADA 104:1398-1409, 2004. With permission.

VLCD, the addition of a small amount of fat to the diet, replacing some of the carbohydrate and protein, may promote gallbladder emptying, reducing the incidence of cholesterol gallstones [23].

4.3.1.1 Liquid Fasts

Liquid diets were developed primarily to induce rapid weight loss by stimulating ketosis. Early formulas were found nutritionally lacking and even led to death in some extreme cases [24]. Under the guidance of an experienced team of weight management providers, full liquid fasts can offer a viable method for weight loss that is rewarding for the patient [25].

Reputable companies, such as Health Management Resources (HMR, Inc., Boston, MA), and Optifast (Novartis Nutrition, Minneapolis, MN), provide products to assist patients in the full (and partial) liquid diet, such as packets of powdered formula the patient prepares themselves, prepackaged entrees, and meal replacement bars. The product composition is low fat, low carbohydrate, and high protein. Typically, the diet consists of five to six liquid meals each day. A physician prescribes these diets with a registered dietitian and a behaviorist focusing on behavior change. All team members provide strong encouragement for adherence to the selected meal plan which benefits compliance [26]. Some side effects of the full liquid diet include constipation or diarrhea, hair loss, reduction in the thermal effect of food leading to feelings of coldness, and muscle cramps possibly due to loss of electrolytes through diuresis.

4.3.1.2 Protein-Sparing Modified Fast (PSMF)

In the early 1980s, Blackburn corroborated findings that a protein-supplemented fast could combat loss of lean body mass during active weight loss [26]. These fasts have been successfully used for safe, rapid weight loss in obese adults as well as severely obese older children and adolescents [27]. Weight loss success is greatest in the heaviest patients and those with the longest adherence to both the PSMF and maintenance program [28]. Although effective in the short term, there is no evidence that long-term PSMF is more beneficial than regular dietary restriction [29].

A PSMF is described as a very-low-calorie (<800 calories) ketogenic diet that achieves a hormonal milieu furthering optimal weight loss and levels of satiety consistent with compliance [30]. True clinical adherence to the PSMF generally is 4 to 16 weeks for adults. It is mandatory that a physician oversees the PSMF patient; when the patient is ready to refeed, a dietitian can help in the transition to a balanced-calorie diet. The PSMF yields a mean weight loss of approximately 4 lb per week in adult patients. Meal plan development for the adult PSMF is outlined in Table 4.5.

TABLE 4.5
Protein-Sparing Modified Fast Guidelines for Adults

High-protein, hypocaloric diet for 12–16 weeks
- 800–1000 kcal
- Protein 1.5 to 2.0g/kg/d (25–75 kcal/oz)
- Avoid high fat protein (100–125 kcal/oz)
- Carbohydrate
  - None during week 1
  - Week 2, add 1/2 head lettuce
  - Week 4, add 10-12g/d as low-starch vegetables (see below)
- 2 L decaffeinated fluid per day
- Supplements
  - Multivitamin with minerals
  - 1000–1200 mg/d calcium
  - 1–2 T/d Milk of Magnesia
  - Monitor serum potassium and supplement 20 mEq/d as needed
- Refeeding (over 3–6 week period) by adding additional vegetables and fruits slowly
- Maintenance diet (36 weeks)
  - Balanced micronutrients
  - 1200 kcal/d

1 g of carbohydrate
1/2 cup Chinese cabbage, raw
1 clove of garlic, raw
1/2 cup spinach, raw
4 radishes, raw
1 tablespoon onion, raw
1/2 cup alfalfa sprouts, raw

2 g of carbohydrate
1/2 cup green cabbage, raw
1 (7 1/2″) celery stick
1/2 cup cucumber, raw
1/2 cup mushrooms, raw
1/2 cup chopped mustard greens, cooked
1/2 cup zucchini, raw

3 g of carbohydrate
1/2 cup broccoli, raw
1/2 cup cauliflower, raw or cooked
1/2 cup eggplant, raw or cooked
1/2 cup sweet peppers, raw or cooked
1/2 cup summer squash, raw
1/2 cup turnip greens, raw

4 g of carbohydrate
1/2 cup asparagus, cooked
1/2 cup bamboo shoots, raw, cooked

TABLE 4.5 (Continued)
Protein-Sparing Modified Fast Guidelines for Adults

1/2 cup broccoli, cooked
1/2 cup cabbage, cooked
1/2 cup kale, cooked
1/2 cup mushrooms, cooked
1/2 cup spinach, cooked
1/2 cup summer squash, cooked
1/2 cup zucchini, cooked
1/2 cup green/yellow beans, cooked

4.3.2 Long-Term Diets — The Long Haul

4.3.2.1 Meal Replacements (HMR, Slim-Fast® Foods)

Using meal replacements has given patients another option for reducing high-fat, high-calorie food choices while maintaining adequate nutritional status. One or two meals each day can be replaced with a commercially available liquid shake, bar, or entree that is nutrient dense but lower in fat and total calories. Caloric needs for the day can be rounded out with a minimum of two to three fruit servings, 2 to 3 cups; vegetables, 5 to 6 oz; lean protein, and one to two starch servings, for a caloric range of 1200 to 1400 cal. Using meal replacements has been proven to be safe and efficacious in achieving and maintaining weight loss [35] and can be accomplished with or without medical supervision. Patients regain a sense of control over their eating behaviors and thereby their self esteem while working through the process of learning how to select healthy food. Many products provide nutrition education and online support. These types of diets may be an option in adolescents, but further studies are needed in this population.

4.3.2.2 Balanced Calorie Deficit Diet (USDA Food Guide Pyramid, DASH)

The Dietary Guidelines for Americans, 2005, have taken a strong stand toward including a variety of fresh fruits and vegetables, whole grains, low-fat protein, and healthy fats into our diets. The USDA Food Guide Pyramid depicts a healthy diet and self-selected calorie level as a simple visual tool. Yet, overweight and obesity still prevail and in weight management centers, health care providers see day to day the difficulties of traversing the barriers patients face in making healthy choices.

Meal planning with a patient is like perusing a map at the onset of a long journey. There are many avenues that could be taken to reach the destination; however, some are practical and efficient roadways while others are longer, more scenic routes. In other words, you choose between a structured meal plan that outlines exchanges in specific serving sizes required at each meal, to liberalized recommendations as identified in the NCEP ATP III Therapeutic Lifestyle Changes (TLC) plan, equivalent to the previously known American Heart Association Step II diets. Paying particular attention to the patient's needs is key to unraveling the mystery of which road to recommend and in deftly changing the route along the way as obstacles appear. Each patient presents a unique opportunity for the provider to identify cognitive, affective, and sensory (kinetic) learning styles; these learning styles will dictate which educational material is most appropriate.

Due to the delicate components involved in successful behavior change, a dietitian should be involved in addressing meal planning regardless of the structure chosen by the patient. A multitude of concepts prevail, including environmental control, appropriate preplanning for grocery shopping, cooking methods, and basic nutrition knowledge. A dietitian using appropriate cognitive behavioral counseling strategies (see Chapter 3) can help to lead the patient toward greater success by moving through barriers and obstacles to change and by allowing the patient the option of choice according to the stage of readiness in which he or she presents.

For those requiring structured meal plans, these are readily available through a multitude of national organizations, such as the American Dietetic Association and American Heart Association. A less structured, yet self-selecting approach that satisfies the provider while instilling greater freedom of choice for a patient who is put off by the rigidity of a meal plan identifying specific foods can be found in the TLC or DASH diets. Building on the concept of Fill Your Plate (Figure 4.1), which

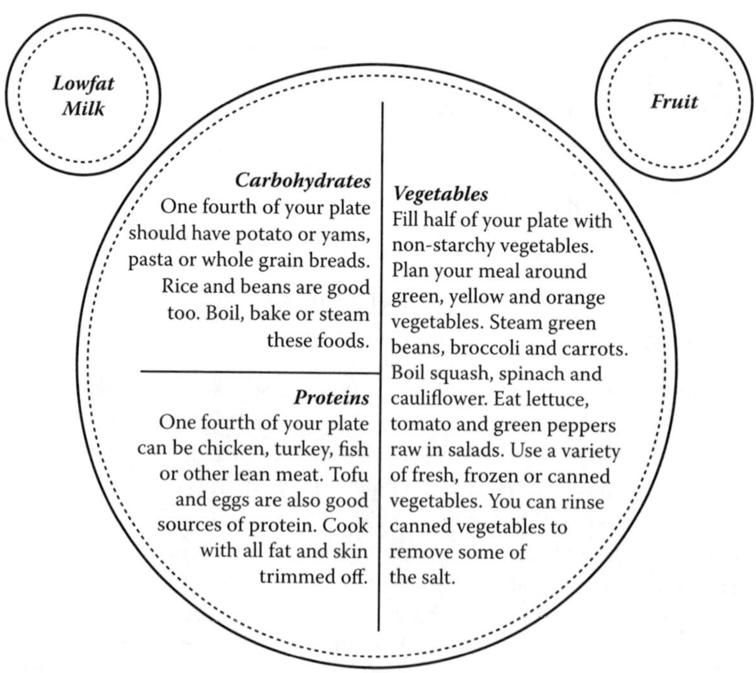

FIGURE 4.1 Meal diagram.

is a simple visual aid that doesn't require counting calories or serving size knowledge. For example, a meal diagram may include one half of the plate for low-carbohydrate vegetables, one fourth for protein, one fourth for a complex carbohydrate or starchy vegetable, and low-fat milk plus fruit.

4.4 RESEARCH AND EVIDENCE-BASED DIETS ACCORDING TO NUTRIENT COMPOSITION

4.4.1 Low-Carbohydrate, High-Fat Diets

Several clinical trials provide evidence that in the short term, a low-carbohydrate, high-fat diet can be beneficial. These data reveal that when compared to a typical low-fat diet in subjects who were compliant to the dietary recommendations, there was greater weight loss and improvements in triglycerides and high-density lipoprotein-cholesterol (HDL-C) at 3 and 6 months. However, at 12 months, the subjects in the low-carbohydrate, high-fat diet group exhibited a higher attrition rate, more noncompliance, and the difference in weight loss between the two groups was not statistically significant [6,32–34]. Three-year unpublished data from Samaha and colleagues reveal that the group consuming low-carbohydrate diets approached their baseline weight, while the low-fat group continued to slowly lose weight [35]. However, the low-carbohydrate, high-fat approach in the short term may be well worth it to achieve greater blood glucose control and triglyceride levels for a patient with diabetes or metabolic syndrome.

4.4.2 Very-Low-Fat, High-Carbohydrate Diets

A therapeutically effective dietary approach for patients with cardiovascular disease who are nearing the stage of necessity for medical intervention such as angioplasty is the very low fat, high-carbohydrate diet popularized by Dr. Dean Ornish. This near-vegetarian diet focuses more on improving health with weight loss as a secondary outcome. The dietary program couples a high intake of legumes, vegetables, fruits, and whole grains, with a minimum of fat-free dairy products and no processed foods or meat, foul, or poultry, with stress reduction that includes meditation, prayer, and yoga. Animal protein, being high in cholesterol, saturated fat, and oxidants, is avoided, and even "good fats," such as nuts, seeds, and avocados, are shunned to maintain a very low-fat approach. While this approach has been documented to be efficacious for those already at a serious level of cardiac illness, it is difficult to follow except for the most committed and motivated and those willing to embrace change resulting from a total lifestyle approach, not just diet [36]. While it is true that saturated fats from animal protein increase cardiovascular risk more than mono- and polyunsaturated fats from vegetable oils, nuts, seeds, and other plant-based fat sources, a 10% fat diet is difficult for many in our meat-eating society who find vegetarian diets unappealing. For weight loss in most Americans, an overall reduction of fat intake to 25 to 30% of daily calories — as well as reducing total caloric intake — is more palatable.

4.4.3 Low Glycemic Index and Glycemic Load

Glycemic index (GI) is a property of carbohydrate-containing foods, which describes the rise of blood glucose after a meal [37]. The GI is based on the glucose index — comparing how quickly foods are digested compared to glucose (or white bread), where the glucose index is set to equal 100. The more rapidly a carbohydrate is digested, absorbed and transformed into glucose, the higher the GI of that carbohydrate. Most starchy carbohydrates including refined grains and potatoes have a high GI, whereas typically fruits, vegetables, and legumes have a lower GI. The GI level of a food is calculated based on the GI and the total amount of carbohydrate. Consumption of foods with a low GI/load has been linked to improved satiety [37]. When compared to a standard reduced-fat diet (55 to 60% carbohydrates and 25 to 30% calories from fat), GI diets (45 to 50% complex carbohydrates, 30 to 35% calories from fat) have proven more successful in decreasing BMI in retrospective or short-term randomized studies [38,40]. Short-term investigations suggest that consumption of low-GI carbohydrates may delay the return of hunger and reduce subsequent energy intake compared to the consumption of higher-GI carbohydrates, which have been linked to excessive hunger and overeating [36]. More research is needed on the long-term effects of a low-GI diet as treatment for obesity. In general, a low-GI diet contains 32 g of fiber (the average American has a daily fiber intake of 10 to 15 g). Of note, the and new dietary reference intakes (DRIs) for fiber are 25 g daily for women and 38 g for men (ages 19 to 50 years).

4.4.4 Low-Fat, High-Fiber Diets

Typically, a low-fat, high-fiber diet, plus physical activity, is the most widely used weight management protocol and is used in non-evidence-based formal dieting groups such as Weight Watchers as well as the evidence-based USDA Dietary Guidelines for Americans, 2005 [41], the USDA Food Guide Pyramid, and the DASH diet.

The DASH diet encourages two or less servings of meat with up to five to nine servings of fruits and vegetables, seven to eight servings of whole grains, and two to three low- or nonfat dairy servings per day. Monounsaturated fat is promoted over saturated fat, and sodium intake is reduced to 2400 mg daily. Two to four servings of legumes and nuts are recommended throughout a 7-day time frame. Sweets are limited to five servings per week and include foods such as sugar, syrup, and jelly. Processed foods usually contain a good amount of sodium and, therefore, are reduced to maintain the daily sodium level [42].

4.4.5 Vegetarian Diets

Counseling vegetarians for weight loss can prove challenging for the patient who does not include soy products in his or her diet. Substituting tofu, soybeans, tempeh, natural peanut butter, or nuts in appropriate portions, and meat analogs with a low carbohydrate percentage for large portions of legumes can be an acceptable approach. One to two servings of legumes daily is acceptable, and lacto- and ovovegetarians can include fat-free dairy products, soymilk or soy yogurt, and eggs or egg whites as protein.

4.4.6 Summary

Weight loss occurs when caloric intake is less than caloric expenditure, and thus there are many diets that can elicit weight loss. The Dietary Guidelines for Americans 2005 [41] recommends a diet rich in fruits and vegetables, whole grains, and lean proteins and for weight loss, to decrease caloric intake while maintaining an adequate nutrient intake. There are many diets that one can choose from for weight loss, and they all seem to work equally well [43]. Adherence to a well-balanced, low calorie diet is key to successful weight loss, and weight maintenance requires a motivated patient who is willing to persist despite powerful hormonal forces created by the calorie deficit geared towards repletion of fat stores.

4.5 WEIGHT LOSS SURGERY — DIETARY STAGES OF ADVANCEMENT

4.5.1 General Guide

For patients who do not respond to the modest or aggressive weight loss approaches listed above, who are motivated as well as psychologically prepared for the lifestyle changes that follow the most aggressive dietary treatment, weight loss surgery can be recommended. The gold standard in most bariatric centers is the Roux-en-Y gastric bypass procedure that combines gastric restriction and intestinal bypass for malabsorption; however, the lap-adjustable gastric banding (LAGB) procedure is becoming increasingly more popular. There are no standardized guidelines for the nutritional care of the weight loss surgery patient; however, the NIH is monitoring bariatric surgery through a recently established Clinical Research Consortium [44], and some states have developed and implemented statewide position statements on this issue, including Massachusetts [45]. Practitioners advance the diet following surgery in a multitude of ways, some having patients remain on liquid, pureed, and soft diets longer than others, largely basing their treatment protocol on the success of their previous patients as well as general recommendations found in the literature. In any event, progression of dietary advancement must be made according to the tolerance level of the patient and type of surgery (Table 4.6).

During the transition from liquids to solids, there are certain guidelines that have proven to be effective regardless of the timing of advancement:

- As the gastric pouch can contain only approximately 30 to 60 mL initially, meals should take 20 min and food should be well chewed to allow for full satiety.
- Avoid drinking liquids during meals.
- Carbonated beverages can cause bloating and distention, therefore should be avoided.
- Sugar-free beverages reduce episodes of dumping syndrome (a condition that happens when the lower end of the jejunum fills too quickly with undigested food from the stomach; in weight loss surgery patients, dumping can be caused by ingestion of sweets and simple carbohydrates).

TABLE 4.6
Dietary Stages of Advancement Post Gastric Surgery

	Stage 1
Food Type	Water
Duration	0–1 day
Begin/End	Post-op day 1
Amount	1–2 oz/hour
Fluid Goal	14–32 oz/day*
	Stage 2
Food Type	Clear Liquids
Duration	1–2 days
Begin	Post-op day 1–2
End	Post-op day 2–3
Amount	2–3 oz/hour
Fluid Goal	32–48 oz/day*
	Stage 3
Food Type	Full Liquids
Duration	6–28 days
Begin	Post-op day 2–4
End	Post-op day 8–32
Amount	3–6 servings of 4–6 oz each per day (minimum 24 oz full liquid and 24 oz clear liquid/day)
Fluid Goal	48 oz/day (no more than 72 oz/day)
Protein Goal	45–80 gm/day
	Stage 4
Food Type	Pureed/Ground/Diced Foods
Duration	21–42 days
Begin	Post-op day 9–33
End	Post-op day 30–76
Amount	2–3 oz pureed/ground/diced food taken 3–5 times/day plus 0–2 8-oz servings full liquids
Fluid Goal	48–72 oz/day
Protein Goal	50–70 gm/day
	Stage 5
Food Type	Low Fat Solids
Duration	Ongoing
Begin	Post-op day 40-147
Amount	Variable; some protocols base this stage on the American Diabetes Association food exchange list
Fluid Goal	48–72 oz/day
Protein Goal	60–80 gm/day

* (Based on 14–16 waking hours)

[a] Non-fat milk, low-fat creamed soups blended with milk, sugar-free pudding/custard

[b] Includes meat, poultry, fish, tofu, and dairy products. Starches, fruit, vegetables excluded except soft fruits/vegetables can be included.

- During the full liquid stage, proteins of high biological value should be included, such as nonfat milk, soups made with milk, and sugar-free puddings; powdered skim milk or powdered egg whites can be added to these liquids to increase the protein level.
- Most protein sources are considered safe; however, beef (especially ground beef), shrimp, scallops, and lobster have been globally difficult for patients to tolerate.
- Make protein first priority at every meal or snack.
- Avoid breads that are doughy, gummy or sticky; dry breads such as toast and crackers are often better tolerated.
- Avoid the peelings, cores, and seeds of fruits and vegetables in the early stages.
- Popcorn, nuts, rice, grapes, cherries, cherry or grape tomatoes, and corn have also been less tolerated and should be avoided.
- Vitamin and mineral deficiencies can occur with these procedures — refer to Chapter 7 for more information regarding multivitamin and mineral supplementation.

4.6 PEDIATRIC AND ADOLESCENT POPULATION

4.6.1 Goals for Treatment of Childhood and Adolescent Overweight

The primary goal of treatment for children and adolescents who are overweight is to achieve and maintain a healthy body weight by promoting beneficial lifestyle behaviors including consumption of a well-balanced diet, increased physical activity, behavior modification, and family involvement [46]. Pediatric weight management goals should be realistic, should focus on small, gradual behavioral changes, and should not attempt to normalize weight [47]. In fact, a goal for many overweight children is long-term weight maintenance that allows for a steady decline in BMI as children grow in height. However, children or adolescents with secondary complications from obesity and a BMI > 95th percentile or higher may benefit from weight loss (Table 4.4). In the treatment of an overweight child or adolescent, where weight loss is the goal, a fairly small change in diet or activity can achieve this goal [48].

4.6.2 Estimating Energy Needs for Children

In free-living children and adolescents, there is no accurate way to determine energy needs. It is widely known that energy needs are most variable in children and depend on basal metabolism, rate of growth, body size, onset of puberty, and physical activity [44]. The Recommended Daily Allowances (RDAs) and the Estimated Energy Requirements (EER) from the Dietary Reference Intakes for Energy (Table 4.8) serve as guides for estimating energy needs of children and adolescents aged 2–20 and 3–18 yr, respectively. As much of the data for children has been estimated, the RDAs and

TABLE 4.7
Treatment Goals for Pediatric Weight Management [46]

Age (yr)	BMI 85–95 Percentile	BMI >95 Percentile	No Complications	Complications
2–7	Yes	—	Maintenance	Maintenance
2–7	—	Yes	Maintenance	Up to 1 lb loss per month
>7	Yes	—	Maintenance	Up to 1 lb loss per month
>7	—	Yes	Up to 1 lb loss per month	Up to 1 lb loss per month

Source: Adapted from Barlow E., Dietz W.H., *Pediatrics*, 102, 1, 1998.

TABLE 4.8
Dietary Reference Intakes for Estimated Energy Requirements (EER) in Children and Adolescents

Estimated Energy Requirements for Boys 3-8 years

$$\text{EER} = 88.5 - (61.9 \times \text{age [yr]}) + \text{PA} \times (26.7 \times \text{weight [kg]} + 903 \times \text{height [m]}) + 20 \text{ kcal}$$

Estimated Energy Requirements for Boys 9-18 years

$$\text{EER} = 88.5 - (61.9 \times \text{age [yr]}) + \text{PA} \times (26.7 \times \text{weight [kg]} + 903 \times \text{height [m]}) + 25 \text{ kcal}$$

Where PA is the Physical Activity Coefficient

PA = 1.00 if physical activity level is estimated to be >1.0 <1.4 (Sedentary)
PA = 1.13 if physical activity level is estimated to be >1.4 <1.6 (Low Active)
PA = 1.26 if physical activity level is estimated to be >1.6 <1.9 (Active)
PA = 1.42 if physical activity level is estimated to be >1.9 <2.5 (Very Active)

Estimated Energy Requirements for Girls 3-8 years

$$\text{EER} = 135.3 - (30.8 \times \text{age [yr]}) + \text{PA} \times (10.0 \times \text{weight [kg]} + 934 \times \text{height [m]}) + 20 \text{ kcal}$$

Estimated Energy Requirements for Girls 9-18 years

$$\text{EER} = 135.3 - (30.8 \times \text{age [yr]}) + \text{PA} \times (10.0 \times \text{weight [kg]} + 934 \times \text{height [m]}) + 25 \text{ kcal}$$

Where PA is the Physical Activity Coefficient

PA = 1.00 if physical activity level is estimated to be > 1.0 < 1.4 (Sedentary)
PA = 1.16 if physical activity level is estimated to be > 1.4 < 1.6 (Low Active)
PA = 1.31 if physical activity level is estimated to be > 1.6 < 1.9 (Active)
PA = 1.56 if physical activity level is estimated to be > 1.9 < 2.5 (Very Active)

Source: Reprinted with permission from DRI: Energy, Carbohydrate, Fiber, Fat, Fatty Acids, Cholesterol, Protein, and Amino Acids © 1996 by the National Academy of Sciences, Courtesy of the National Academies Press, Washington, D.C.

DRIs are meant to apply to groups, not individual children, as they cannot be used as a measure of adequacy for a given child. Therefore, much attention is focused on the child's or adolescent's dietary intake and activity level. Children's weight loss or maintenance may be reached by a 125 to 150 kcal deficit in sedentary children and 200 to 500 kcal deficit in older children. This may be accomplished by removing as little as 8 oz of juice from the diet (Table 4.9).

TABLE 4.9
Example of Usual Daily Intake of an 8-Year-Old Boy

	Meal	Calories
Breakfast	1½ cup sugared cereal	
	8 oz 2% milk	
	10 oz orange juice	482
Snack	8 oz fruit punch	
	20 mini-cheese crackers	240
Lunch	2 slices wheat bread	
	2 slices ham	
	1 slice American cheese	
	1 tsp yellow mustard	
	1 apple	
	8 oz 1% milk	
	4 oz fruit juice	588
After-school snack	2 slices wheat bread	
	1 tbsp peanut butter	
	8 oz fruit juice	350
Dinner	1 cup mashed potatoes with margarine	
	2 baked chicken legs (6 oz)	
	½ cup corn	
	8 oz 2% milk	622
Total Daily Calories*		2,282

Suggested Modifications to Daily Intake

Limit juice to 8 oz per day. This would significantly decrease the total caloric intake as this boy was consuming 30 oz of fruit juice per day

Choose 1% low fat milk or nonfat milk instead of 2% milk

Decrease portion of meat at dinner to 1 serving (1 leg); recommend leaner cuts of meat (such as chicken breast)

Monitor starch portion of dinner meal (potato and corn are both starchy vegetables)

Increase intake of fruits and vegetables at meals and snacks

*Compare total calories consumed with the DRI's EER for an 8-year-old boy of 1,453 calories per day.

Approximate values for each food can be found on the American Diabetes Association's website at www.diabetes.org.)

4.6.3 Conventional Diets for Treating Pediatric Overweight

An effective nutrition care plan for treating overweight children and adolescents can be developed through the interview process (Figure 4.10). The care plan includes dietary modification, increasing physical activity, behavior modification, and family involvement.

The dietary goals for the treatment of overweight children and adolescents should focus on a healthy intake of fruits, vegetables, whole grains, low-fat dairy products, legumes, fish, and lean meat. These foods should be consumed via regular

TABLE 4.10
Pediatric Weight Management: Obtaining a Diet and Physical Activity History; Suggested Questions for Health Care Providers

Beverages

How much juice or soda is the child drinking? What type of beverage does the child bring for school lunch or snack? Does the child drink water or flavored water? What type of milk does the family consume?

High Fat/High Sugar Foods

What type of snack foods does the child choose? How often does the child consume dessert? How often does the child consume fast foods? How often does the child consume fried foods? What type of fat does the family use when cooking?

Portion Sizes

Who portions the child's foods at dinner? What is used to determine what portion the child will receive (spoon, cup, etc.)? Are portions appropriate for age using the palm of the child's hand?

Whole Grains, Fruits and Vegetables

What type of cereal and bread does the child most consume? How often does the child consume whole grain products (cereal, bread, rice)? How often are fruits and vegetables offered at meals? Does the child consume these foods when offered?

Meal Patterns

Does the child skip any meals? Is breakfast offered at home or at school? Does the child bring a snack to school? Is lunch prepared at home or bought at school? Is a snack offered after school? Does the family eat meals together? How often are family meals? Are family meals structured? Does the child eat in front of the TV?

Activity

How often does the child participate in a structured activity (sports, camp, etc.)? Does the child participate in school gym, if offered? How many hours a day does the child participate in active play? Does the child have any limitations to participating in physical activity?

Sedentary Behavior

How many hours of TV or video play does the child engage in daily? Is TV watching monitored?

Sleep Habits

Does the child have a regular bedtime? Is bedtime different on the weekends? Is there a TV in the child's bedroom? Does the child fall asleep with the TV on?

Source: Adapted from Collins, F., Johnson, S.L., and Krebs, N.F. Screen for and treat overweight in 2–5 year olds? Yes! *Contemporary Pediatrics*, 21:10, 60–74.

well-balanced meals and snacks. The USDA's Dietary Guidelines for Americans, 2005, and the recently published American Heart Association's Dietary Recommendations encompass the appropriate modality in which to achieve these goals. It is important to stress that changes in the diet will result in improved health and that these changes are permanent and not a temporary meal plan for rapid weight loss [50]. Some strategies for dietary and lifestyle modifications are:

- *Limit sugar-sweetened beverages including soft drinks and fruit juices:* Sugar-sweetened beverages are a concentrated source of excess calories in the diets of children, adolescents, and adults. Limiting these beverages to 4 to 6 oz/day for children 1 to 6 years of age and 8 to 12 oz/day for children 7 to 18 years of age will significantly decrease daily total calorie intake [51]. Increasing consumption of plain or flavored water or low-fat milk can be an amenable substitution to soda and juice.
- *Avoid desserts or high-sugar/high-fat snack foods*: To reduce feelings of deprivation in children and adolescents, begin to limit these foods one at a time. Also, when limiting foods, provide alternative choices. For example, if limiting ice cream, suggest low-fat frozen yogurt or low-fat flavored yogurt with fruit.
- *Select appropriate portion sizes*: Recommend using the child's palm of hand for appropriate portions. As the child's nutrition requirements change with growth, so does the portion. This is a quick and easy tool for parents to remember. Another guide for monitoring portions is the American Diabetes Association's "Fill Your Plate" guide to healthy eating. This guide focuses on dividing one's plate into three sections: vegetables, lean protein, and carbohydrates. Consumption of vegetables is the largest, at one half the plate. Carbohydrates and lean protein share the other half, with one fourth of the plate each. Vegetables with a higher carbohydrate count, such as corn, peas, and potatoes should be given much attention, as these should be included in the carbohydrate versus the vegetable portion of the plate. Figure 4.2 is an adaptation of the American Diabetes Association's "Fill Your Plate" guide to healthy eating used to educate parents and children about portion control.
- *Increase consumption of high-nutrient dense foods*: Such as fruits and vegetables. A great way to increase the fruit or vegetable content of a child's diet is to increase portions of fruits and vegetables at meals. For example, at dinner, suggest filling half the plate with vegetables while the parents do as well. Even choose one or more types of vegetables to add color and many nutrients.
- *Limit the amount of saturated fat in the diet*: The major sources of saturated fat in the diets of children are full-fat milk and cheese and fatty meats. Suggest choosing 1% low-fat milk or nonfat milk, lean meats such as skinless chicken breast, lean beef, and fish. Monitor the use of butter or lard in the cooking process.
- *Encourage the intake of whole grains*: Decrease the amount of enriched flour foods in the child's diet as whole grains provide a great source of

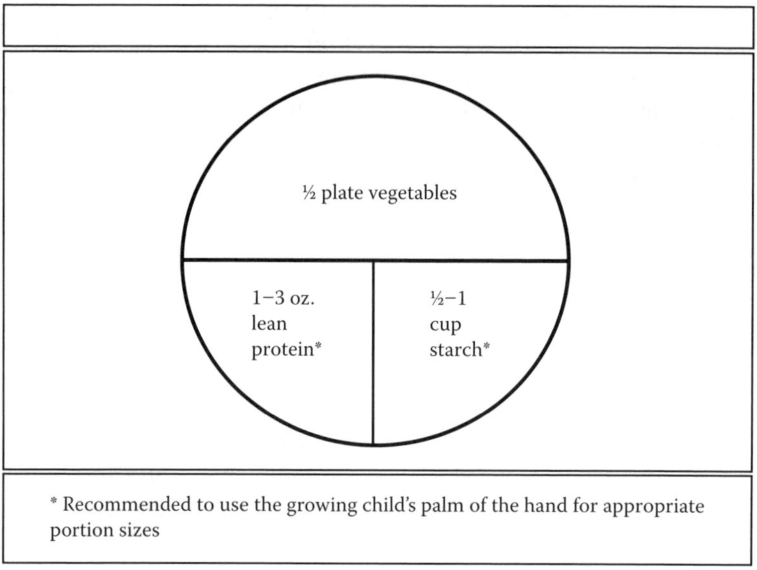

FIGURE 4.2 Suggested portion plate for children. For further portion size information, see Chapter 11, Table 11.20.

satiety-promoting fiber, especially when decreasing the fat content of the diet. Choose whole grain cereals, breads, rice, and pastas.

- *Importance of meal patterns and structured eating*: Routine eating is a key tool for understanding hunger and satiety signals. Both children and adults often have lost their ability to tune into their internal signals of hunger and fullness. It is well known that children and adolescents often have irregular meal patterns and often skip one or two meals each day, most often breakfast. Suggest a small breakfast in the morning to "start their engines," such as a piece of fruit with a low-fat yogurt, and then build to a more balanced breakfast. Encourage them to bring their lunch to school or pack snacks when they know they will be away from home.
- *Limit TV watching, especially in the evening*: Children's television-viewing habits have been associated with an increased risk for obesity, poor eating habits, and low activity levels [52,53]. Extended and frequent television viewing may decrease the time and opportunity for physical activity and family interaction. The American Academy of Pediatrics recommends introducing TV after 2 yr of age and limiting television viewing and video time to 1 to 2 h/day for all children and adolescents.
- *Television viewing in the evening*: This, especially in the context of having a television set in the child's bedroom, has been associated with increased bedtime resistance and increased sleep-onset delay [53]. It is recommended that there be no TV, computer, or video games as well as distracting toys in the bedroom.

- *Implement bedtime routines:* Children require a minimum of 9 h of restful sleep each night. Encourage parents to provide a consistent bedtime each night to promote a restful sleep cycle. To avoid a delay in the onset of sleep, children should develop bedtime rituals such as bathing or brushing teeth before bedtime.
- *Encourage family involvement in meal preparation and having a family dinner*: Behavioral approaches to the treatment of overweight children and adolescents need to be conducted with family support and professional counseling. Many parents of overweight children also struggle with overweight and obesity. When parents make healthy eating and physical activity a family priority, they do not treat their overweight children differently than the rest of the family by placing them on diets or exercise programs outside of the regular family routine [54,55]. Key components to this family approach include nutrition education on lifestyle behaviors, modification of the home/school environment, and motivation to change by modeling behaviors and contracting [47]. The first step in developing a healthy family lifestyle is for parents to examine their own behavior and recognize how it influences their children. Parents who participate in weight control and lose weight can enhance weight loss and maintenance efforts of their offspring. It has been demonstrated that the long-term effectiveness of a weight control program is significantly improved when the intervention is directed at the parents as well as the child, rather than aimed at the child alone [56,57]. However, much of the research in this area has been conducted in homogeneous and motivated groups and did not include individual treatment and rarely included adolescents and minorities [53]. Still, many behavioral approaches used with adults have been successfully applied to children and adolescents. Such strategies include:
  - Self-monitoring of food intake and physical activity
  - Taking more time to eat in a relaxed atmosphere
  - Eating less often — reducing grazing
  - Restricting eating to the dining room table (no TV, etc.)
  - Using nonfood rewards and incentives for desirable behaviors. (Table 4.11 includes suggested tips for implementing dietary recommendations for children and adolescents)

The NHLBI promotes behavior therapy as a useful adjunct when incorporated into treatment for weight loss and weight maintenance. As there is suggestive evidence that a patient's motivation for change is a key component of weight management, providers need to assess his or her readiness to change to make the appropriate recommendations. A combination of behavior therapy plus physical activity and a low-calorie diet can make weight change a manageable task for parents and their children.

An alternative teaching tool used in diet modification for children is the "Stoplight" diet (Table 4.12). This tool, developed by Epstein et al., has been successfully used in the treatment of childhood overweight in preschool and preadolescent children [58]. The Stoplight Diet for Parents and children is based on the four-food

TABLE 4.11
Suggested Dietary Modifications for Childhood and Adolescent Overweight

Decrease sugar intake, including sugar-sweetened drinks and juices. Limit intake to 8 oz or less per day. Flavored waters or sugar free drinks are favorable substitutions to sugary beverages.
Avoid high-sugar and high-fat snack foods.
Consume fruits and vegetables daily (monitor for added salt and sugar found in canned and frozen products).
To increase vegetable and fruit consumption at meals, encourage portioning $^1/_2$ of plate with fruit or vegetable, $^1/_4$ of plate with starch, and $^1/_4$ of plate with lean meat.
Use the child's palm of hand to monitor portion sizes at meals and snacks. Portions sizes will increase with growth.
Choose whole grain breads, cereals, pasta and rice
- Choose a cereal with greater than 4 grams of fiber and less than 200 calories per serving.
- Products should have "whole grain" as the first ingredient on the food label.

Monitor fat intake
- Choose skinless, boneless chicken, lean cuts of meat, fish and low fat (1% fat) or nonfat dairy products.
- Use unsaturated oils, such as canola and safflower, in place of trans fats or saturated fats, such as butter.
- Limit intake of cream or cheesy sauces.

For further information go to www.cdc.gov.

groups and divides foods into three categories: green, yellow, and red. Green foods are lower in calories, lower in fat, and typically high in fiber, such as nonstarchy vegetables. Green foods can be consumed freely. Yellow foods have an increased nutrient density than green foods and include most fruits and starches such as potatoes, bread, and pasta. Yellow foods should be limited in daily dietary intake using appropriate portion sizes. Red foods are high in fat and sugar, such as ice cream and cookies, as well as commercially prepared bakery items and bread, such as biscuits and croissants, and should be consumed rarely. Along the same lines, offering children and adolescents foods that have a lower GI can prove effective in the prevention of weight gain, weight loss where warranted, and increase satiety and overall satisfaction (see Table 4.13, Glycemic Index Diet for Children).

4.6.4 Aggressive Weight Loss Approaches

The very-low-calorie PSMF can be used in adolescents for a shorter duration than in adults (4–12 weeks). In growing individuals, although not commonly used in prepubertal children, the PSMF is designed to maximize weight loss, preserve

TABLE 4.12
Stoplight Diet for Children

Green Foods	
Non-starchy vegetables	Asparagus, beans (Italian, green, wax), broccoli, carrots, cauliflower, collards, cucumbers, eggplant, mushrooms, peppers, salad, spinach, squash, tomatoes
Vegetable juice	Tomato, V-8
Yellow Foods	
Fruits	Apple, banana, cantaloupe, grapefruit, lemon, mango, orange, peach, pear, plum, strawberries, watermelon
Fruit juices	Apple, orange, pineapple, grapefruit
Starchy vegetables	Artichokes, beans (garbanzo, lentil, pinto, navy), corn, peas, potato (baked, boiled, mashed), pumpkin
Milk/dairy	Nonfat or low fat (1%) cheese, milk and yogurt
Grains	bread (white, whole-grain), English muffin, unsweetened cereal (oatmeal, bran, wheat and corn flakes), pasta, rice (white and brown)
Meat/protein	Eggs, fish (nonfried and unbreaded), shrimp, scallops, tuna, chicken breast and drumstick, turkey
Nonfried	Lean cuts of beef, lamb, pork, veal, hot dog, peanut butter
Red Foods	
Fruits	Avocado
Dried	Prunes, date, figs, raisins
Fruit juices	Cranberry, grape, prune
Starchy, fried or creamy vegetables	Refried or baked beans, au gratin or scalloped potatoes, french fries, tater tots
Milk/dairy	Whole or 2% milk and yogurt, chocolate milk or hot cocoa made with 2% milk, ice cream
Grains	Pastries, doughnuts, cornbread, waffles, muffin, french toast, sugared cereals, fried rice
Meat/protein	Eggs (fried or prepared with fat)
Fried	Fish, shellfish, chicken, duck, goose, corned beef, sausage, bacon, bologna, salami
Nuts	Almonds, cashews, peanuts, walnuts, macadamia, pecans

Source: Epstein, L.H. and Squires, S. *The Stoplight Diet for Children: An Eight-Week Program for Parents and Children.* Boston: Little, Brown and Company, 1988. Reprinted with permission from Lipincott, Williams & Wilkins.

mineral balance, and achieve positive nitrogen balance, thereby conserving lean muscle mass (Figure 4.14) [47]. Overweight adolescents using PSMF showed successful short-term weight reduction [59]; however long-term data reveals mixed results of 25 to 48% of maintained weight loss after a one-year follow-up [59–60]. At 15-month follow-up, maintenance of weight loss was similar to that of a less restrictive approach [60].

TABLE 4.13
Glycemic Index Diet for Children

Food	Favorable	Less Favorable
Concentrated sweets	Sugar-free, low-fat pudding	Candy, cakes, cookies, frozen yogurt, ice cream, jams, jellies, pies, syrup, sugar (white, brown or powdered)
Fruits	Apple, orange, pear, grapes, lemon, kiwi, peach, plum	Banana, cranberries, watermelon, all dried fruits (prunes, raisins, figs)
Grains	Barley, pumpernickel, rye or whole kernel (flourless) bread, all-bran cereals	Bagels, enriched breads and bread products, chips, cornbread, couscous, crackers, croutons, doughnuts, English muffins, granola, pasta, pancakes, popcorn, pretzels, rice (all types), tortillas
Legumes	Black beans, black-eyed peas, butter beans, chickpeas (garbanzo), kidney beans, lentils, navy beans, soybeans, lima beans	
Meats	Lean poultry, fish, and red meat (using low-fat cooking methods)	Processed meats such as sausage and bacon
	Firm tofu, tempeh, and seitan	
Milk/Dairy	1% and 2% milk, yogurt and cheese	Nonfat milk, yogurt and cheese
Vegetables	Artichoke, asparagus, broccoli, beans (wax or green), Brussels sprouts, cauliflower, cucumber, eggplant, lettuce, mushrooms, onions, peppers, spinach, tomatoes	Acorn squash, beets, carrots, corn, peas, potatoes, sweet potatoes, yams

Read the food label to make sure there are no added sugars to the canned foods. There are a few items such as doughnuts that have a lower glycemic index than bagels but would not be considered a favorable choice due to their high saturated and trans fat content.

For complete list of foods refer to: Foster-Powell K, Holt SH, Brand-Miller JC. International table of glycemic index and glycemic load values. Am. J. Clin. Nutr. Jul;76(1):5-56, 2002.

4.7 CONCLUSION

In today's climate of multiple weight management options, we must keep our focus toward evidence-based, safe, efficacious recommendations. While it is true that one diet does not fit all, the deciding bell rings with finality that the goal we should be seeking to accomplish is prevention of weight gain. For those who have yet to succeed in this endeavor, we must recognize that obesity is a disease that deserves lifelong treatment and that, as providers, we must be acquainted with the multiple genres of weight loss modalities available and familiar enough with our patient to distinguish the appropriate intervention for their readiness to change.

TABLE 4.14
Protein-Sparing Modified Fast Diet for Children and Adolescents

High-Protein, Hypocaloric Diet for 12 Weeks

600-800 kcal
Protein 2g/kg/d (maximum 100g/d; approximately 50% of calories)
    13–20 oz/d lean meat or substitute
Fat approximately 30–40% of calories
Carbohydrate 10–20% of calories
    As low-starch vegetables, may include one fruit
Ad Libitum: tea, bouillon, pickles, spices, mustard
2 L of water per day

Supplements
Multivitamin with minerals
Elemental calcium supplement to meet the Recommended Daily Intake
Monitor serum potassium and supplement as needed

Maintenance Diet (36 Week)

Balanced Micronutrients
1,200 kcals/d

Source: Reprinted with Permission. Lenders, C. and Hoppin, A. Management and Treatment of Obesity. In: *Nutrition in Pediatrics: Basic Science and Clinical Applications,* 3rd ed., Walker, W., Watkins, J., Duggan, C., Eds., B.C. Decker, Ch. 54: 929, 2003.

As stated earlier, research implies that popular or fad diets do not work for the long term. In most popular diets, attrition is high, adherence low, and weight loss is entirely due to a reduction in total caloric intake. Lifestyle, BMI, dietary preferences, and cardiovascular risk factors must be taken into account when recommending a dietary protocol for weight loss, whether the dictated approach is more aggressive, such as fasting, the use of pharmacotherapy, or weight loss surgery, or less invasive like a planned dietary approach along with behavior change. Compliance and adherence to diet, and calories reduced below daily need, are the best predictors of long-term success in weight changes, not the macronutrient content [59], and can be achieved by employing a team approach and cognitive behavioral therapy.

REFERENCES

1. Foster, G.D., Wadden, T.A., Makris, A.P., Davidson, D., Sanderson, R.S., Allison, D.B., Kessler, A., Primary care physicians' attitudes about obesity and its treatment, *Obes. Res.*, 11(10), 1168, 2003.
2. Puhl, R., Brownell, K.D., Bias, discrimination, and obesity, *Obes. Res.*, 9(12), 788, 2001.
3. Wang, S.S., Brownell, K.D., Wadden, T.A., The influence of the stigma of obesity on overweight individuals, *Int. J. Obes. Relat. Metab. Disord.: J. Int. Assoc. Study Obes.,* 28(10), 1333–1337, 2004.

4. Schwartz, M.B., Chambliss, H.O., Brownell, K.D., Blair, S.N., Billington, C., Weight bias among health professionals specializing in obesity, *Obes. Res.,* 11(9), 1033–1039, 2003.
5. World Health Organization, Obesity, preventing and managing the global epidemic: Report of a WHO consultation on obesity, Geneva, Switzerland: WHO Technical Report Series-894, 2000.
6. Foster, G.D., Wyatt, H.R., Hill, J.O., McGuckin, B.G., Brill, C., Mohammed, B.S., Szapary, P.O., Rader, D.J., Edman, J.S., Klein, S., A randomized trial of a low-carbohydrate diet for obesity, *N. Engl. J. Med.,* 348(21), 2082–2090, 2003.
7. Field, A., Austin, S.B., Taylor, C.B., Malspeis, S.M., Rosner, B., Rockett, H., Gillman, M.W., Colditz, G.A., Relation between dieting and weight change among preadolescents and adolescents, *Pediatrics*, 112, 900, 2003.
8. Ness-Abramof, R., Apovian, C.A., An update on medical therapy for obesity, *Nutr. Clin. Pract.,* 18, 145–156, 2003.
9. Steward H.L., Bethea M.C., Andrews S.S., Balart L.A., *Sugar Busters*!, Ballantine Publishing, New York, 1995.
10. Eades, M.R., Eades, M.D., *Protein Power*, New York, Bantam Books, 1999.
11. Atkins, R.C., *Dr. Atkins' New Diet Revolution,* New York: Rev. Ed. Avon Books, Inc., 1998.
12. Stice, E., Cameron, R.P., Killen, J.D., Hayward, C., Taylor, C.B., Naturalistic weight-reduction efforts prospectively predict growth in relative weight and onset of obesity among female adolescents, *J. Consult. Clin. Psychol.,* 67, 967, 1999.
13. Wadden, T.A., Sternberg, J.A., Letizia, K.A., Stunkard, A.J., Foster, G.D., Treatment of obesity by very low calorie diet, behavior therapy and their combinations: a five-year perspective, *Int. J. Obes. Relat. Metab. Disord.,* 13(suppl 2), S39–S46, 1989.
14. Phelan, S., Hill, J.O., Lang, W., Dibello, J.R., Wing, R.R., Recovery from relapse among successful weight maintainers, *Am. J. Clin. Nutr.*, 78, 1079–1084, 2003.
15. US Dept of Agriculture: The food guide pyramid, Washington, DC: USDA, Home and Garden Bull 252, 1992.
16. American Diabetes Association, The American Dietetic Association: Exchange Lists for Weight Maintenance, Alexandria, VA: America Diabetes Association, 1995.
17. US Dept of Agriculture: Dietary guidelines for Americans, 2005, Washington, DC: USDA Dept of Health and Human Services, 2005, from http://www.nhlbi.nih.gov/health/ public/heart/hbp/dash/, accessed on June 28, 2005.
18. Saper, R.B., Eisenberg, D.M., Phillips, R.S., Common dietary supplements for weight loss, *Am. Fam. Phys.,* 70(9), 1731–1738, 2004.
19. Bray, G.A., The expert weighs in, *Obes. Manage.,* 1(1), 6–8, 2005.
20. Wadden, T.A., Brownell, K.D., Foster, G.D., Obesity: responding to the global epidemic, *J. Consult. Clin. Psychol.,* 70(3), 510–525, 2002.
21. Orzano, A.J., Scott, J.G., Diagnosis and treatment of obesity in adults: an applied evidence-based review, *J. Am. Board Fam. Pract.,* 17(5), 359–369.
22. Bryner, R.W., Ullrich, I.H., Sauers, J., Donley, D., Hornsby, G., Kolar, M., Yeater, R., Effects of resistance vs. aerobic training combined with an 800 calorie liquid diet on lean body mass and resting metabolic rate, *J. Am. Coll. Nutr.,* 18(2), 115–121, 1999.
23. Festi, D., Colecchia, A., Orsini, M., Sangermano, A., Sottili, S., Simoni, P., Mazzella, G., Villanova, N., Bazzoli, F., Lapenna, D., Petroni, M.L., Pavesi, S., Neri, M., Roda, E., Gallbladder motility and gallstone formation in obese patients following very low calorie diets. Use it (fat) to lose it (well), *Int. J. Obes. Rel. Metab. Dis.: J. Int. Assoc. Study Obes.*, 22, 592–600, 1998.

24. Panzer, C., Apovian, C.M., Aggressive diets and lipid responses, *Curr. Cardiol. Rep.*, 6, 464–473, 2004.
25. Ahmed, W., Flynn, M.A., Alpert, M.A., Cardiovascular complications of weight reduction diets, *Am. J. Med. Sci.*, 321, 280–284, 2001.
26. Blackburn, G.L., Protein requirements with very low calorie diets, *Postgrd. Med. J.*, 60(Suppl 3):59-65, 1984.
27. Merritt, R.J., Bistrian, B.R., Blackburn, G.L., Consequences of modified fasting in obese pediatric and adolescent patients, *J. Pediatr.*, 96(1):13-19, 1980.
28. Palgi, A., Read, J.L., Greenberg, I., Hoefer, M.A., Bistrian, B.R., Blackburn, G.L., Multidisciplinary treatment of obesity with a protein-sparing modified fast: Results in 668 outpatients, *Am. J. Public Health*, 75(10):1190-1194, 1985.
29. Stallings, V.A., Archibald, E.H., Pencharz, P.B., Harrison, J.E., Bell, L.E., One-year follow-up of weight, total body potassium, and total body nitrogen in obese adolescents treated with the protein-sparing modified fast. *Am. J. Clin. Nutr.*, 48(1):91-94, 1988.
30. Blackburn, G.L., Bevis, L.C., The obesity epidemic: prevention and treatment of the metabolic syndrome, Medscape Clinical Update: Diabetes and Endocrinology CME Center, September 18, 2003. http://www.medscape,com/viewprogram/2015.
31. Flechtner-Mors, M., Ditschuneit, H.H., Johnson, T.D., Suchard, M.A., Adler, G., Metabolic and weight loss effects of long-term dietary intervention in obese patients: four-year results, *Obes. Res.*, 8(5), 399–402, 2000.
32. Stern, L., Iqbal, N., Seshadri, P., Chicano, K.L., Daily, D.A., McGrory, J., Williams, M., Gracely, E.J., Samaha, F.F., The effects of low-carbohydrate versus conventional weight loss diets in severely obese adults: one-year follow-up of a randomized trial, *Ann. Intern. Med.*, 140, 778–785, 2004.
33. Samaha, F.F., Iqbal, N., Seshadri, P., Chicano, K.L., Daily, D.A., McGrory, J., Williams, T., Williams, M., Gracely, E.J., Stern, L., A low-carbohydrate as compared with a low-fat diet in severe obesity, *N. Engl. J. Med.*, 348, 2074–2081, 2003.
34. Brehm, B.J., Seeley, R.J., Daniels, S.R., D'Alessio, D.A., A randomized trial comparing a very low carbohydrate diet and a calorie-restricted low fat diet on body weight and cardiovascular risk factors in healthy women, *J. Clin. Endocrinol. Metabol.*, 88, 1617–1623, 2003.
35. Samaha, F., Effect of cardiovascular risks and metabolic syndrome, 2005, unpublished data.
36. Ornish, D., Scherwitz, L.W., Billings, J.H., Brown, S.E., Gould, K.L., Merritt, T.A., Sparler, S., Armstrong, W.T., Ports, T,A., Kirkeeide, R.L., Hogeboom, C., Brand, R.J., Intensive lifestyle changes for reversal of coronary heart disease, *JAMA*, 280, 2001–2007, 1998.
37. Roberts, S.B., Glycemic index and satiety, *Nutr. Clin. Care*, 6(1), 20–26, 2003.
38. Ludwig, D.S., Majzoub, J.A., Al-Zaharani, A., Dallal, G.E., Blanco, I., Roberts, S.B., High glycemic index foods, overeating and obesity, *Pediatrics*, 103(3), 26e, 1999.
39. Spieth, L.E., Harnish, J.D., Lenders, C.M., Raezer, L.B., Pereira, M.A., Hangen, S., Ludwig, D.S., A low-glycemic index diet in the treatment of pediatric obesity, *Arch. Pediatr. Adolesc. Med.*, 154(9), 947, 2000.
40. Ebbeling, C.B., Leidig, M.M., Sinclair, K.B., Hangen, J.P., Ludwig, D.S., A reduced-glycemic load in the treatment of adolescent obesity, *Arch. Pediatr. Adolesc. Med.*, 157(8), 725, 2003.
41. Dietary Guidelines for Americans, 2005, Department of Health and Human Services (HHS) and the Department of Agriculture (USDA), January 12, 2005, from http://www. health.gov/dietaryguidelines/, accessed on July 4, 2005.

42. Appel, L.J., Brands, M.W., Daniels, S.R., Karanja, N., Elmer, P.J., Sacks, F.M., American Heart Association, Dietary approaches to prevent and treat hypertension: a scientific statement from the American Heart Association, *Hypertension*, 47, 296–308, 2006.
43. Dansinger, M.L., Gleason, J.A., Griffith, J.L., Selker, H.P., Schaefer, E.J. Comparison of the Atkins, Ornish, Weight Watchers, and Zone diets for weight loss and heart disease risk reduction. *JAMA* 2005; 293:43-53.
44. Bariatric Surgery Clinical Research Consortium (RFA), Available at: http://www.niddk. nih.gov/fund/crfo/may2002council/rfac502_1.htm, accessed July 4, 2005.
45. Saltzman, E., Anderson, W., Apovian, C.M., Boulton, H., Chamberlain, A., Cullum-Dugan, D., Cummings, S., Hatchigian, E., Hodges, B., Keroack, C.R., Pettus, M., Thomason, P., Veglia, L., Young, L.S., Criteria for patient selection and multidisciplinary evaluation and treatment of the weight loss surgery patient, *Obes. Res.*, 13, 234–243, 2005.
46. Barlow, E., Dietz, W.H., Obesity evaluation and treatment: expert committee recommendations, *Pediatrics*, 102, 1, 1998.
47. Mullen, M.C., Shield, J. Eds., *Childhood and Adolescent Overweight: The Health Professional's Guide to Identification, Treatment and Prevention*, American Dietetic Association 2004.
48. Gidding, S.S., Dennison, B.A., Birch, L.L., Daniels, S.R., Gilman, M.W., Lichtenstein, A.H., Rattay, K.T., Steinberger, J., Stettler, N., Van Horn, L., American Heart Association; American Academy of Pediatrics, Dietary recommendations for children and adolescents: a guide for practitioners: consensus statement from the American Heart Association, *Circulation*, 27, 112(13), 2061–2075, 2005.
49. *Pediatric Nutrition Handbook*, Fourth Edition, Committee on Nutrition, American Academy of Pediatrics 1998.
50. American Academy of Pediatrics (www.appp.org/).
51. Locard, E., Mamelle, N., Billette, A., et al., Risk factors of obesity in a 5 year old population parental versus environmental factors, *Int. J. Obes. Relat. Metab. Dis.*, 16, 721–729, 1992.
52. Durant, R.H., The relationship among television watching, physical activity, and body composition of young children, *Pediatrics*, 94, 441–455, 1994.
53. Owens, J., Maxim, R., McGuinn, M., Nobile, C., Msall, M., Alario, A., Television-viewing habits and sleep disturbance in school children, *Pediatrics*, 104, 27, 1999.
54. Epstein, L.H., Family-based behavioral intervention for obese children, *Int. J. Obes. Relat. Metab. Disord.*, 20, S14, 1996.
55. Epstein, L.H., Valoski, A., Winf, R.R., Ten year follow-up of behavioral, family-based treatment or obese children, *JAMA*, 264, 2519–2523, 1990.
56. Golan, M., Weizman, A., Apter, A., Fainaru, M., Parents as the exclusive agents of change in the treatment of childhood obesity, *Am. J. Clin. Nutr.*, 67, 1130–1138, 1998.
57. Summerbell, C.D., Ashton, V., Campbell, K.J., Edmunds, L., Kelly, S., Waters, E., Interventions for treating obesity in children, *Cochrane Database Syst. Rev.*, 2, 2004.
58. Epstein, H., Myers, M.D., Raynnor, H.A., Saelens, B.E., Treatment of pediatric obesity, *Pediatrics*, 101(3), 554, 1998.
59. Stallings, V.A., Archibald, E.H., Pencharz, P.B., Harrison, J.E., Bell, L.E., One-year follow-up of weight, total body potassium, and total body nitrogen in obese adolescents treated with the protein-sparing modified fast, *Am. J. Clin. Nutr.*, 48, 91, 1988.

60. Brown, M.R., Klish, W.J., Hollander, J., Campbell, M.A., Forbes, G.B., A high protein, low calorie liquid diet in the treatment of very obese adolescents; long-term effect on lean body mass, *Am. J. Clin. Nutr.*, 38, 20, 1983.
61. Figueroa-Colon, R., von Almen, T.K., Franklin, F.A., Schuftan, C., Suskind, R.M., Comparison of two hypocaloric diets in obese children, *Am. J. Dis. Child.*, 147, 160, 1993.
62. Dansinger, M.L., Gleason, J.A., Griffith, J.L., Seiker, H.P., Schaefer, E.J., Comparison of the Atkins, Ornish, Weight Watchers, and Zone diets for weight loss and heart disease risk reduction: a randomized trial, *JAMA*, 293(1), 43–53, 2005.

5 Exercise Therapy for the Overweight Adult

John M. Jakicic, Amy D. Otto, and Kristen Polzien

CONTENTS

5.1 INTRODUCTION

Current estimates of the prevalence of overweight (body mass index [BMI] $\geq$ 25.0 kg/m^2) and obesity (BMI $\geq$ 30.0 kg/m^2) in adults is 65% and 30%, respectively [1]. These prevalence rates are of concern because of their demonstrated association with numerous chronic conditions such as cardiovascular disease, diabetes, and various forms of cancer [2]. Therefore, it is critical to understand factors that contribute to enhancing the prevention and treatment of excess body weight.

Ultimately, the management of body weight is dependent on energy balance, which includes the balance between energy intake and energy expenditure. To prevent weight gain and to sustain weight loss, theoretically, energy expenditure needs to be equivalent to energy intake. However, to reduce the prevalence of overweight and obesity, it is necessary to elicit an energy imbalance that results in an energy deficit in which energy expenditure exceeds energy intake. Energy expenditure includes resting energy expenditure, the thermic effect of meals, and nondiscretionary forms of physical activity to perform activities of daily living, but the most variable component of energy expenditure is discretionary leisure-time physical activity (LTPA). Increasing LTPA in the form of structured exercise, lifestyle activity, and other forms of activity can contribute to an increase in energy expenditure and result in an energy deficit. Thus, it is important to understand the impact of an increase in energy expenditure resulting from LTPA on weight loss, prevention of weight gain, and prevention of weight regain following weight loss.

5.2 PHYSICAL ACTIVITY RECOMMENDATIONS FOR THE PREVENTION OF WEIGHT GAIN

The increasing prevalence of overweight and obesity warrants the need for interventions to prevent weight gain. Because of its impact on energy expenditure, which can affect energy balance, physical activity may significantly contribute to the prevention of weight gain. This hypothesis is supported by data from prospective observational studies. Data from the Pound of Prevention study supported this hypothesis and demonstrated that an increase in energy expenditure from physical activity may have contributed to the prevention of weight gain in adults [3]. Results from the Harvard Alumni Study have demonstrated that individuals participating in levels of physical activity that are consistent with the current public health guidelines (30 min of moderate intensity physical activity on most days of the week) had lower body weight than individuals not reporting this level of physical activity [4]. DiPietro et al. reported that a modest increase in fitness, which most likely is a result of an increase in physical activity, prevented weight gain across a 4-year period in adults in the Aerobic Center Longitudinal Study [5]. These data provide support for the inclusion of physical activity in efforts to prevent or minimize weight gain.

It is important to translate these findings from cross-sectional and observational studies to effective interventions for the prevention of weight gain. The recently completed STRIDDE Study reported that control subjects gained weight, whereas those who participated in exercise had modest decreases in body weight and measures of body fatness, and this appears to occur in a dose–response manner [6]. Moreover, an ongoing clinical trial in our laboratory examines the role of physical activity in the prevention of weight gain in moderately overweight (BMI = 25.0 to 29.9 kg/m^2) adults. Unpublished initial results from this study demonstrate that 150 to 300 min/wk of physical activity without a recommendation to reduce energy intake results in an average of 1 to 2 kg of weight loss (1–2% reduction in body weight) across 6 to 18 mo. However, a significant predictor of prevention of weight gain in this study is the magnitude of increase in cardiorespiratory fitness.

These data may suggest that physical activity performed at a sufficient dose and intensity to significantly increase cardiorespiratory fitness may be important in preventing weight gain and will potentially result in a modest reduction in body weight. This is an important consideration for clinicians who treat and counsel individuals at risk for weight gain, which can result in an increase in the risk of chronic disease. Initially, these individuals should be counseled to participate in at least 150 min/week of moderate-intensity physical activity, as it appears that this may be sufficient to reduce risk of chronic disease and may prevent weight gain.

If weight gain continues, the amount of physical activity may need to be increased gradually to between 150 and 300 min/week, and this level can be determined by monitoring the point at which body weight gain ceases. It needs to be emphasized that although physical activity can assist in weight gain prevention, this does not allow an individual to consume an unlimited amount of energy in the form of food, as ultimately a positive energy imbalance will result in weight gain. These recommendations are consistent with recent dietary guidelines, which state that to manage body weight and prevent gradual, unhealthy body weight gain in adulthood, an individual should "engage in approximately 60 min of moderate- to vigorous-intensity activity on most days of the week while not exceeding caloric intake requirements" [7].

5.3 PHYSICAL ACTIVITY RECOMMENDATIONS FOR WEIGHT LOSS

Typical behavioral weight loss interventions focus on altering energy balance by reducing energy intake through modifications in eating behavior and increasing energy expenditure through an increase in physical activity. When combined, modification to both eating and physical activity behaviors has been shown to result in an approximately 10% reduction in body weight within the initial 6 months of a weight loss intervention [2,8]. However, it is important to understand the potential contribution of each of these behaviors to weight loss.

It has been consistently demonstrated that <10% of initial weight loss results from an increase in physical activity, with the remaining weight loss likely resulting from a decrease in energy intake. For example, Wing et al. [9] reported a 10.4% weight loss from the combination of diet plus exercise, 9.1% weight loss from diet alone, and 2.1% weight loss from exercise alone across a 6-month weight loss intervention. Similar results were reported by Hagan et al. [10] across a 12-week weight loss intervention. Reductions in body weight were 11.4%, 8.4%, and 0.3% in males and 7.5%, 5.5%, and 0.6% in females participating in diet plus exercise, diet alone, or exercise alone, respectively [10]. These findings are consistent with the review of the literature conducted for the clinical guidelines developed by the National Institutes of Health [2], and suggest that physical activity may independently have a small to modest effect on initial weight loss in overweight and obese adults.

These findings do not suggest that reductions in energy intake are more important than an increase in energy expenditure from physical activity for weight loss. Rather, to maximize initial weight loss, clinicians recommending an increase in physical activity should also consider dietary recommendations to modify energy intake. There is a growing body of literature to suggest that improvements in cardiorespiratory fitness resulting from an increase in physical activity can improve health-related outcomes independent of body weight. Barlow et al. [11] have confirmed that higher levels of cardiorespiratory fitness are associated with reduced health risk in women, independent of body weight. Lee et al. [12], Wei et al. [13], and Farrell et al. [14] reported similar findings for men. In a sample of men with type 2 diabetes, Church et al. [15] reported that cardiorespiratory fitness reduces all-cause mortality independent of body weight. However, these studies typically did not include data from a sufficient number of individuals with a BMI > 35 kg/m^2, which may indicate that these results are only generalizable to individuals classified as overweight (BMI: 25–29.9 kg/m^2) and individuals with Class I obesity (30–34.9 kg/m^2). Stevens et al. [16] reported that there is no interaction between fitness and excess body weight in men and women, suggesting that excess body weight can negatively impact health, regardless of fitness level. However, it may be that increasing physical activity can improve health outcomes in overweight and obese adults either through the direct impact on risk factors or indirectly by enhancing body weight control.

A continuing challenge for clinicians is how best to assist patients with the maintenance of weight loss in the long term. According to data from weight loss interventions, approximately 33 to 50% of initial weight loss can be regained in the ensuing 12 to 18 mo [8]. This is most likely a result of the inability to sustain an adequate balance between energy intake and energy expenditure. For example, McGuire et al. [17] reported that individuals in the National Weight Control Registry who reported regain of body weight also reported an increase in energy intake and a decrease in energy expenditure. Jakicic et al. [18] reported that successful long-term weight loss was achieved through a constellation of behaviors, which included maintaining both a reduced energy intake and high levels of energy expenditure from physical activity. Thus, it appears that physical activity is an important factor in the prevention of weight regain, and therefore it is relevant for clinicians to understand the appropriate doses of physical activity necessary to achieve this goal.

To sustain weight loss in adulthood, the 2005 U.S. Dietary Guidelines recommend participation in at least 60 to 90 min of daily moderate-intensity physical activity while not exceeding caloric intake requirements [7]. This recommendation is consistent with previous recommendations from the American College of Sports Medicine [19], the Institute of Medicine [20], and the International Association for the Study of Obesity [21]. These recommendations are based on a growing body of scientific literature in this area of study. Data from our laboratory have demonstrated that maintaining approximately 250 to 300 min per week of at least moderate-intensity physical activity improves weight loss at 12 [22] and 18 mo [23]. Preliminary analyses of current data also demonstrate that approximately 300 min of physical activity per week is important for maintaining approximately a 12 to 14% weight loss for a period of 24 mo [24]. These results are consistent with results of other studies that have supported the need for similar levels of physical activity to successfully sustain weight loss in the long term [25–27]. Thus, when appropriate, clinicians should consider gradually progressing individuals to these levels of physical activity, in combination with maintaining an appropriate level of energy intake, to maximize long-term weight loss and to prevent weight regain.

5.4 IMPACT OF ALTERNATIVE MODES OF PHYSICAL ACTIVITY ON WEIGHT LOSS

The majority of clinical trials have incorporated aerobic forms of physical activity (i.e., brisk walking) into the weight loss interventions. This may be a result of a number of factors that include preferences of the individual; Jakicic et al. [22] confirmed this by reporting that approximately 80 to 90% of activity sessions reported by overweight adults engaged in a weight loss program were in the form of brisk walking. Despite these findings, there is an interest in alternative forms of physical activity in the management of body weight.

5.4.1 Resistance Exercise

Findings with regard to the benefits of resistance exercise in overweight and obese adults are mixed. In a review of the literature, Donnelly et al. [28] concluded that resistance exercise does not appear to improve weight loss when compared to other forms of physical activity. Preliminary analysis from a 6-month intervention conducted in our laboratory has demonstrated that the addition of resistance exercise to a traditional behavioral weight loss intervention did not result in improved weight loss [29]. Although the majority of studies conducted in this area have been relatively short in duration (6 mo), the results of the few long-term studies published to date have also demonstrated no significant improvement in weight loss with the addition of resistance exercise to a standard behavioral weight loss intervention [30]. This may be a result of the lack of adherence to resistance exercise in the long term [30].

Despite resistance exercise not demonstrating an improvement in weight loss, there is some evidence that resistance exercise may impact other health-related outcomes. Jurca et al. [31] demonstrated, in a sample of participants from the Aerobics Center Longitudinal Study, that resistance exercise may reduce all-cause mortality. However, Jannsen et al. [32] reported that resistance exercise did not improve selected risk factors related to metabolic control when compared to weight loss alone, with changes in visceral fat related to changes in risk factors. Thus, changes in visceral adiposity may be one of the physiological mechanisms by which resistance exercise may impact metabolic risk factors and the onset of disease, and this will require further research.

Resistance exercise has clearly been demonstrated to improve muscular strength [33,34], and it has been proposed that this may improve physical function and quality of life of overweight and obese adults [35]. Thus, there may be benefits of resistance exercise that occur regardless of the impact on body weight, and these should be considered when developing a physical activity program for overweight adults. However, it remains unclear how best to increase adoption and maintenance of resistance exercise, and this is an important and necessary consideration to realize the potential benefits of this form of physical activity.

5.4.2 Yoga

A currently popular form of physical activity is yoga. There are a variety of forms of yoga, with each form including differentiated factors such as the type of movement patterns that are performed. Despite the popularity of this form of physical activity, there has been limited research in this area. Using preliminary data from a study conducted in our research center, we found no significant increase in weight loss across a 6 to 12 month intervention when yoga was added to a standard behavioral weight loss program [29]. However, additional studies are needed to confirm these findings and further examine possible body fat loss. Despite the lack of evidence to support the use of yoga to improve weight loss, there may be other benefits of yoga that support the inclusion of this form of physical activity for overweight adults. There is some evidence that various forms of yoga can maintain the range of motion, improve physical function, and reduce pain [36,37], and this may improve health-related quality of life. However, despite these potential benefits, clinicians should be mindful of the limitations of yoga in improving weight loss beyond what is achievable in standard behavioral weight loss interventions.

5.4.3 Aquatic Activity

Because excess body weight increases the force placed on weight-bearing joints of the body, which can potentially result in musculoskeletal injury, a common recommendation is for overweight adults to consider aquatic forms of physical activity. However, there are limited data on the acceptance of aquatic forms of physical activity by overweight and obese adults, and there are limited data on whether aquatic forms of physical activity improve weight loss outcomes. Preliminary evidence from our laboratory appears to indicate that overweight adults report that they enjoy this form of physical activity [38]. However, this does not appear to result in an improvement in weight loss compared to a standard behavioral weight loss program [39]. Potential limitations are the need for an individual to have access to a pool to perform this type of physical activity and to feel comfortable exercising in water. These factors should be considered when recommending this form of physical activity to overweight and obese adults.

5.5 CONSIDERATIONS TO ENHANCE PHYSICAL ACTIVITY PARTICIPATION

Despite the potential importance of physical activity in weight gain prevention, enhancement of initial weight loss, or prevention of weight regain, long-term adherence to physical activity recommendations is a challenge. Thus, it is important for clinicians to understand potential strategies that can be used to improve energy expenditure from physical activity.

5.5.1 Intermittent Exercise

The public health recommendations for physical activity published in 1995 by the Centers for Disease Control and Prevention and the American College of Sports Medicine suggested that health benefits of physical activity could be realized if sufficient levels of physical activity were accumulated throughout the day. This suggests that individuals do not need to perform physical activity in continuous bouts of 30 to 60 min to realize the potential health benefits. It has been demonstrated that intermittent forms of physical activity can increase cardiorespiratory fitness [40] and improve selected risk factors [41]. Jakicic et al. [23,42] reported that the accumulation of physical activity across intermittent periods throughout the day (i.e., three 10-min activity sessions) can be a strategy to improve physical activity participation in previously sedentary overweight adults during the initial 6 months of an intervention. Thus, the accumulation of physical activity should be considered as an alternative intervention approach to facilitate the adoption of physical activity in previously sedentary, overweight adults. Because this strategy does not appear to improve the ability to sustain adequate levels of physical activity compared to traditional forms of exercise, this could be used as an alternative strategy that may facilitate participation in physical activity during periods when there are barriers to participation in more traditional durations of physical activity (i.e., 30 to 60 continuous minutes).

5.5.2 Lifestyle Approaches to Increasing Physical Activity

Levine et al. [43] have demonstrated that overweight adults sit for greater periods of time throughout the day compared to normal weight adults. This may have implications for overall energy expenditure differences between these individuals, and this could impact body weight. Thus, it may be beneficial for individuals to seek opportunities to become more physically active in their daily lifestyle, and this may occur in the form of reducing the reliance on motorized forms of transportation and automation of common daily and occupational tasks. Studies that have examined recommendations to increase lifestyle forms of physical activity have demonstrated changes in fitness and body weight that are similar to what is observed with structured exercise [44,45]. However, to date, these studies have failed to report the specific pattern and modes of physical activity, and therefore it is difficult to understand how individuals interpret these recommendations and whether this simply results in the adoption of structured periods of exercise. Research is needed to better understand the role of lifestyle physical activity on body weight regulation. Despite the need for more research in this area, it is likely that overweight and obese adults can benefit from reducing periods of sedentary behavior and increasing periods of activity throughout the day, regardless of the initial impact on body weight.

A potentially useful tool that may assist in promoting an increase in lifestyle forms of physical activity is a pedometer. Pedometers are relatively inexpensive and can be used to promote an increase in movement throughout the day. It appears that a sedentary adult accumulates approximately 3000 to 5000 steps throughout the day, and for every 2000 to 2500 steps, an individual walks the equivalent of 1 mile. Thus, recommending a progressive increase in physical activity that results in a total of 10,000 steps per day would be the equivalent of adding at least 2 miles of walking per day, which is consistent with current public health guidelines to reduce the risk of chronic disease [7,46,47]. Moreover, the accumulation of at least 10,000 steps per day may be associated with improvements in health-related parameters [48]. To promote weight loss, it has been suggested that it may be necessary to progressively increase daily steps to levels above 10,000 steps per day [49].

5.6 SUMMARY

Obesity is a significant public health problem that results in an increase in the risk for numerous chronic diseases and significantly increases healthcare costs [2]. It is important to develop interventions to prevent weight gain, enhance weight loss, and improve the long-term maintenance of weight loss. Examination of the scientific literature demonstrates the importance of increasing physical activity in weight control efforts. There is evidence that adequate levels of physical activity minimize weight gain, and when used in combination with a reduction in energy intake can enhance weight loss. Of importance is the evidence to support the need for adequate levels of physical activity to sustain weight loss in the long term. It appears that progression to approximately 300 min of physical activity per week may be needed to achieve this goal. However, there is limited evidence that alternative forms of physical activity such as resistance exercise, yoga, or aquatic exercise improve weight loss outcomes compared to traditional forms of physical activity commonly included in behavioral programs. This may indicate that the mode of physical activity is not important for weight control provided that a sufficient dose of physical activity is performed. The challenge continues to be the ability to develop interventions that promote the long-term maintenance of adequate levels of physical activity to promote weight control. There is a need to develop effective strategies that promote sufficient participation in physical activity to enhance both weight control and health-related outcomes in overweight and obese adults.

ACKNOWLEDGMENTS

Dr. Jakicic, Dr. Otto, and Dr. Polzien were supported by research funding from the National Institutes of Health (HL70257, HL67826, DK066150). Dr. Jakicic is on the scientific advisory boards for the Coca-Cola Beverage Institute for Health and Wellness, the Calorie Control Council, BodyMedia, Inc., and One Rock Technologies, Inc.

REFERENCES

1. Hedley, A.A., Ogden, C.L., Johnson, C.L., Carroll, M.D., Curtin, L.R., Flegal, K.M., Prevalence of overweight and obesity among U.S. children, adolescents, and adults, 1999–2002, *JAMA,* 291, 2847–2850, 2004.
2. National Institutes of Health, National Heart, Lung, and Blood Institute, Clinical guidelines on the identification, evaluation, and treatment of overweight and obesity in adults — The evidence report, *Obes. Res.,* 6(2), 1998.
3. Sherwood, N.E., Jeffery, R.W., French, S.A., Hannan, P.J., Murray, D.M., Predictors of weight gain in the Pound of Prevention study, *Int. J. Obes.,* 24, 395–403, 2000.
4. Lee, I-M., Paffenbarger, R., Associations of light, moderate, and vigorous intensity physical activity with longevity: The Harvard Alumni Health Study, *Am. J. Epidemiol.,* 151(3), 293–299, 2000.
5. DiPietro, L., Kohl, H.W., Barlow, C.E., Blair, S.N., Improvements in cardiorespiratory fitness attenuate age-related weight gain in healthy men and women: the Aerobics Center Longitudinal Study, *Int. J. Obes.,* 22, 55–62, 1998.

6. Slentz, C.A., Duscha, M.S., Johnson, J.L., et al., Effects of the amount of exercise on body weight, body composition, and measures of central obesity. STRIDDE — A randomized controlled study, *Arch. Int. Med.,* 164, 31–39, 2004.
7. Department of Health and Human Services and U.S. Department of Agriculture, *Dietary Guidelines for Americans*, www.healthierus.gov/dietaryguidelines, 2005.
8. Wing, R.R., Behavioral weight control, in *Handbook of Obesity Treatment*, Wadden, T.A., Stunkard, A.J., Eds., The Guilford Press, New York, 301–316, 2002.
9. Wing, R.R., Venditti, E.M., Jakicic, J.M., Polley, B.A., Lang, W., Lifestyle intervention in overweight individuals with a family history of diabetes, *Diab. Care,* 21(3), 350–359, 1998.
10. Hagan, R.D., Upton, S.J., Wong, L., Whittam, J., The effects of aerobic conditioning and/or calorie restriction in overweight men and women, *Med. Sci. Sports Exerc.,* 18(1), 87–94, 1986.
11. Barlow, C.E., Kohl, H.W., Gibbons, L.W., Blair, S.N., Physical activity, mortality, and obesity, *Int. J. Obes.,* 19, S41–S44, 1995.
12. Lee, S., Kuk, J.I., Katzmarzyk, P.T., Blair, S.N., Church, T.S., Ross, R., Cardiorespiratory fitness attenuates metabolic risk independent of subcutaneous and visceral fat in men, *Diab. Care,* 28, 895–901, 2005.
13. Wei, M., Kampert, J., Barlow, C.E., et al., Relationship between low cardiorespiratory fitness and mortality in normal-weight, overweight, and obese men, *JAMA,* 282(16), 1547–1553, 1999.
14. Farrell, S.W., Braun, L., Barlow, C.E., Cheng, Y.J., Blair, S.N., The relation of body mass index, cardiorespiratory fitness, and all-cause mortality in women, *Obes. Res.,* 10(6), 417–423, 2002.
15. Church, T.S., LaMonte, M.J., Barlow, C.E., Blair, S.N., Cardiorespiratory fitness and body mass index as predictors of cardiovascular disease mortality among men with diabetes, *Arch. Intern. Med.,* 165, 2114–2120, 2005.
16. Stevens, J., Cai, J., Evenson, K.R., Thomas, R., Fitness and fatness as predictors of mortality from all causes and from cardiovascular disease in men and women in the lipid research clinics study, *Am. J. Epidemiol.,* 156(9), 832–841, 2002.
17. McGuire, M.T., Wing, R.R., Klem, M.L., Lang, W., Hill, J.O., What predicts weight regain in a group of successful weight losers? *J. Consult. Clin. Psychol.,* 67(2), 177–185, 1999.
18. Jakicic, J.M., Wing, R.R., Winters-Hart, C., Relationship of physical activity to eating behaviors and weight loss in women, *Med. Sci. Sports Exerc.,* 34(10), 1653–1659, 2002.
19. Jakicic, J.M., Clark, K., Coleman, E., et al., American College of Sports Medicine position stand: appropriate intervention strategies for weight loss and prevention of weight regain for adults, *Med. Sci. Sports Exerc.,* 33(12), 2145–2156, 2001.
20. Institute of Medicine, Dietary Reference Intakes for Energy, Carbohydrates, Fiber, Fat, Protein and Amino Acids (Macronutrients): A Report of the Panel on Macronutrients, Subcommittees on Upper Reference Levels of Nutrients and Interpretation and Uses of Dietary Reference Intakes, and the Standing Committee on the Scientific Evaluation of Dietary Reference Intakes, The National Academies Press, Washington, D.C., 2002.
21. Saris, W.H.M., Blair, S.N., van Baak, M.A., et al., How much physical activity is enough to prevent unhealthy weight gain? Outcome of the I.A.S.O. 1st Stock Conference and Consensus Statement, *Obes. Rev.,* 4, 101–114, 2003.
22. Jakicic, J.M., Marcus, B.H., Gallagher, K.I., Napolitano, M., Lang, W., Effect of exercise duration and intensity on weight loss in overweight, sedentary women. A randomized trial, *JAMA,* 290, 1323–1330, 2003.

23. Jakicic, J.M., Winters, C., Lang, W., Wing, R.R., Effects of intermittent exercise and use of home exercise equipment on adherence, weight loss, and fitness in overweight women: a randomized trial, *JAMA,* 282(16), 1554–1560, 1999.
24. Jakicic, J.M., Marcus, B., Lang, W., Effect of varying doses of exercise on 24-month weight loss in overweight adults, *Obes. Res.,* 13(Suppl), A24, 2005.
25. Jeffery, R.W., Wing, R.R., Sherwood, N.E., Tate, D.F., Physical activity and weight loss: does prescribing higher physical activity goals improve outcome? *Am. J. Clin. Nutr.,* 78(4), 684–689, 2003.
26. Klem, M.L., Wing, R.R., McGuire, M.T., Seagle, H.M., Hill, J.O., A descriptive study of individuals successful at long-term maintenance of substantial weight loss, *Am. J. Clin. Nutr.,* 66, 239–246, 1997.
27. Schoeller, D.A., Shay, K., Kushner, R.F., How much physical activity is needed to minimize weight gain in previously obese women, *Am. J. Clin. Nutr.,* 66, 551–556, 1997.
28. Donnelly, J.E., Jakicic, J.M., Pronk, N.P., et al., Is resistance exercise effective for weight management? *Evid. Based Prev. Med.,* 1(1), 21–29, 2004.
29. Gallagher, K.I., Jakicic, J.M., Otto, A.D., Mohr, C.R., Thomas, E., Examination of twelve month changes in body weight and body composition following alternative forms of exercise, *Med. Sci. Sports Exerc.,* 37(5), Suppl, S339, 2005.
30. Wadden, T.A., Vogt, R.A., Andersen, R.E., Exercise in the treatment of obesity: effects of four interventions on body composition, resting energy expenditure, appetite, and mood, *J. Consult. Clin. Psychol.,* 65, 269–277, 1997.
31. Jurca, R., LaMonte, M.J., Church, T.S., et al., Association of muscle strength and aerobic fitness with metabolic syndrome in men, *Med. Sci. Sports Exerc.,* 36(8), 1301–1307, 2004.
32. Jannsen, I., Fortier, A., Hudson, R., Ross, R., Effects of an energy-restrictive diet with or without exercise on abdominal fat, intermuscular fat, and metabolic risk factors in obese women, *Diab. Care,* 25(3), 431–438, 2002.
33. Kraemer, W.J., Volek, J.S., Clark, K.L., et al., Physiological adaptations to a weight-loss dietary regimen and exercise programs in women, *J. Appl. Physiol.,* 83(1), 270–279, 1997.
34. Kraemer, W.J., Volek, J.S., Clark, K.L., et al., Influence of exercise training on physiological and performance changes with weight loss in men, *Med. Sci. Sports Exerc.,* 31, 1320–1329, 1999.
35. Jakicic, J.M., Physical activity considerations for the treatment and prevention of obesity, *Am. J. Clin. Nutr.,* 82(1 Suppl), 226S–229S, 2005.
36. Oken, B.S., Zajdel, D., Kishiyama, S., et al., Randomized, controlled, six-month trial of yoga in healthy seniors: effects on cognition and quality of life, *Altern. Ther. Health Med.,* 12(1), 40–47, 2006.
37. Williams, K.A., Petronis, J., Smith, D., et al., Effect of Iyengar yoga therapy for chronic low back pain, *Pain,* 115, 107–117, 2005.
38. Otto, A.D., Nagle, E.F., Jakicic, J.M., et al., Comparison of physical activity enjoyment during aquatic exercise in overweight women, *Med. Sci. Sports Exerc.,* 35(5), Suppl, 2003.
39. Nagle, E.F., Otto, A.D., Jakicic, J.M., Robertson, R.J., Goss, F.L., Ranalli, J.L., Effects of aquatic plus walking exercise on weight loss and function in sedentary obese females, *Med. Sci. Sports Exerc.,* 35(5), Suppl, 2003.
40. DeBusk, R., Stenestrand, U., Sheehan, M., Haskell, W., Training effects of long versus short bouts of exercise in healthy subjects, *Am. J. Cardiol.,* 65, 1010–1013, 1990.

41. Ebisu, T., Splitting the distances of endurance training: on cardiovascular endurance and blood lipids, *Jap. J. Phys. Educ.,* 30, 37–43, 1985.
42. Jakicic, J.M., Wing, R.R., Butler, B.A., Robertson, R.J., Prescribing exercise in multiple short bouts versus one continuous bout: effects on adherence, cardiorespiratory fitness, and weight loss in overweight women, *Int. J. Obes.,* 19, 893–901, 1995.
43. Levine, J.A., Lanningham-Foster, L.M., McCrady, S.K., et al., Interindividual variation in posture allocation: possible role in human obesity, *Science,* 307(5709), 584–586, 2005.
44. Andersen, R., Wadden, T., Bartlett, S., Zemel, B., Verde, T., Franckowiak, S., Effects of lifestyle activity vs. structured aerobic exercise in obese women: a randomized trial, *JAMA,* 281, 335–340, 1999.
45. Dunn, A., Marcus, B., Kampert, J., Garcia, M., Kohl, I.I.I.H., Blair, S., Comparison of lifestyle and structured interventions to increase physical activity and cardiorespiratory fitness, *JAMA,* 281, 327–334, 1999.
46. Pate, R.R., Pratt, M., Blair, S.N., et al., Physical activity and public health: a recommendation from the Centers for Disease and Prevention and the American College of Sports Medicine, *JAMA,* 273(5), 402–407, 1995.
47. US Department of Health and Human Services, *Physical Activity and Health: A Report of the Surgeon General,* US Department of Health and Human Services, Centers for Disease Control and Prevention, National Center for Chronic Disease Prevention and Health Promotion, Atlanta, GA, 1996.
48. Tudor-Locke, C., Bassett, D.R., How many steps/day are enough? Preliminary pedometer indices for public health, *Sports Med.,* 34(1), 1–8, 2004.
49. Yamanouchi, K., Takashi, T., Chikada, K., et al., Daily walking combined with diet therapy is a useful means for obese, N.I.DDM patients not only to reduce body weight but also to improve insulin sensitivity, *Diab. Care,* 18(6), 775–778, 1995.

6 Pharmacologic Therapy for Obesity and Overweight in Adults and Adolescents

Marie Thearle and Louis J. Aronne

CONTENTS

6.1 INTRODUCTION

Before initiating medical therapy, obesity must be understood as a lifelong, chronic, and relapsing disease that rarely responds completely to lifestyle modifications. Obesity is the accumulation of excess adipose tissue associated with an increased risk for diabetes mellitus, hypertension, dyslipidemia, stroke, gallbladder disease, sleep apnea, osteoarthritis, and certain cancers. The prevalence of obesity is rising in the U.S., with an estimated 64% of Americans classified as overweight or obese in 2000 [1]. Potential contributing factors to the increase in obesity include easy access to highly palatable and energy-dense foods, a relatively sedentary lifestyle, and a genetic legacy to preferentially store energy. Much of our evolutionary history involved surviving starvation such that, once adipose tissue accumulates, homeostatic neuroendocrine mechanisms resist attempts to diminish the supply of excess energy. When hypocaloric diets alone are used to reduce weight, a counter-regulatory increase in appetite and decrease in resting energy expenditure occur in an attempt to return the body to its former weight [2]. These metabolic changes make long-term maintenance of weight loss difficult to achieve. Pharmacologic therapy is frequently needed as an adjunct to lifestyle modifications for successful weight loss and maintenance.

During the history of pharmacologic treatment for obesity, most medications have been associated with side effects, abuse, and weight regain despite ongoing treatment — characteristics that have led most practitioners to steer clear of prescribing them. Some of the first attempts to treat obesity occurred in the 1800s with thyroid extract, which led to symptoms and consequences of hyperthyroidism [3]. Later, the use of amphetamine led to addiction and caused several deaths [3]. More recently, fenfluramine and dexfenfluramine were withdrawn from the market due to associated primary pulmonary hypertension and valvulopathy [4].

Many patients have unrealistic expectations about weight loss and anticipate satisfactory cosmetic results in addition to improved health outcomes [5]. A meta-analysis of modern medications used to treat obesity demonstrated that no single medication led to an average weight loss greater than 4 kg over that seen with behavioral changes. In addition, weight loss tends to plateau after 6 mo and further treatment is aimed mostly at maintenance of the reduced weight [6]. However, despite this seemingly modest amount of additional weight loss, small changes in body mass index (BMI), an estimation of percent body fat, have been associated with improvements in obesity-related complications [7]. A small reduction in BMI may also lead to a longer life span, although no studies have directly determined the effect of obesity treatment on mortality [8].

Many physicians and patients are resistant to pharmacologic treatment of obesity and hold the new antiobesity pharmaceuticals to unrealistic standards of safety and efficacy. While safety is of utmost importance with any drug, it is important to note that many diseases are treated with medications that carry risk, because it is believed that the benefit to the patient is greater than the risk. The same standards should apply to antiobesity drugs. The key is to treat the patients at the greatest medical risk in order to reduce morbidity and mortality.

6.2 INITIATING TREATMENT

Guidelines issued by the National Institutes of Health (NIH) support the paradigm of obesity as a chronic disease and recommend weight loss to improve the health of obese patients and overweight patients with comorbidities [9]. Due to the convenience of measurement, BMI, which is the body weight in kilograms divided by the height in meters squared, is currently used to define the degree of obesity. Overweight is defined as a BMI greater than 25, obesity as a BMI greater than 30, and extreme obesity as a BMI greater than 40. The mainstay of obesity treatment remains behavioral modification [5]. However, if lifestyle changes are unsuccessful after a 6-mo trial, pharmacological treatment should be considered. Pharmacotherapy is appropriate in patients who are at risk from their obesity, have no contraindications to the medication, are committed to losing weight, and understand the risks, success rates, and need for chronic treatment. It should be emphasized that a patient's commitment to weight loss is a major determinant of future success. If the patient is ambivalent about losing weight, weight maintenance should be emphasized and the complications of obesity should be managed.

Pharmacologic therapy for weight loss can be directed toward reducing appetite, altering nutrient absorption, or increasing thermogenesis. Although, the only medications currently approved for long-term use are sibutramine (Meridia, Abbott Laboratories, Abbott Park, IL) and orlistat (Xenical, Hoffman-LaRoche, Nutley, NJ) (Table 6.1), pharmaceutical companies have made new treatments for obesity a top

TABLE 6.1
Weight Loss Drugs FDA Approved for Long-Term Use

Drug	Dose	Mode of Action	Weight Loss Expected beyond Lifestyle Changes after 1 yr	Adverse Effects	Suggestions for Deciding Which Obese Patients Are Appropriate for the Drug
Orlistat	120 mg 3 times a day before meals	Inhibits pancreatic lipase to decrease fat absorption	4.3 kg	Gastrointestinal symptoms, decreased absorption of fat-soluble vitamins	Associated hypertension, associated dyslipidemia, difficulty removing high-fat foods from diet, frequent habit of eating at restaurants
Sibutramine	Start with 10 mg once a day; increase or decrease by 5 mg, as needed	Norepinephrine, serotonin, and dopamine reuptake inhibitor	2.7 kg	Can increase heart rate and blood pressure; dry mouth, insomnia, constipation, headache	Binge eating, frequent feelings of hunger, erratic eating habits, preoccupation with food

priority and many potential therapies are in various stages of clinical testing. Medication use is indicated in obese patients with either a BMI greater than 30 or a BMI greater than 27 with two or more associated comorbidities including sleep apnea, nonalcoholic fatty liver disease, polycystic ovarian syndrome, gout, diabetes, dyslipidemia, hypertension, or osteoarthritis [9]. Pharmacological treatment is also recommended in women with a waist circumference greater than 35 in (88 cm) or men with a waist circumference greater than 40 in. (102 cm) and two or more associated comorbidities [9]. Obesity treatment with pharmacotherapy is contraindicated during pregnancy.

It is important to emphasize that a weight loss of only 5 to 10% of initial weight is associated with improvements in cardiovascular risk factors [10] and obesity-related comorbidities [7]. Such benefits with modest weight loss are likely because of a greater decrease in visceral fat — the fat depots primarily associated with the risk of developing medical complications. Any medication is associated with side effects and these should be explained to the patient in the context of a benefit-to-risk assessment. Patients should also understand that there is a large amount of variability in responses to weight loss medications, in part, due to patient compliance and, in part, due to individual differences. The NIH guidelines recommend that if a chosen medication does not lead to a 2 kg weight loss in the first month of treatment, the dose should be adjusted or the medication should be discontinued [9]. The maximum weight loss can be expected to occur after about 6 mo of treatment [11]. Further treatment with the medication will be mainly for weight maintenance rather than additional weight loss.

In summary, pharmacotherapy for obesity is indicated in patients with either a BMI greater than 30, or a BMI greater than 27 with two or more associated comorbidities, as well as in women with a waist circumference greater than 35 in. (88 cm) or men with a waist circumference greater than 40 in (102 cm) with two or more associated comorbidities. If a medication does not lead to a 2 kg weight loss in the first month of treatment, the dose should be adjusted or the medication should be discontinued.

6.3 CURRENTLY APPROVED MEDICATIONS FOR WEIGHT LOSS

6.3.1 SIBUTRAMINE

Sibutramine (Meridia, Reductil) was originally developed as an antidepressant but was unsuccessful at improving mood. However, it was found to lead to weight loss via decreased appetite and increased satiety and has been approved for long-term treatment of obesity since 1997. Sibutramine is a beta-phenethylamine [12] that is metabolized by the liver cytochrome P450 (3A4) system to its active metabolites, which inhibit reuptake of serotonin, norepinephrine, and, to a lesser degree, dopamine. Because the half-lives of the active metabolites are 14 to 16 hr, steady state levels are not obtained until after 4 d. These neurotransmitters are anorexigenic peptides and are probably a causal factor for reduced feelings of hunger and food anticipation as well as increased satiety [13] seen with sibutramine administration.

In rodents, sibutramine decreases total caloric intake and specifically decreases consumption of carbohydrate- and fat-rich foods [14]. Sibutramine may also increase thermogenesis [13,15].

More than ten prospective, randomized, controlled trials have been done with sibutramine, all of which have supported its efficacy [16]. These trials have included people of Caucasian, Hispanic, and African-American backgrounds. The trials have included up to a thousand participants and have lasted from 3 mo to 1 yr. Most trials included a run-in period of 2 to 4 weeks to assess for "responders" to sibutramine. People who do not lose 2 kg or 2% of their weight in the first month are unlikely to lose weight with further treatment or escalating doses [12]. Despite high attrition rates, each study has shown significantly greater weight loss with sibutramine at doses greater than 10 mg/d vs. placebo. Both weight loss and occurrence of adverse events appear to be dose related [12,17]. A meta-analysis of three trials of at least 1-yr duration showed that treatment with sibutramine led to a 4.3 kg or 4.6% additional weight loss above that seen with placebo alone [18]. Thirty-four percent more participants on sibutramine lost more than 5% of their original body weight compared to those on placebo and 15% more participants lost more than 10% of their original body weight than in the placebo treated group. Weight loss usually plateaus after 6 mo of treatment but continued treatment is required for maintenance [19–21].

Sibutramine has also been found to be useful for maintaining diet-induced weight loss. Seventy-five percent of patients treated with sibutramine for a year after a very-low-calorie diet sustained 100% of the weight they lost compared to 42% on placebo [22]. In a crossover study, sibutramine led to further decreases in weight after weight loss from lifestyle changes had stabilized. However; sibutramine was more effective if it was initiated earlier in weight loss attempts [19]. In these studies, weight gain occurred with cessation of sibutramine, emphasizing the need for continued pharmacological treatment. In studies addressing the physiologic effects of sibutramine on resting energy expenditure, 15 mg a day of sibutramine offsets the expected decrease in energy expenditure, which usually occurs with diet-induced weight loss [13,15]. After adjustment for body weight, energy expenditure was only 0.8% less on sibutramine following significant weight loss compared to 3.8% less on placebo. No dietary or physical activity changes were made in patients participating in this study [13]. Similar findings were seen in studies where patients were instructed to reduce their caloric intake [15]. The ability of sibutramine to limit the normal decrease in resting energy expenditure after weight loss likely contributes to its effect on weight maintenance.

Reductions in cardiovascular risk factors occur in association with sibutramine-mediated weight loss. Improvements in cholesterol, low-density lipoprotein (LDL), very-low-density lipoprotein (VLDL), insulin, and uric acid can be explained entirely by the amount of weight lost [20,21,23–25]. High-density lipoprotein (HDL) and triglyceride levels improve to a greater extent than expected by the quantity of weight lost [21,22,25]. HDL levels were particularly notable in the Sibutramine Trial of Obesity Reduction and Maintenance (STORM) as they rose 20% in the sibutramine group vs. 12% in the placebo group after weight had stabilized [21]. With weight loss, waist circumference and waist-to-hip ratio also decrease, which may indicate a greater reduction in visceral fat as compared to subcutaneous fat. Loss of visceral fat may be associated with improvements in insulin sensitivity [25]. In nondiabetic obese patients, insulin sensitivity, as measured by the homeostasis model (HOMA) for the assessment of insulin resistance, has been shown to improve with weight loss induced by sibutramine [26].

When sibutramine was studied in type 2 diabetic patients, glucose control improved as shown by decreases in hemoglobin A_{1C}, fasting insulin, and glucose levels [24,25,27]. No additional adverse effects were noted with use in diabetic patients compared to nondiabetic patients. Sibutramine has been used safely in patients on sulfonylureas [24,25], metformin [25,27], and insulin [24].

Obesity is a rapidly growing problem in children and adolescents. While sibutramine is not approved for use in adolescents less than 16 yr of age and most studies have been done in adults, two studies have shown efficacy in adolescents [28,29]. Significantly greater amounts of weight loss were seen in both studies. In one study, no adverse effects were seen [29], but in the second, treatment had to be reduced or discontinued in 44% of the participants on sibutramine due to elevations in blood pressure or heart rate [28]. At this time, any use of sibutramine in adolescents and children is off label, especially since suicide risk is not clear.

The most common adverse effects in clinical trials have been dry mouth, constipation, and insomnia, presumably related to noradrenergic effects. To date, no association with the valvular heart disease that occurred with fenfluramine has been found with use of sibutramine [30]. Sibutramine is contraindicated in patients with associated renal impairment, liver dysfunction, uncontrolled hypertension, or cardiovascular disease. As sibutramine inhibits serotonin reuptake, it should not be used with other serotonin reuptake inhibitors or monoamine oxidase inhibitors as the serotonin syndrome can occur. Sibutramine is associated with increases in systolic blood pressure by 4 mm of mercury (mmHg) and diastolic blood pressure by 2 to 4 mmHg as well as increases in heart rate by 4 beats/min [12,21–23]. The elevations in blood pressure and pulse rate can be highly variable, but can be managed by decreasing or discontinuing the medication. In patients who lose more than 5% of their original weight, blood pressure and heart rate are more likely to be stable or reduced. In the STORM trial, 3% of patients had to be withdrawn from the study over 2 yr due to increases in blood pressure [21]. When sibutramine has been evaluated for cardiovascular safety, it has been decided that the risk/benefit ratio of sibutramine in obesity warranted its further use. Sibutramine has been found to be both safe and efficacious in people with controlled hypertension on angiotensin-converting enzyme inhibitors [31], beta blockers [32], and calcium channel blockers [33]. In 224 hypertensive patients followed for 1 yr on sibutramine, 5.3% developed hypertension, requiring discontinuation of the drug, compared to 1.4% of patients on placebo. However, 40% of patients on sibutramine lost more than 5% of their body weight vs. 9% of patients on placebo, and improvements were seen in triglycerides, HDL, LDL, total cholesterol, and uric acid [33]. A small study investigating the use of 25 mg of metoprolol to prevent adverse effects during treatment with sibutramine found that addition of metoprolol increased patient compliance and decreased the incidence of side effects without altering weight loss efficacy [34]. It is recommended that blood pressure and pulse rate be monitored regularly in all patients on sibutramine.

In summary, sibutramine should be started at a dose of 10 mg a day orally for treatment of obesity. Subsequently, the dose can be increased or decreased by 5 mg a day depending on efficacy and tolerance. A weight loss of about 4 kg over that seen with lifestyle changes can be expected. Sibutramine is best used in patients who complain of frequent feelings of hunger and overeating at meals. Adverse effects can include dry mouth, constipation, and insomnia as well as elevations in blood pressure and heart rate, which should be monitored regularly. The use of sibutramine is contraindicated in individuals with uncontrolled hypertension or cardiovascular disease or with concomitant use of monoamine oxidase inhibitors or serotonin reuptake inhibitors.

6.3.2 Orlistat

Orlistat (Xenical) is an inhibitor of gastrointestinal lipases including pancreatic lipase. It has been approved for use in the treatment of obesity since 1999. At a dose of 120 mg given 3 times a day, orlistat prevents 30% of dietary fat absorption, thereby reducing both caloric and fat intake. Higher doses of orlistat do not lead to additional weight loss [35]. Less than 1% of orlistat is absorbed systemically, resulting in a very good safety profile. Predictably, orlistat treatment leads to reduced resting energy expenditure after weight loss. However, no excess decrease is seen compared to dietary therapy alone [36]. Of note, a second lipase inhibitor, ATL-962, has completed phase II clinical trials [37].

A number of prospective, randomized, placebo-controlled trials have been done, demonstrating the efficacy and safety of orlistat. All studies administered orlistat or placebo in association with a hypocaloric diet containing only 30% of calories from fat. A meta-analysis of 11 one-yr-long trials found that participants treated with orlistat lost 2.7 kg (or about 3%) more than those treated with placebo [18]. An additional 21% of participants taking orlistat lost 5% of their initial body weight compared to the placebo group and 12% more patients treated with orlistat achieved a weight loss of at least 10% compared with placebo [18]. When orlistat treatment is discontinued, weight reaccumulates. Weight gain also tends to recur after a year of therapy; however, continued treatment with orlistat slows the rate of regain. In the second year of treatment, patients who continue on an orlistat regimen regain half as much weight as patients who stop the drug [38,39]. The best predictor of persistent weight loss after 2 yr of treatment is loss of more than 5% of initial body weight in the first 12 weeks [40].

Orlistat has also been found to be useful in preventing weight regain in patients who successfully lost weight using a hypocaloric diet. While patients receiving placebo regained 56% of weight lost, orlistat-treated patients regained only 33%. Twenty-three percent of treated patients maintained all of their weight loss vs. only 16% in the placebo group [41]. In a small study, orlistat did not lead to additional weight loss when given to patients who had successfully lost weight with sibutramine [42].

Successful weight loss with orlistat results in significant improvements in cardiovascular risk factors including lipid profile, blood pressure, waist circumference, fasting insulin, and glucose levels [38,39,43–46]. Orlistat lowers LDL and cholesterol levels independent from the reductions expected with weight loss alone [38,46]. Treatment with orlistat for 1 yr decreased total cholesterol by an additional 5.6% and LDL by an extra 9% beyond reductions seen with placebo treatment [44]. In obese, hypercholesterolemic patients treated with orlistat for 6 mo, total cholesterol was reduced 6% compared to an increase of 3% in the placebo group and LDL was decreased 11% vs. 1% in the placebo group. The percentage of patients who achieved at least a 10% reduction in LDL was 54% in the orlistat-treated group in contrast to 25% in the placebo group [46]. In patients with uncontrolled hypertension, a year of treatment with orlistat led to a fall in diastolic blood pressure (DBP). An additional 14% of treated patients, as compared to patients taking placebo, achieved either a DBP less than 90 mmHg or a reduction in DBP of 10 mmHg. In the same study, an additional 12% of treated patients attained a 30% reduction in cardiovascular risk [10] compared to those given placebo. The greatest reductions in hypertension and hypercholesterolemia are seen in the patients who lose more than 5% of their weight in the first 3 mo [47]. A case series has been reported, which showed histopathological improvement of nonalcoholic steatohepatitis with weight loss, following orlistat treatment [48]. Orlistat has also been implicated in a preferential loss of visceral fat [49].

Orlistat can be effective in the treatment of insulin-resistant states. In a meta-analysis, 23% more patients with impaired glucose tolerance, who were treated with orlistat instead of placebo, had normal glucose utilization after 2 yr. Half as many patients treated with orlistat progressed to a diabetic state [45]. Despite high attrition rates, the Xenical in the Prevention of Diabetes in Obese Subjects (XENDOS) study demonstrated a 37% risk reduction for the development of diabetes with treatment of orlistat over 4 yr in patients with preexisting impaired glucose tolerance [50]. Orlistat treatment has been shown to lead to improved glycemic control in patients with diabetes [51–53]. In patients treated with metformin [51] or insulin [52], addition of orlistat for 1 yr led to improvements in fasting glucose and hemoglobin A_{1C}. Further, a greater percentage of treated patients achieved a reduction in medication requirements [51,52].

Xenical was approved for use in adolescents aged 12 to 16 in late 2003. In phase III trials with more than 500 adolescents, orlistat treatment was reported to lead to a decrease in BMI and, specifically, a decrease in fat mass without affecting the growth of bone or fat-free mass. Adverse effects were reported to be similar to those seen in adults. A small published study has also shown weight loss benefits with orlistat [54]. Studies addressing the safety of orlistat in adolescents have found good safety profiles. However, lower vitamin D levels have been found even when patients were treated with a multivitamin [55,56]. Therefore, vitamin D levels should be monitored in adolescents treated with orlistat and supplements of vitamin D may be needed.

As orlistat is not absorbed systemically; all of its side effects result from its mode of action. Orlistat is contraindicated in people with malabsorptive syndromes and cholestasis. Mild to moderate gastrointestinal side effects are seen in 60 to 80% of patients and include oily spotting, liquid stools, fecal urgency, flatulence, and abdominal cramping. Side effects increase with higher fat intake. While many patients have adverse effects initially, they are usually self-limited, probably because people adjust their diet to make orlistat more tolerable [39]. It is important to educate patients about the need to limit dietary fat to prevent side effects. Psyllium mucilloid given once a day has also been shown to be helpful in reducing side effects [57]. A multivitamin supplement should be taken 2 hours before or after a dose of orlistat as orlistat can impair absorption of fat-soluble vitamins. In a study evaluating the effects of orlistat on bone without vitamin D supplementation, bone density did not change more than expected after 1 yr of treatment; however, an increase in bone resorption markers did occur [58]. Orlistat is safe to administer with most other medications. No changes in the absorption or efficacy of glyburide, oral contraceptives, digoxin, nifedepine, or dilantin were seen when given with orlistat and no more than the usual monitoring is advised. Caution and careful monitoring should be exercised when prescribing orlistat with concomitant use of warfarin or cyclosporine due to the possibility of vitamin K depletion in the former and decreased serum levels in the latter. Rates of cholelithiasis and nephrolithiasis were not increased with orlistat treatment [44].

In summary, orlistat should be used at a dose of 120 mg three times a day orally with meals for the treatment of obesity. An additional weight loss of about 3 kg above that seen with lifestyle changes only can be expected. The best results are likely to be seen in those patients who lose more than 5% of their body weight in the first 12 weeks. Orlistat is a good choice in those patients who frequently eat at restaurants, have difficulty adhering to a low-fat diet, and have concurrent hypertension, diabetes, or hypercholesterolemia. Side effects, which are due to the mode of action, include oily spotting, liquid stools, fecal urgency, flatulence, and abdominal cramping. Because of these effects, orlistat is not very popular among adolescents. A multivitamin supplement containing fat-soluble vitamins should be taken two hours before or after the medication. Orlistat is contraindicated in people with malabsorptive syndromes and cholestasis.

6.3.3 Noradrenergic Agents

Phentermine (Ionamin, Fastin, Adipex) and diethylproprion (Tenuate) are Schedule IV noradrenergic agents, which act via central catecholamine mechanisms to cause appetite suppression for 12 to 14 hr. Phentermine, the most commonly prescribed agent in this class, has been approved for the short-term treatment of obesity since 1959, at a dose of 15 to 30 mg given in the morning. Tolerance and tachyphylaxis tend to develop after use for a few weeks. Studies show a weight loss of 2 to 10 kg above that seen in placebo [11]. Side effects include insomnia, dry mouth, restlessness, constipation, euphoria, nervousness as well as increased pulse rate and blood pressure. Psychosis has been reported in association with treatment. The use of noradrenergic agents is contraindicated in patients with cardiovascular disease, hypertension, hyperthyroidism, or a history of drug abuse, or in those taking monoamine oxidase inhibitors. No large-scale, long-term studies of weight loss have been performed. If these drugs are used for more than 3 mo, patients should be informed that such use has not been studied.

6.4 MEDICATIONS IN CLINICAL TRIALS AND OFF-LABEL USE OF MEDICATIONS

A large number of drugs and peptides are in the early stages of evaluation for benefit in obesity and have been tested in preclinical and clinical trials. We will review the drugs that have been approved for other indications but studied for weight loss effects and which are occasionally used by obesity experts for the treatment of obesity off-label. In addition, we will briefly review the drugs currently under evaluation in clinical trials.

6.4.1 Antiepileptic Drugs

Two Food and Drug Administration (FDA)-approved antiepilepsy drugs, zonisamide (Zonegran) and topiramate (Topamax), have been evaluated for weight loss benefits. Both were noted to lead to weight loss in antiseizure trials [59,60]. The mechanism by which either leads to weight loss remains unclear.

Topiramate blocks voltage-dependent sodium and calcium channels, which is believed to account for its antiepileptic properties. In addition, it antagonizes glutamate kainite receptor and enhances γ–aminobutyric acid (GABA) activity. Glutamate has been implicated as an orexigenic agent and antagonism may account for the weight loss effects of topiramate. In a randomized, placebo-controlled trial, 60 weeks of treatment with 192 mg/d topiramate led to a 7.6 kg of additional weight loss in the treatment group compared to the placebo group. Forty-three percent more subjects in the treatment group lost at least 5% of their initial weight and 34% lost more than 10% of their body weight. Associated improvements in blood pressure and glucose tolerance were also seen [61]. Topiramate may be especially useful in patients who suffer from binge eating disorder [62]. Because of the frequency of patients who experience an adverse effect including at least one mild to moderate neurologic event such as paresthesia, memory difficulties, concentration problems, nervousness, depression and language problems, phase III trials of topiramate use in obesity were halted by the manufacturing company pending development of an extended-release version of topiramate [61]. A small number of patients in that study reported suicidal ideation. Because many of these adverse events occur early in treatment and resolve with cessation of treatment, topiramate is occasionally used off-label with the patient's permission. Topiramate may be useful in patients with frequent feelings of hunger and a history of binge eating but should not be used in patients with a history of depression. In addition to monitoring for neurologic effects, serum bicarbonate levels should be checked before initiating therapy and periodically thereafter, as topiramate is a weak carbonic anhydrase inhibitor and hyperchloremic acidosis may occur [61,63].

Similar to topiramate, zonisamide antagonizes sodium and calcium channels. However, it also has serotonergic and dopaminergic activity, which is thought to contribute to its ability to stimulate weight loss. In a small randomized placebo-controlled trial, treatment with zonisamide over 4 mo led to 5 kg of additional weight loss over placebo. Forty-seven percent more treated patients lost greater than 5% of their original weight compared to the placebo group. In an optional single blind extension of the same trial for a further 16 weeks, the average weight loss increased by a further 3.1 kg in the treated group. Major side effects were fatigue, which occurred in 30% of the treatment group and a small, but significant, increase in serum creatinine. The increase in creatinine occurred in the first 16 weeks and no further increases were seen in the second half of the study [64]. In antiepileptic studies of zonisamide, somnolence was also noted to be a side effect [59]. Longer and larger-scale studies will be needed to further assess the efficacy and safety of these drugs.

6.4.2 Metformin

Metformin (Glucophage), approved for treatment of type 2 diabetes, activates AMP-activated protein kinase (AMPK), which leads to inhibition of liver gluconeogenesis and stimulation of glucose uptake by muscle [65]. In the large Diabetes Prevention Program Research Trial, metformin was compared to placebo or lifestyle intervention as a means to prevent the development of diabetes in nondiabetic patients with impaired glucose tolerance. Although less successful than lifestyle changes such as exercise and a hypocaloric diet, treatment with metformin decreased the incidence of diabetes by 31% over an average follow-up of 2.8 yr. Treatment with metformin was also associated with a 2.1 kg weight loss [66]. Similar results were observed in adolescents with elevated insulin levels [67]. Metformin has been approved by the FDA for use in adolescents with type 2 diabetes. Although it is unlikely that metformin will stand alone as a treatment for obesity, it may be a useful adjunctive therapy in insulin-resistant obese patients to prevent the development of diabetes and should be first-line therapy in the obese diabetic patient.

6.4.3 Bupropion

Bupropion (Wellbutrin, Zyban) is approved for treatment of depression and as a smoking cessation aid but has also been found to facilitate weight loss. Bupropion acts to inhibit norepinephrine and dopamine reuptake in the central nervous system, which may facilitate weight loss. In a 24-week randomized, placebo-controlled study, bupropion led to a 1.7% greater weight loss than placebo at 300 mg/d and a 3.7% greater weight loss at 400 mg/d. Thirty-seven percent more participants who were treated with 400 mg/d of bupropion vs. placebo lost at least 5% of their initial body weight and 26% more patients lost greater than 10% of their initial body weight. In a 24-week extension of this study, some weight regain occurred but the average weight loss with at least 300 mg/d bupropion remained about 5% of initial body weight [68]. A comparable study in obese patients with depressive symptoms showed similar results [69]. In both studies, there was no increase in adverse effects; however, there is a known 0.4% risk of seizure at a dose of 400 mg/d. Bupropion may be a useful adjunct to assist weight loss efforts in obese patients who have depressive symptoms.

6.4.4 Ciliary Neurotrophic Factor Analog

Recombinant human CNTF (Axokine) is in stage III clinical trials. It was originally developed as a potential treatment for amyotrophic lateral sclerosis (ALS).

Although ineffective in treating ALS, CNTF was noted to cause weight loss in these studies [70]. Subsequently, the receptor for CNTF has been found to share similarities with the leptin receptor. Leptin is a hormone released from fat cells, which conveys a message of energy availability to the hypothalamus. Leptin deficiency leads to severe obesity [71]. Leptin acts via its receptor to activate a Janus kinase/signal transduction and translation (JAK/STAT) system, which ultimately leads to decreased expression of neuropeptide Y (NPY), a potent appetite stimulant, and increased expression of anorexigenic neuropeptides [72]. Leptin has been unsuccessful at inducing weight loss as most obese individuals already have high circulating concentrations of leptin and may be considered leptin resistant. However, CNTF is able to bypass the leptin system by independent activation of the JAK/STAT system. It has been found to reduce food intake in both leptin-responsive and leptin-resistant rodents [73]. In leptin-resistant mice, treatment also led to significant improvements in hyperinsulinemia and hypercholesterolemia [74]. Cessation of CNTF, unlike discontinuation of a hypocaloric diet, did not result in overeating or rebound weight gain, which suggested that CNTF has the ability to lower the hypothalamic body weight set point [73]. The continued effects after the drug is stopped have raised some concerns about possible long-term central nervous system effects [75].

The efficacy of Axokine, a truncated form of CNTF (rhvCNTF), was limited by the development of antibodies in 70% of the participants. An initial published 12-week study with 173 participants demonstrated an additional weight loss of 3 kg beyond that seen in the placebo group at the optimal dose of 1 μg/kg, given subcutaneously. Preliminary results indicated that patients were able to maintain their weight loss for up to 1 yr after stopping the study drug. The most common adverse reactions were nausea, cough, musculoskeletal pain, and injection site reactions [76]. Despite these initial studies, the phase III trial indicated more modest results limited by the formation of anti-rhvCNTF antibodies. After 1 yr of treatment with rhvCNTF, participants had lost an additional 1.6 kg compared to those receiving placebo. Seven percent more subjects on rhvCNTF instead of placebo lost more than 5% of their initial body weight. In those 30% of participants who did not develop antibodies, weight loss was 2.9 kg beyond that seen with placebo. RhvCNTF treatment was associated with decreases in blood pressure, triglycerides, waist circumference, and insulin resistance [77]. Further studies are in progress.

6.4.5 Cannabinoid Receptor Antagonists

Endocannabinoids stimulate food intake through cannabinoid receptors (CB1) in the hypothalamus. Endogenous agonists of the CB1 receptor, anandamide and 2-arachidonoyl glycerol, have been shown to stimulate feeding and to be upregulated in genetically obese leptin-deficient rodents [78]. Reversal of leptin deficiency reduces these endocannabinoids [79]. In addition, the drug marinol, a CB1 agonist, is approved to treat the cachexia of cancer and AIDS. Mice without an active CB1 receptor have decreased adiposity on a standard diet, are resistant to diet-induced obesity, and have poor feeding efficiency, and there is a suggestion that they have an increased metabolic rate on a high-fat diet [80].

An antagonist of the CB1 receptor, SR141716 or rimonabant (Acomplia), was initially developed to attenuate the effects of marijuana [81]. Rimonabant has been found to suppress food intake in genetically obese and diet-induced obese animals [82,83]. Although tolerance quickly developed to the anorexic effects of rimonabant in treated diet-induced obese mice, the rodents maintained a 20% weight loss and a 50% decrease in body fat over 5 weeks [84]. Upon withdrawal of the drug, weight gain recurs [83]. In phase II trials, rimonabant was reported to lead to an additional weight loss of 2.9 kg compared to placebo at a dose of 20 mg/d for 16 weeks, with only minor gastrointestinal side effects [85]. Further results from phase II trials indicate that an additional 34% of subjects lost greater than 10% of their body weight with 1 yr of treatment compared to placebo [75]. In a randomized, placebo-controlled phase III trial (the Rimonabant in Obesity lipids trial), rimonabant was reported to improve lipid profiles [86]. The results of other completed phase III trials for rimonabant are pending. Side effects may include nausea, vomiting, anxiety, and depressed mood. One case of multiple sclerosis was reported [87].

6.4.6 Human Growth Hormone Fragment

When growth hormone (GH) is given to patients with GH deficiency, it leads to decreased adiposity and improved lean muscle mass; but these effects are not seen when obese patients without GH deficiency are treated with growth hormone [88]. However, a synthetic C-terminal fragment of human GH (hGH), AOD9604, has been developed, which does not interact with the GH receptor. AOD9604 was found to reduce body weight by stimulating lipolysis in leptin deficient-mice without development of the anabolic side effects of hGH, which include hyperglycemia and cell proliferation [89]. Phase I randomized, placebo-controlled clinical trials have been completed in a small group of obese males, demonstrating that oral doses of AOD9604 are safe over a 3-week period in humans. AOD9604 was also noted to cause a 0.5 kg weight loss over the 3 weeks as compared to placebo [90]. Initial reports of phase II trials are that over a 12-week period, 1 mg/d of AOD9604 led to a weight loss of 2 kg over that seen with placebo, without severe side effects.

6.4.7 5-HT$_{2C}$ Agonist

Serotonin (5-HT) is a neurotransmitter thought to be important in weight homeostasis. Mice without a 5-HT$_{2C}$ receptor are obese due to hyperphagia and are prone to seizures [91]. Activation of the 5-HT$_{2C}$ receptor causes hypophagia and increased energy expenditure in obese rodents, which leads to significant weight loss [92,93]. One of the 5-HT$_{2C}$ receptor agonists, APD356, was shown to decrease fat mass and improve lipid profiles in animals [94]. In phase I trials, APD356 given over 14 d was reported as well tolerated with some side effects, which include headache, nausea, and vomiting. Echocardiograms done after the 2-week period showed no change in heart valves, although long-term studies will need to be done to demonstrate the safety of these drugs. A dose of 10 mg/d was found to reduce meal size in participants. Phase II trials are now under way.

6.4.8 Cholecystokinin-α Agonist

Cholecystokinin (CCK) is a peptide hormone released by the small intestine in response to intraluminal digestive products. The CCK-A receptor is expressed in both the alimentary tract and the hypothalamus. CCK acts to stimulate pancreatic secretion, gallbladder contraction, and intestinal motility; inhibits gastric emptying, and contributes to feelings of post-meal satiety through the CCK-A receptors in the brain. When given to rodents and humans, an orally active CCK-A receptor agonist decreases food intake. Phase II trials with orally active CCK agonists are being conducted [95].

6.4.9 P57

P57 is a steroidal glycoside extracted from the South African cactus, *Hoodia gordonii*. This cactus has a history of anorectic properties and recently has been found to cause weight loss. In animals, P57 has been reported to cause hypophagia, decreased body weight, and resistance to a high-fat diet [96]. In phase I clinical trials, treatment with P57 was reported to lead to a 30% decrease in caloric intake by participants. P57 may lead to weight loss by increasing Adenosine triphosphate (ATP) levels in the hypothalamus [97]. P57 is now in phase II clinical trials.

6.4.10 Peptide $YY_{3\text{-}36}$

Peptide $YY_{3\text{-}36}$ (PYY) is released by endocrine cells in the distal small bowel and colon after a meal and acts to signal satiety and decrease food intake through a gut-hypothalamic pathway. PYY acts as an "ileal brake" to suppress gastric motility, signal satiety, and promote meal termination. The amount of PYY secreted postprandially is in direct response to the number of calories ingested. Compared to lean individuals, obese people exhibit a blunted postprandial PYY response. It is unclear if the blunted PYY response seen in the obese is a result or a cause of the obesity. Two hours after an infusion of PYY, lean and obese subjects reported decreased appetite and ate 30% less at a buffet meal than those subjects who had received a saline infusion [98]. Total caloric intake over the next 24 hr was also decreased in the patients who had received the PYY infusion. Clinical trials of intranasal PYY are under way. Early reports of a 1-week trial of 100 μg of intranasal PYY given three times a day indicated that PYY was well tolerated and reduced food intake, leading to a 0.6 kg weight loss over the week. Common side effects were nausea, headache, and dizziness [99].

6.4.11 Oleoyl Estrone

Like leptin, oleoyl estrone is produced by adipose tissue and its levels are related to the degree of adiposity. When administered to obese animals, oleoyl estrone results in decreased caloric intake and maintenance of energy expenditure despite the loss of fat stores [100]. Oleoyl estrone appears to reduce fat mass primarily by decreasing adipocyte size and number [101]. When oleoyl estrone was given in combination with sibutramine to rodents, the effects were synergistic, resulting in a greater weight loss than that achieved when using either drug alone [102]. Phase I clinical trials have recently been initiated with oleoyl estrone.

In summary, there are a number of drugs in clinical trials, as well as drugs approved for other uses being tested for possible effects on weight loss. The safety and efficacy, as well as the practicality of using these drugs, have yet to be determined. However, there are a number of promising possibilities, giving hope that the pharmacologic repertoire available to treat obesity will increase in the near future.

6.5 FUTURE TARGETS

The elucidation of neuroendocrine pathways regulating body weight and energy homeostasis has resulted in a large number of peptides and drugs in preclinical and clinical trials. Leptin was one of the first hormones tested in clinical trials but the results were disappointing because most obese individuals already have high leptin levels and are leptin resistant. Leptin is secreted by adipocytes and affects the synthetic pathways of both anorectic and orexigenic peptides. Manipulation of the leptin-signalling pathways may be an alternative approach to inducing weight loss. For example, central leptin resistance has been reported to involve suppression of cytokine signaling-3 (SOCS3). Therefore, SOCS3 inhibitors may be able to overcome leptin resistance [75].

The expression of orexigenic peptides produced in the hypothalamus, such as neuropeptide Y (NPY) and agouti-related protein, is downregulated by leptin. Leptin also increases the expression of anorectic peptides in the hypothalamus, including cocaine- and-amphetamine-regulated transcript (CART) and α–MSH, a peptide produced after posttranslational cleavage of the proopiomelanocortin polyprotein. In addition, a small protein called beacon was recently discovered in animals prone to obesity and insulin resistance. Infusion of beacon leads to elevations in NPY levels and an increase in food intake and body weight [103]. Manipulation of these pathways to inhibit production or activity of orexigenic peptides or to increase levels of anorectic peptides may prove to be useful in managing obesity. For example, NPY receptor antagonists are in the early stages of evaluation for obesity treatment.

Alternatively, activation of the receptors for anorectic peptides may be a future option. One possible pharmacologic target that has been identified is a receptor for α–MSH. There are five different receptors for α–MSH. Two of these, the melanocortin 3 and 4 receptors (MC3R and MC4R), are expressed in the brain. Mice without the MC4R are hyperphagic and obese. Mice without the MC3R have increased adiposity due to decreased energy expenditure without significant changes in food intake. Stimulation of MC4R leads to reduced food intake and increased energy expenditure. An intranasal MC4R agonist led to a 0.8 kg weight loss in lean humans over 6 weeks [104] but results have not yet been duplicated in obese humans. The MC4R is a particularly promising option because although human obesity is likely to have polygenic causes, mutations in the MC4R have been reported in about 4% of humans with morbid obesity. These mutations are associated with early onset of obesity, hyperinsulinemia, and tall stature.

At the intracellular level, the actions of leptin and insulin converge to decrease food intake and restrict body weight. As a negative regulator of both insulin and leptin, protein tyrosine phosphatase 1B (PTP1B) has been identified as a protein that may be inhibited for the treatment of obesity and insulin resistance. Mice without an active PTP1B gene have increased insulin sensitivity in liver and skeletal muscle, have low adiposity, and are resistant to diet-induced obesity. Genetically obese rodents treated with a PTP1B inhibitor had lower body weights and decreased adiposity over 6 weeks compared to controls. PTP1B inhibitors are under initial evaluation for use in obesity and diabetes.

Another orexigenic molecule in the hypothalamus, which influences energy homeostatis, is melanin-concentrating hormone (MCH). MCH levels are increased in states of leptin deficiency, including fasting. Mice without an MCH gene are lean due to hypophagia and increased energy expenditure. In diet-induced obese rodents, an MCH antagonist led to a reduction in body weight over a 4-week period [105]. Such MCH antagonists may prove useful in treating obese humans. There are other hypothalamic hormones, which are involved in energy homeostasis; but most of these have multiple effects throughout the body and manipulation of these molecules to produce weight loss is likely to have undesirable side effects.

Another area in which a rapid increase in knowledge has led to possible therapeutic options is the understanding of neurohormones secreted by the gastrointestinal tract. PYY and CCK have already been mentioned as molecules that may become a pharmacologic option. Ghrelin is a peptide secreted by oxyntic cells in the gastric fundus. Ghrelin concentrations increase preprandially and decrease after food intake. Ghrelin may be one of the causal factors in the sensation of hunger. Infusion of ghrelin in humans results in an increase in both appetite and food intake. When individuals have achieved a hypocaloric induced weight loss, plasma ghrelin levels are found to be higher. This may be a factor in the increased hunger seen after weight loss, which contributes to the difficulty maintaining weight loss. Because obese individuals tend to have reduced ghrelin concentrations, it is unclear if ghrelin is a cause of obesity. However, a ghrelin antagonist remains an interesting possibility, especially to assist with weight maintenance following weight loss.

The small intestine releases molecules that are involved in meal termination and the signaling of satiety. For example, oxyntomodulin and glucagon-like peptide 1 (GLP-1) are released postprandially from the same intestinal cells that secrete PYY. An infusion of oxyntomodulin in humans suppresses appetite and reduces food intake over a 12-hr period. GLP-1 is an insulin secretagogue but has also been shown to decrease gastric motility, reduce short-term food intake, and increase satiety in both lean and obese individuals. The effects of both these peptides may be through interactions with the GLP-1 receptor. GLP-1 is inactivated by the enzyme dipeptidyl peptidase IV (DPP-IV). Long-acting GLP-1 agonists and DPP-IV inhibitors have been developed for the treatment of type 2 diabetes. Pramlintide, a synthetic analog of amylin, and exenatide, a long-acting GLP-1 agonist, have both been shown to reduce body weight. The use of these GLP-1 agonists in obese rodents reduced food intake and fat deposition, in addition to improving glucose tolerance [106]. Mice without a functional DPP-IV enzyme are resistant to diet-induced obesity and development of impaired glucose tolerance [107]. The GLP-1 agonists and DPP-IV inhibitors may become therapeutic options for obesity, in addition to type 2 diabetes.

Gastric inhibitory polypeptide (GIP) is released from the duodenum in response to absorption of fat or glucose. Rodents on a high-fat diet have hypersecretion of GIP and increased fat deposition, leading to insulin resistance. Mice without a GIP receptor are protected from both diet-induced obesity and associated insulin resistance.

Adiponectin is a hormone secreted by adipocytes, which increases fatty acid oxidation in muscle, and reduces fat accumulation without altering food intake. It also leads to improved insulin sensitivity and reduced atherosclerosis and has anti-inflammatory properties. Adiponectin levels are inversely related to the degree of adiposity. Mice lacking adiponectin have early onset diet-induced insulin resistance while mice overexpressing adiponectin are resistant to diet-induced obesity and have improved insulin sensitivity [108]. Active investigation into the possible therapeutic options using adiponectin is ongoing.

Concentrations of glucocorticoids may also regulate fat metabolism, especially at the intracellular level. Although levels of glucocorticoids are not elevated in most obese individuals, the action of glucocorticoids locally on adipose tissue and skeletal muscle may be enhanced due to elevated enzyme activity of 11β-hydroxy steroid dehydrogenase type I (11βHSD1). Mice without functional 11βHSD1 are protected from accumulation of visceral fat and insulin resistance. Mice with fat-specific overexpression of 11βHSD1 develop visceral obesity with insulin and leptin resistance, dyslipidemia, and hypertension. Obese humans with the metabolic syndrome of obesity, insulin resistance, hypertension, and dyslipidemia also have increased 11βHSD1 enzyme activity at the adipocyte level. Inhibition of 11βHSD1 is a potential treatment option for the metabolic syndrome.

Other pharmacologic options include targeting the synthesis and oxidation of fatty acids. Carnitine palmitoyltransferase1 (CPT1) is the enzyme that controls the rate-limiting step for the oxidation of fatty acids. Fatty acid synthase is involved in the synthesis of fatty acids. Fatty acid synthase inhibitors have been developed, which result in anorexia and decreased body fat. One of these peptides, C75, is an inhibitor of fatty acid synthase and a stimulator of CPT1. Lean and obese mice treated with C75 have profound weight loss and decreased food intake, perhaps because of an increase in fatty acid oxidation. These mice lost body fat and demonstrated a reversal of hepatic steatosis [109].

An aminosterol that increases fatty oxidation and inhibits hepatic triglyceride synthesis has also been found. Treatment of genetically obese mice with this aminosterol leads to an increase in energy expenditure, a decrease in food intake, weight loss, and a reversal of hepatic steatosis [110]. Stearoyl-coenzyme A desaturase (SCD) is a lipogenic enzyme that synthesizes monounsaturated fatty acids. Mice without SCD1 have decreased fat mass and increased insulin sensitivity and are protected from diet-induced obesity due to increased energy expenditure. In these mice, fatty acid oxidation is increased at the same time that lipid storage is decreased [111]. Interestingly, mice without SCD1 also have low levels of PTP1B in muscle [112]. While leptin-deficient mice are markedly obese, combining leptin deficiency with an inactive SCD1 enzyme in mice leads to rodents that are less obese and have increased energy expenditure [113]. This indicates that inhibiting SCD1 may bypass leptin resistance.

In the past, thyroid hormone has been an unsuccessful treatment for obesity due to its unacceptable cardiovascular side effects. Two thyroid receptors have now been found. The alpha receptor (TRα) appears to regulate heart rate, while the beta receptor (TRβ) regulates metabolic rate. In animals, a selective TRβ agonist led to increased energy expenditure, with a minimal increase in heart rate. Over 1 week, the TRβ agonist led to weight loss up to 7% as well as a reduction in cholesterol levels [114]. Further preclinical testing is being done on these molecules.

Given that treatment with a single medication leads to a weight loss plateau after about 6 mo, it is likely that therapy with more than one medication will be necessary in order to achieve maximum weight loss goals. Synergy has already been demonstrated in rodent studies. For example, rodents receiving both a CB1 receptor antagonist and α–MSH had a greater suppression of appetite than rodents receiving only one medication [115]. In the future, targeting both appetite and energy expenditure will probably lead to the greatest effects on weight. It has been suggested that the current state of medication availability for obesity is similar to the status of hypertension treatment a few decades ago [116]. Few medications were available, limited efficacy was possible with monotherapy, and understanding of the underlying mechanisms of disease was in the early stages. As more medications become available, our ability to treat obesity will expand. At some point, the prevention and treatment of obesity will obviate the need to treat the complications of obesity.

The future of the pharmacologic treatment of obesity is promising, with many new drugs in the early stages of development. Most importantly, the rapid growth in our understanding of weight-regulating mechanisms will allow us to select more specific targets and permit us to design effective drug combinations. A summary of potential therapeutic targets is included in Table 6.2.

TABLE 6.2
Potential Targets for New Obesity Treatments

Stimulators	Inhibitors
Serotonin (5-HT_{2C} receptor)	NPY Y1 and Y5 receptors
Leptin receptor	Ghrelin
PYY_{3-36}	MCH receptor
MC3 receptor	DPP-IV
MC4 receptor	Agouti-related protein
α-MSH	11βHSD1
CART receptor	SCD1
CCK-A receptor	Fatty acid synthase
GLP-1 receptor	GIP
Adiponectin	SOCS3
CNTF	PTP1B
Cocaine- and amphetamine-regulated transcript	—
Oxyntomodulin	—
Human GH fragment	—
CPT1	—
TRβ	—

6.6 MEDICATIONS THAT MAY CAUSE WEIGHT GAIN AND POSSIBLE ALTERNATIVES

Many commonly prescribed medications cause weight gain as a side effect, including neuropsychiatric medications, steroids, and diabetes medications. Before considering the use of antiobesity medications, a patient's drug regimen should be reviewed and the possibility of switching any medications that cause weight gain should be considered. For example, sulfonylureas, thiazolidinediones, and insulin tend to cause weight gain. While good diabetic control is of importance, metformin should be considered as the first-line drug in the obese diabetic as it may induce weight loss, improve body composition, and improve the lipid profile. The alpha-glucosidase inhibitors acarbose and miglitol may also induce weight loss. In addition, as described above, orlistat and sibutramine can lead to improvements in hemoglobin A_{1C} levels in diabetics. Similarly, antihistamines can cause weight gain and alternatives such as intranasal fluticasone or decongestants should be considered whenever possible. Alpha and beta blockers used for treating hypertension may lead to increased weight. Alternative therapies for hypertension, which do not cause weight gain, include calcium channel blockers, diuretics, and angiotensin-converting enzyme inhibitors.

Steroid hormones including oral contraceptives, progestational steroids, and glucocorticoids can lead to large amounts of weight gain. Substitutions in this category are more difficult to find, but whenever possible, alternatives such as barrier contraceptives instead of oral contraceptives should be used in the morbidly obese patient. Likewise, if possible, nonsteroidal anti-inflammatory drugs or inhaled steroids should be used instead of glucocorticoids. Other common medications leading to large amounts of weight gain are psychiatric medications. For instance, most antidepressants and such antipsychotics as olanzapine and clozapine have been associated with weight gain and obesity-related comorbidities. As described earlier, bupropion may induce weight loss and should be used as initial therapy in an obese person with depression. Ziprasodone and aripiperazole are antipsychotics that can be used and are weight neutral. Many antiepileptics and mood stabilizers also cause weight gain and a change to zonisamide or topiramate can lead to normalization of body weight. When initiating any therapy in an obese patient, the weight gain side effects of medications should be considered. Further, in initiating a weight loss plan, medication changes may lead to dramatic effects.

6.7 CONCLUSIONS

As lifestyle modification has had limited success in treating the obesity epidemic, we need more effective and safe pharmacotherapy for obesity treatment. The only currently approved long-term pharmacologic treatments for obesity are sibutramine and orlistat. They provide greater weight loss than that seen with dieting alone, and a greater percentage of patients receiving medical treatment achieve weight losses of more than 5% of their initial body weight, which is the minimum amount associated with improvements in blood pressure, insulin sensitivity, and dyslipidemia. Still, the only medical intervention that achieves dramatic, sustained weight loss is gastric bypass surgery, discussed in Chapter 7. However, our knowledge about the complicated pathways regulating energy intake and energy expenditure is increasing rapidly. In the next decade, there should be exciting new advances in obesity management. Therapies specifically targeting homeostatic pathways such as the gut-hypothalamic axis, anorexic and orexigenic hormone receptors in the hypothalamus, and central and peripheral nutrient-sensing pathways are possible. Counter-regulatory mechanisms such as increased hunger and decreased energy expenditure, which occur with weight loss, as well as the downregulation of the targeted receptors will have to be overcome. However, with increased knowledge will come increased possibilities and one anticipates that with multidrug therapy targeting different regulatory elements, effective, long-term weight loss will become possible with pharmacologic treatment.

REFERENCES

1. Flegal KM, Carroll MD, Ogden CL, Johnson CL. Prevalence and trends in obesity among US adults, 1999–2000. *JAMA.* 2002;288(14):1723–1727.
2. Rosenbaum M, Leibel RL, Hirsch J. Obesity. *N Engl J Med.* 1997;337(6): 396–407.
3. Bray GA, Greenway FL. Current and potential drugs for treatment of obesity. *Endocr Rev.* 1999;20(6):805–875.
4. From the Centers for Disease Control and Prevention. Cardiac valvulopathy associated with exposure to fenfluramine or dexfenfluramine: US Department of Health and Human Services interim public health recommendations, 1997. *JAMA.* Dec 3 1997;278(21):1729–1731.
5. Wadden TA, Berkowitz RI, Sarwer DB, Prus-Wisniewski R, Steinberg C. Benefits of lifestyle modification in the pharmacologic treatment of obesity: a randomized trial. *Arch Intern Med.* 2001;161(2):218–227.
6. Haddock CK, Poston WS, Dill PL, Foreyt JP, Ericsson M. Pharmacotherapy for obesity: a quantitative analysis of four decades of published randomized clinical trials. *Int J Obes Relat Metab Disord.* 2002;26(2):262–273.
7. Goldstein DJ. Beneficial health effects of modest weight loss. *Int J Obes Relat Metab Disord.* 1992;16(6):397–415.
8. Allison DB, Fontaine KR, Manson JE, Stevens J, VanItallie TB. Annual deaths attributable to obesity in the United States. *JAMA.* 1999;282(16):1530–1538.
9. National Institutes of Health, National Heart Lung and Blood Institute, and North American Association for the Study of Obesity: The practical guide: identification, evaluation, and treatment of overweight and obesity in adults. Bethesda, MD: NIH; 2000.
10. Bakris G, Calhoun D, Egan B, Hellmann C, Dolker M, Kingma I. Orlistat improves blood pressure control in obese subjects with treated but inadequately controlled hypertension. *J Hypertens.* 2002;20(11):2257–2267.
11. Yanovski SZ, Yanovski JA. Obesity. *N Engl J Med.* Feb 21 2002;346(8):591–602.
12. Bray GA, Blackburn GL, Ferguson JM, et al. Sibutramine produces dose-related weight loss. *Obes Res.* 1999;7(2):189–198.
13. Hansen DL, Toubro S, Stock MJ, Macdonald IA, Astrup A. The effect of sibutramine on energy expenditure and appetite during chronic treatment without dietary restriction. *Int J Obes Relat Metab Disord.* 1999;23(10):1016–1024.

14. LeBlanc M, Thibault L. Effect of sibutramine on macronutrient selection in male and female rats. *Physiol Behav.* 2003;80(2–3):243–252.
15. Walsh KM, Leen E, Lean ME. The effect of sibutramine on resting energy expenditure and adrenaline-induced thermogenesis in obese females. *Int J Obes Relat Metab Disord.* 1999;23(10):1009–1015.
16. Thearle M, Aronne LJ. Obesity and pharmacologic therapy. *Endocrinol Metab Clin North Am.* 2003;32(4):1005–1024.
17. Hanotin C, Thomas F, Jones SP, Leutenegger E, Drouin P. Efficacy and tolerability of sibutramine in obese patients: a dose-ranging study. *Int J Obes Relat Metab Disord.* 1998;22(1):32–38.
18. Padwal R, Li SK, Lau DC. Long-term pharmacotherapy for overweight and obesity: a systematic review and meta-analysis of randomized controlled trials. *Int J Obes Relat Metab Disord.* 2003;27(12):1437–1446.
19. Fanghanel G, Cortinas L, Sanchez-Reyes L, Berber A. Second phase of a double-blind study clinical trial on sibutramine for the treatment of patients suffering essential obesity: 6 months after treatment cross-over. *Int J Obes Relat Metab Disord.* 2001; 25(5):741–747.
20. Wirth A, Krause J. Long-term weight loss with sibutramine: a randomized controlled trial. *JAMA.* 2001;286(11):1331–1339.
21. James WP, Astrup A, Finer N, et al. Effect of sibutramine on weight maintenance after weight loss: a randomised trial. STORM Study Group. Sibutramine Trial of Obesity Reduction and Maintenance. *Lancet.* 2000;356(9248): 2119–2125.
22. Apfelbaum M, Vague P, Ziegler O, Hanotin C, Thomas F, Leutenegger E. Long-term maintenance of weight loss after a very-low-calorie diet: a randomized blinded trial of the efficacy and tolerability of sibutramine. *Am J Med.* 1999; 106(2): 179–184.
23. Fanghanel G, Cortinas L, Sanchez-Reyes L, Berber A. A clinical trial of the use of sibutramine for the treatment of patients suffering essential obesity. *Int J Obes Relat Metab Disord.* 2000;24(2):144–150.
24. Finer N, Bloom SR, Frost GS, Banks LM, Griffiths J. Sibutramine is effective for weight loss and diabetic control in obesity with type 2 diabetes: a randomised, double-blind, placebo-controlled study. *Diabetes Obes Metab.* 2000;2(2):105–112.
25. Fujioka K, Seaton TB, Rowe E, et al. Weight loss with sibutramine improves glycaemic control and other metabolic parameters in obese patients with type 2 diabetes mellitus. *Diabetes Obes Metab.* 2000;2(3):175–187.
26. Gokcel A, Gumurdulu Y, Karakose H, et al. Evaluation of the safety and efficacy of sibutramine, orlistat and metformin in the treatment of obesity. *Diabetes Obes Metab.* 2002;4(1):49–55.
27. McNulty SJ, Ur E, Williams G. A randomized trial of sibutramine in the management of obese type 2 diabetic patients treated with metformin. *Diabetes Care.* 2003;26(1):125–131.
28. Berkowitz RI, Wadden TA, Tershakovec AM, Cronquist JL. Behavior therapy and sibutramine for the treatment of adolescent obesity: a randomized controlled trial. *JAMA.* 2003;289(14):1805–1812.
29. Godoy-Matos A, Carraro L, Vieira A, et al. Treatment of obese adolescents with sibutramine: a randomized, double-blind, controlled study. *J Clin Endocrinol Metab.* 2004.
30. Bach DS, Rissanen AM, Mendel CM, et al. Absence of cardiac valve dysfunction in obese patients treated with sibutramine. *Obes Res.* 1999;7(4):363–369.

31. McMahon FG, Weinstein SP, Rowe E, Ernst KR, Johnson F, Fujioka K. Sibutramine is safe and effective for weight loss in obese patients whose hypertension is well controlled with angiotensin-converting enzyme inhibitors. *J Hum Hypertens.* 2002;16(1):5–11.
32. Sramek JJ, Leibowitz MT, Weinstein SP, et al. Efficacy and safety of sibutramine for weight loss in obese patients with hypertension well controlled by beta-adrenergic blocking agents: a placebo-controlled, double-blind, randomised trial. *J Hum Hypertens.* 2002;16(1):13–19.
33. McMahon FG, Fujioka K, Singh BN, et al. Efficacy and safety of sibutramine in obese white and African American patients with hypertension: a 1-year, double-blind, placebo-controlled, multicenter trial. *Arch Intern Med.* 24 2000;160(14):2185–2191.
34. Ersoz HO, Ukinc K, Baykan M, et al. Effect of low-dose metoprolol in combination with sibutramine therapy in normotensive obese patients: a randomized controlled study. *Int J Obes Relat Metab Disord.* 2004; 28(3):378–383.
35. Van Gaal LF, Broom JI, Enzi G, Toplak H. Efficacy and tolerability of orlistat in the treatment of obesity: a 6-month dose-ranging study. Orlistat Dose-Ranging Study Group. *Eur J Clin Pharmacol.* 1998;54(2):125–132.
36. Karhunen L, Franssila-Kallunki A, Rissanen P, et al. Effect of orlistat treatment on body composition and resting energy expenditure during a two-year weight-reduction programme in obese Finns. *Int J Obes Relat Metab Disord.* 2000;24(12):1567–1572.
37. Kopelman P, Bryson AM, Palmer RM. Efficacy and tolerability of ATL-962, a lipase inhibitor, in obese patients. Paper presented at 13th European Congress on Obesity (ECO); May 26–29, 2004.
38. Davidson MH, Hauptman J, DiGirolamo M, et al. Weight control and risk factor reduction in obese subjects treated for 2 years with orlistat: a randomized controlled trial. *JAMA.* 1999;281(3):235–242.
39. Sjostrom L, Rissanen A, Andersen T, et al. Randomised placebo-controlled trial of orlistat for weight loss and prevention of weight regain in obese patients. European Multicentre Orlistat Study Group. *Lancet.* 1998;352(9123):167–172.
40. Rissanen A, Lean M, Rossner S, Segal KR, Sjostrom L. Predictive value of early weight loss in obesity management with orlistat: an evidence-based assessment of prescribing guidelines. *Int J Obes Relat Metab Disord.* 2003;27(1):103–109.
41. Hill JO, Hauptman J, Anderson JW, et al. Orlistat, a lipase inhibitor, for weight maintenance after conventional dieting: a 1-y study. *Am J Clin Nutr.* 1999;69(6):1108–1116.
42. Wadden TA, Berkowitz RI, Womble LG, Sarwer DB, Arnold ME, Steinberg CM. Effects of sibutramine plus orlistat in obese women following 1 year of treatment by sibutramine alone: a placebo-controlled trial. *Obes Res.* 2000;8(6):431–437.
43. Krempf M, Louvet JP, Allanic H, Miloradovich T, Joubert JM, Attali JR. Weight reduction and long-term maintenance after 18 months treatment with orlistat for obesity. *Int J Obes Relat Metab Disord.* 2003;27(5):591–597.
44. Finer N, James WP, Kopelman PG, Lean ME, Williams G. One-year treatment of obesity: a randomized, double-blind, placebo-controlled, multicentre study of orlistat, a gastrointestinal lipase inhibitor. *Int J Obes Relat Metab Disord.* 2000;24(3):306–313.
45. Heymsfield SB, Segal KR, Hauptman J, et al. Effects of weight loss with orlistat on glucose tolerance and progression to type 2 diabetes in obese adults. *Arch Intern Med.* 2000;160(9):1321–1326.
46. Muls E, Kolanowski J, Scheen A, Van Gaal L. The effects of orlistat on weight and on serum lipids in obese patients with hypercholesterolemia: a randomized, double-blind, placebo-controlled, multicentre study. *Int J Obes Relat Metab Disord.* 2001;25(11):1713–1721.

47. Guy-Grand B, Drouin P, Eschwege E, Gin H, Joubert JM, Valensi P. Effects of orlistat on obesity-related diseases – a six-month randomized trial. *Diabetes Obes Metab.* 2004;6(5):375–383.
48. Harrison SA, Ramrakhiani S, Brunt EM, Anbari MA, Cortese C, Bacon BR. Orlistat in the treatment of NASH: a case series. *Am J Gastroenterol.* 2003;98(4):926–930.
49. Tiikkainen M, Bergholm R, Rissanen A, et al. Effects of equal weight loss with orlistat and placebo on body fat and serum fatty acid composition and insulin resistance in obese women. *Am J Clin Nutr.* 2004;79(1):22–30.
50. Torgerson JS, Hauptman J, Boldrin MN, Sjostrom L. XENical in the prevention of diabetes in obese subjects (XENDOS) study: a randomized study of orlistat as an adjunct to lifestyle changes for the prevention of type 2 diabetes in obese patients. *Diabetes Care.* 2004;27(1):155–161.
51. Miles JM, Leiter L, Hollander P, et al. Effect of orlistat in overweight and obese patients with type 2 diabetes treated with metformin. *Diabetes Care.* 2002; 25(7):1123–1128.
52. Kelley DE, Bray GA, Pi-Sunyer FX, et al. Clinical efficacy of orlistat therapy in overweight and obese patients with insulin-treated type 2 diabetes: a 1-year randomized controlled trial. *Diabetes Care.* 2002;25(6):1033–1041.
53. Halpern A, Mancini MC, Suplicy H, et al. Latin-American trial of orlistat for weight loss and improvement in glycaemic profile in obese diabetic patients. *Diabetes Obes Metab.* 2003;5(3):180–188.
54. Ozkan B, Bereket A, Turan S, Keskin S. Addition of orlistat to conventional treatment in adolescents with severe obesity. *Eur J Pediatr.* 2004;163(12):738–741.
55. McDuffie JR, Calis KA, Booth SL, Uwaifo GI, Yanovski JA. Effects of orlistat on fat-soluble vitamins in obese adolescents. *Pharmacotherapy.* 2002;22(7): 814–822.
56. McDuffie JR, Calis KA, Uwaifo GI, et al. Three-month tolerability of orlistat in adolescents with obesity-related comorbid conditions. *Obes Res.* 2002;10(7):642–650.
57. Cavaliere H, Floriano I, Medeiros-Neto G. Gastrointestinal side effects of orlistat may be prevented by concomitant prescription of natural fibers (psyllium mucilloid). *Int J Obes Relat Metab Disord.* 2001;25(7):1095–1099.
58. Gotfredsen A, Westergren Hendel H, Andersen T. Influence of orlistat on bone turnover and body composition. *Int J Obes Relat Metab Disord.* 2001;25(8):1154–1160.
59. Faught E, Ayala R, Montouris GG, Leppik IE. Randomized controlled trial of zonisamide for the treatment of refractory partial-onset seizures. *Neurology.* 2001;57(10): 1774–1779.
60. Elterman RD, Glauser TA, Wyllie E, Reife R, Wu SC, Pledger G. A double-blind, randomized trial of topiramate as adjunctive therapy for partial-onset seizures in children. Topiramate YP Study Group. *Neurology.* 1999;52(7): 1338–1344.
61. Wilding J, Van Gaal L, Rissanen A, Vercruysse F, Fitchet M. A randomized double-blind placebo-controlled study of the long-term efficacy and safety of topiramate in the treatment of obese subjects. *Int J Obes Relat Metab Disord.* 2004;28(11):1399–1410.
62. McElroy SL, Arnold LM, Shapira NA, et al. Topiramate in the treatment of binge eating disorder associated with obesity: a randomized, placebo-controlled trial. *Am J Psychiatry.* 2003;160(2):255–261.
63. Bray GA, Hollander P, Klein S, et al. A 6-month randomized, placebo-controlled, dose-ranging trial of topiramate for weight loss in obesity. *Obes Res.* 2003;11(6): 722–733.
64. Gadde KM, Franciscy DM, Wagner HR, 2nd, Krishnan KR. Zonisamide for weight loss in obese adults: a randomized controlled trial. *JAMA.* 2003;289(14):1820–1825.

65. Zhou G, Myers R, Li Y, et al. Role of AMP-activated protein kinase in mechanism of metformin action. *J Clin Invest.* 2001;108(8):1167–1174.
66. Knowler WC, Barrett-Connor E, Fowler SE, et al. Reduction in the incidence of type 2 diabetes with lifestyle intervention or metformin. *N Engl J Med.* 2002; 346(6): 393–403.
67. Freemark M, Bursey D. The effects of metformin on body mass index and glucose tolerance in obese adolescents with fasting hyperinsulinemia and a family history of type 2 diabetes. *Pediatrics.* 2001;107(4):55–66.
68. Anderson JW, Greenway FL, Fujioka K, Gadde KM, McKenney J, O'Neil PM. Bupropion SR enhances weight loss: a 48-week double-blind, placebo-controlled trial. *Obes Res.* 2002;10(7):633–641.
69. Jain AK, Kaplan RA, Gadde KM, et al. Bupropion SR vs. placebo for weight loss in obese patients with depressive symptoms. *Obes Res.* 2002;10(10): 1049–1056.
70. Anonymous.A double-blind placebo-controlled clinical trial of subcutaneous recombinant human ciliary neurotrophic factor (rHCNTF) in amyotrophic lateral sclerosis. ALS CNTF Treatment Study Group. *Neurology.* 1996;46(5):1244–1249.
71. Halaas JL, Gajiwala KS, Maffei M, et al. Weight-reducing effects of the plasma protein encoded by the obese gene. *Science.* 1995;269(5223):543–546.
72. Muraoka O, Xu B, Tsurumaki T, Akira S, Yamaguchi T, Higuchi H. Leptin-induced transactivation of NPY gene promoter mediated by JAK1, JAK2 and STAT3 in the neural cell lines. *Neurochem Int.* 2003;42(7):591–601.
73. Lambert PD, Anderson KD, Sleeman MW, et al. Ciliary neurotrophic factor activates leptin-like pathways and reduces body fat, without cachexia or rebound weight gain, even in leptin-resistant obesity. *Proc Natl Acad Sci U.S.A.* 2001;98(8):4652–4657.
74. Sleeman MW, Garcia K, Liu R, et al. Ciliary neurotrophic factor improves diabetic parameters and hepatic steatosis and increases basal metabolic rate in db/db mice. *Proc Natl Acad Sci U.S.A.* 2003;100(24):14297–14302.
75. Korner J, Aronne LJ. Pharmacological approaches to weight reduction: therapeutic targets. *J Clin Endocrinol Metab.* 2004;89(6):2616–2621.
76. Ettinger MP, Littlejohn TW, Schwartz SL, et al. Recombinant variant of ciliary neurotrophic factor for weight loss in obese adults: a randomized, dose-ranging study. *JAMA.* 2003;289(14):1826–1832.
77. Weinstein S, Tardiff B, Bays H, Guler H, Aronne L. Weight loss with recombinant human variant ciliary neurotrophic factor (rhvCNTF [AXOKINE®]) improves glycemic control in overweight/obese subjects, especially in those with abnormal glycemic parameters at baseline. Paper presented at American Diabetes Association: 64th Scientific Sessions (ADA); June 4–8, 2004.
78. Williams CM, Kirkham TC. Observational analysis of feeding induced by Delta9-THC and anandamide. *Physiol Behav.* 2002;76(2):241–250.
79. Di Marzo V, Goparaju SK, Wang L, et al. Leptin-regulated endocannabinoids are involved in maintaining food intake. *Nature.* 2001;410(6830):822–825.
80. Ravinet Trillou C, Delgorge C, Menet C, Arnone M, Soubrie P. CB1 cannabinoid receptor knockout in mice leads to leanness, resistance to diet-induced obesity and enhanced leptin sensitivity. *Int J Obes Relat Metab Disord.* 2004;28(4): 640–648.
81. Huestis MA, Gorelick DA, Heishman SJ, et al. Blockade of effects of smoked marijuana by the CB1-selective cannabinoid receptor antagonist SR141716. *Arch Gen Psychiatry.* 2001;58(4):322–328.
82. Kirkham TC. Endogenous cannabinoids: a new target in the treatment of obesity. *Am J Physiol Regul Integr Comp Physiol.* 2003;284(2):R343–344.

83. Colombo G, Agabio R, Diaz G, Lobina C, Reali R, Gessa GL. Appetite suppression and weight loss after the cannabinoid antagonist SR 141716. *Life Sci.* 1998;63(8):PL113–117.
84. Ravinet Trillou C, Arnone M, Delgorge C, et al. Anti-obesity effect of SR141716, a CB1 receptor antagonist, in diet-induced obese mice. *Am J Physiol Regul Integr Comp Physiol.* 2003;284(2):R345–353.
85. Jensen M, Abu-Lebdeh H, Geohas J, et al. The selective CB1-receptor antagonist rimonabant reduces body weight and waist circumference in obese subjects. Paper presented at 13th European Congress on Obesity (ECO); May 26–9, 2004.
86. Pi-Sunyer X. Clinical design of the studies of weight reduction and metabolic effects with rimonabant: the RIO (rimonabant in obesity) program. Paper presented at North American Association for the Study of Obesity (NAASO) Annual Meeting; November 14–18, 2004.
87. van Oosten BW, Killestein J, Mathus-Vliegen EM, Polman CH. Multiple sclerosis following treatment with a cannabinoid receptor-1 antagonist. *Mult Scler.* 2004;10(3): 330–331.
88. Shadid S, Jensen MD. Effects of growth hormone administration in human obesity. *Obes Res.* 2003;11(2):170–175.
89. Heffernan M, Summers RJ, Thorburn A, et al. The effects of human GH and its lipolytic fragment (AOD9604) on lipid metabolism following chronic treatment in obese mice and beta(3)-AR knock-out mice. *Endocrinology.* 2001;142(12):5182–5189.
90. Herd C. Safety and tolerability of anti-obesity compound AOD9604 in obese men — Results from a phase IIa, double-blind placebo controlled study. Paper presented at North American Association for the Study of Obesity; October 11–15, 2003.
91. Tecott LH, Sun LM, Akana SF, et al. Eating disorder and epilepsy in mice lacking 5-HT2c serotonin receptors. *Nature.* 1995;374(6522):542–546.
92. Hayashi A, Sonoda R, Kimura Y, et al. Antiobesity effect of YM348, a novel 5-HT2C receptor agonist, in Zucker rats. *Brain Res.* 2004;1011(2):221–227.
93. Dunlop J, Sabb AL, Mazandarani H, et al. WAY-163909 ((7bR,10aR)-1,2,3,4,8,9,10,10a-octahydro-7bH-cyclopenta-[b][1,4]diazepino[6,7,1hi]indole); a novel 5-HT2C receptor selective agonist with anorectic activity. *J Pharmacol Exp Ther.* 2005.
94. Bjenning C. Increased sensitivity in female obesity-prone rats to the weight loss effect of APD356, a selective 5-HT2C agonist. Paper presented at North American Association for the Study of Obesity (NAASO); 14–18, 2004.
95. Szewczyk JR, Laudeman C. CCK1R agonists: a promising target for the pharmacological treatment of obesity. *Curr Top Med Chem.* 2003;3(8):837–854.
96. Halford J. The plant extract P57, reduces food intake and body weight gain in rats offered normal or highly palatable diets. Paper presented at North American Association for the Study of Obesity (NAASO); 14–18, 2004.
97. MacLean DB. Studies on the anorectant mechanism of a plant steroidal glycoside: increased ATP production or content in the hypothalamus may be a signal for the energy sensing of satiety. Paper presented at Endocrine Society Annual Meeting (ENDO); June 19–22, 2003.
98. Batterham RL, Cohen MA, Ellis SM, et al. Inhibition of food intake in obese subjects by peptide YY3-36. *N Engl J Med.* 2003;349(10):941–948.
99. Brandt G. Intranasal peptide YY 3-36: phase I dose ranging and dose sequencing studies. Paper presented at North American Association for the Study of Obesity (NAASO); November 14–18, 2004.
100. Lopez-Marti J, Diaz-Silva M, Salas A, et al. Oleoyl-estrone induces the massive loss of body weight in Zucker fa/fa rats fed a high-energy hyperlipidic diet. *J Nutr Biochem.* 2000;11(11–12):530–535.

101. Remesar X, Fernandez-Lopez JA, Blay MT, et al. Effect of oral oleoyl-estrone on adipose tissue composition in male rats. *Int J Obes Relat Metab Disord.* 2002;26(8): 1092–1102.
102. Firestone L. Additive effects of combined treatment of overweight rats with oleoyl-estrone, and dexfenfluramine, sibutramine or phentermine. Paper presented at North American Association for the Study of Obesity (NAASO); November 14–18, 2004.
103. Collier GR, McMillan JS, Windmill K, et al. Beacon: a novel gene involved in the regulation of energy balance. *Diabetes.* 2000;49(11):1766–1771.
104. Fehm HL, Smolnik R, Kern W, McGregor GP, Bickel U, Born J. The melanocortin melanocyte-stimulating hormone/adrenocorticotropin(4-10) decreases body fat in humans. *J Clin Endocrinol Metab.* 2001;86(3):1144–1148.
105. Borowsky B, Durkin MM, Ogozalek K, et al. Antidepressant, anxiolytic and anorectic effects of a melanin-concentrating hormone-1 receptor antagonist. *Nat Med.* 2002; 8(8):825–830.
106. Szayna M, Doyle ME, Betkey JA, et al. Exendin-4 decelerates food intake, weight gain, and fat deposition in Zucker rats. *Endocrinology.* 2000;141(6):1936–1941.
107. Conarello SL, Li Z, Ronan J, et al. Mice lacking dipeptidyl peptidase IV are protected against obesity and insulin resistance. *Proc Natl Acad Sci U.S.A.* 2003; 100(11): 6825–6830.
108. Shklyaev S, Aslanidi G, Tennant M, et al. Sustained peripheral expression of transgene adiponectin offsets the development of diet-induced obesity in rats. *Proc Natl Acad Sci U.S.A.* 2003;100(24):14217–14222.
109. Thupari JN, Kim EK, Moran TH, Ronnett GV, Kuhajda FP. Chronic C75 treatment of diet-induced obese mice increases fat oxidation and reduces food intake to reduce adipose mass. *Am J Physiol Endocrinol Metab.* 2004;287(1):E97–E104.
110. Takahashi N, Qi Y, Patel HR, Ahima RS. A novel aminosterol reverses diabetes and fatty liver disease in obese mice. *J Hepatol.* 2004;41(3):391–398.
111. Ntambi JM, Miyazaki M, Stoehr JP, et al. Loss of stearoyl-CoA desaturase-1 function protects mice against adiposity. *Proc Natl Acad Sci U.S.A.* 2002;99(17): 11482–11486.
112. Rahman SM, Dobrzyn A, Dobrzyn P, Lee SH, Miyazaki M, Ntambi JM. Stearoyl-CoA desaturase 1 deficiency elevates insulin-signaling components and down-regulates protein-tyrosine phosphatase 1B in muscle. *Proc Natl Acad Sci U.S.A.* 2003; 100(19):11110–11115.
113. Cohen P, Miyazaki M, Socci ND, et al. Role for stearoyl-CoA desaturase-1 in leptin-mediated weight loss. *Science.* 2002;297(5579):240–243.
114. Grover GJ, Mellstrom K, Ye L, et al. Selective thyroid hormone receptor-beta activation: a strategy for reduction of weight, cholesterol, and lipoprotein (a) with reduced cardiovascular liability. *Proc Natl Acad Sci U.S.A.* 2003;100(17): 10067–10072.
115. Verty AN, McFarlane JR, McGregor IS, Mallet PE. Evidence for an interaction between CB1 cannabinoid and melanocortin MCR-4 receptors in regulating food intake. *Endocrinology.* 2004;145(7):3224–3231.
116. Bray GA, Tartaglia LA. Medicinal strategies in the treatment of obesity. *Nature.* 2000;404(6778):672–677.

7 Surgical Treatment of Obesity

Alene J. Wright, Ranjan Sudan, and R. Armour Forse

CONTENTS

7.1 INTRODUCTION

Obesity has become a national epidemic in the U.S. The age-adjusted prevalence of overweight adults has increased from 55.9%, according to reports in 1988 to 1994, to 64.5%, according to reports from 1999 to 2000. More strikingly, the prevalence of extreme obesity has increased from 2.9 to 4.7% in the same period [1]. The health consequences of obesity are staggering. Not only is the risk of premature death increased twofold in the morbidly obese, but obesity is associated with an increased rate of multiple serious medical conditions, including hypertension, type 2 diabetes mellitus, cholelithiasis, cancers of the breast, colon, and uterus, infertility, wound infections, arthritis, and pulmonary disease [2].

Surgical treatment of morbid obesity is not a new concept; however, a recent increase in the number of individuals pursuing this treatment can be attributed to a combination of media attention, development of laparoscopic procedures, extreme obesity, and failure of nonoperative traditional treatments in the superobese, among other factors. The number of bariatric surgical procedures performed annually has increased from 16,000 in the early 1990s to approximately 103,000 in 2003 [3].

Current indications for surgery were established in 1991 by a National Institutes of Health (NIH) consensus panel. For adults, a body mass index (BMI) (a measurement of a patient's weight in relation to his or her height) that is ≥ 40 kg/m^2 — or ≥ 35 kg/m^2 with serious, coexisting conditions such as coronary heart disease or other atherosclerotic diseases, type 2 diabetes, sleep apnea, and other associated obesity-related diseases including gynecological abnormalities, osteoarthritis, gallstones, and stress incontinence — is an indication for bariatric surgery. In addition, most bariatric centers agree that a patient must also have previously attempted weight loss through nonsurgical means and failed before pursuing weight loss surgery [4].

7.2 EVALUATING THE POTENTIAL BARIATRIC PATIENT

The evaluation of a patient who is interested in bariatric surgery is complex and exhaustive. A multidisciplinary approach, including evaluations by the surgeon as well as a nutrition specialist and a psychologist, is quickly becoming the standard for the recommendation of the potential bariatric patient. In addition to meeting the above-mentioned NIH guidelines for surgery for morbid obesity, the patient must be an acceptable operative risk, as these are elective operative procedures. Contraindications to bariatric surgical procedures have traditionally excluded patients with psychosis, substance abuse, and major organ failure.

Preoperative evaluation usually includes the patient's complete medical history and a full physical examination to identify other potential risk factors including, but not limited to, hypertension, type 2 diabetes, and hypoventilation syndrome. Many programs utilize psychological and nutritional evaluations as well. A dietitian conducts a thorough evaluation of the patient's relationship with food and eating behaviors. Basic laboratory data and specialized laboratory tests are individualized.

The bariatric team must obtain a thorough informed consent from the patient. A social support network for the patient is also encouraged, as the process of surgery and weight loss can be emotionally challenging. Many centers, therefore, offer support groups and informational sessions for current or prospective patients. Often, potential patients are also required to attend preoperative informational sessions that detail surgical options, risks, benefits, side effects, and expected weight loss. Preoperative education should emphasize permanent dietary and lifestyle modifications that are essential to successful long-term weight loss.

7.3 PROCEDURES FOR WEIGHT LOSS

Bariatric procedures can be classified into restrictive, malabsorptive, or combination procedures. Purely malabsorptive procedures induce weight loss by decreasing the length of the small intestine that is exposed to the nutrient stream. The purely restrictive procedures limit the volume of food that an individual can eat and induce satiety earlier. Combined malabsorptive and restrictive procedures currently seem to be the ideal formula for maximizing weight loss; these procedures have been extensively developed during the last decade, especially as minimally invasive procedures. Lastly, some novel weight loss procedures are in the experimental stage.

7.3.1 Malabsorptive Procedures

In 1953, Kremen and colleagues (from the University of Minnesota) performed the first reported surgical bypass procedure to induce weight loss — the jejunoileal bypass (JIB). They reported the procedure in 1954 [5]. As summarized elsewhere [6,7], prior to this, Varco of the University of Minnesota had performed a similar procedure, and Dr. Vicktor Henrikkson in Sweden had completely resected a portion of small intestine to achieve a similar result.

The JIB (Figure 7.1) originally involved an end-to-end jejunoileostomy, with a separate ileocecostomy for drainage of the bypassed segment. Further evolution of

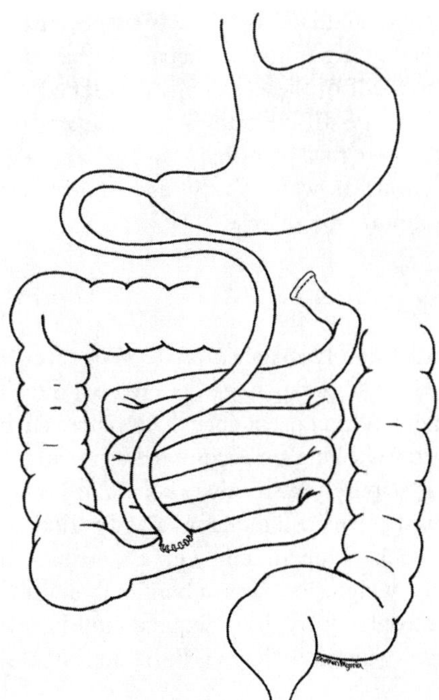

FIGURE 7.1 Jejunoileal bypass. (Sherman Bigovnia, Boston University School of Medicine.)

the JIB in the 1960s included an anastomosis near the ileocecal valve in the terminal ileum, instead of the colon, in the form of an end-to-side jejunoileostomy by Sherman et al. as well as Payne and DeWind as reviewed elsewhere [6].

Weight loss was dramatic with the original JIB; however, reversal was all but assured secondary to the electrolyte imbalance, uncontrolled diarrhea, and liver failure seen in most patients. Reversal almost universally resulted in weight regain. A one-stage procedure, as refined by Payne and DeWind, consisting of an anastomosis of the proximal 35 cm of the jejunum to the terminal ileum, 10 cm from the ileocecal valve, was developed in the hope of ameliorating some of the most severe side effects. Surprisingly, almost 10% of the revised procedures failed to achieve significant weight loss, probably because of the reflux of nutrients into the patient's bypassed ileum [6].

Further modification by Arch and Buchwald, in which 40 cm of the jejunum was anastomosed to 4 cm of the ileum, proved of particular benefit to hyperlipidemic patients. On average, 3 mo postoperatively, cholesterol levels were reduced by 90%, and triglycerides by 96% [6]. In a larger trial called the Program on the Surgical Control of the Hyperlipidemias (POSCH), reductions were more modest but cholesterol levels were, on average, 23% lower at 5 yr post-JIB [8]. (Secondary subgroup analysis of the major clinical end points in the POSCH included overall mortality, atherosclerotic coronary heart disease (ACHD) mortality, and ACHD mortality or myocardial infarction were encouraging [8].) Even with newer modifications of this procedure, diarrhea was still very problematic and common within 30 min of ingestion of a meal.

The JIB was largely abandoned by the 1980s because of concerns regarding hepatic consequences, including fulminant hepatic failure and death in up to 5% of patients. As many as one half of these patients developed cirrhosis within 25 yr of undergoing a variation of the JIB. Findings from several retrospective long-term studies include an increased risk of urinary calculi and electrolyte abnormalities [9,10]. These complications as well as arthralgia, fever, and cutaneous eruptions may be the result of autoimmune disease [11].

7.3.2 Restrictive Procedures

With the complications of purely malabsorptive procedures, a new type of surgery for weight loss emerged, as surgeons hoped to create a more physiologic operation to reduce long-term metabolic consequences. As reviewed elsewhere, Mason and Ito (1971), who had been working on a combined gastric-bypass procedure in the 1960s, performed the first purely restrictive procedure for weight loss in the form of a horizontal gastroplasty. This technique involved partial stapling of the stomach, creating a smaller stomach compartment with a narrow outlet along the greater curvature. Unfortunately, weight loss was suboptimal and difficult to maintain with either the horizontal gastroplasty or the subsequent modifications by others — which included the divided gastroplasty, vertical vs. horizontal staple lines, and partitioning [6].

Surgeons further developed the restrictive procedure to improve weight loss and the maintenance of the loss. In the early 1980s, Fabito and Laws independently used reinforcement of the gastric outlet as a means of maintaining a small aperture into the remaining stomach to maintain restriction. Although it has been reported that patients who were able to maintain small aperture sizes and intact staple lines experience good long-term weight loss; MacLean et al [12,13] reported that almost 50% had disrupted staple lines, stenosis, or aperature enlargement.

Whether it was seromuscular reinforcement, a silastic ring, or even mesh, multiple variations that combined some form of gastroplasty with a reinforced outlet emerged. The most well known of these procedures, the vertical banded gastroplasty (VBG) — originally developed by Mason and modified by Eckhout, Willbanks, and Moore — is still performed in select situations today. The basic premise involved making a through-and-through hole in both layers of the stomach to create a window through which a stapler could be passed to make a small, usually vertical, gastric pouch. The outlet was then reinforced with either a silastic ring or even mesh [6].

The laparoscopic era in the early 1990s also heralded in the ability to perform this procedure minimally invasively. However, it was found that the polypropylene mesh tended to cause excessive granulation tissue and, even, obstruction [11]. Erosion of the band into the stomach also occurred [14].

The concept of adding a band to the distal part of the gastroplasty led other surgeons to develop pure "band" procedures for restriction, which, theoretically, would restrict the stomach but would not have the additional risk associated with cutting or stapling the stomach. In the early 1980s, Molina employed the use of a nonadjustable mesh band; however, that procedure was abandoned for lack of long-term data showing substantial weight loss. Kuzmak and Hellers conceptualized an adjustable band that could be insufflated with saline or desufflated to add or subtract restriction with a subcutaneous port system (Figure 7.2) [11]. This procedure is now

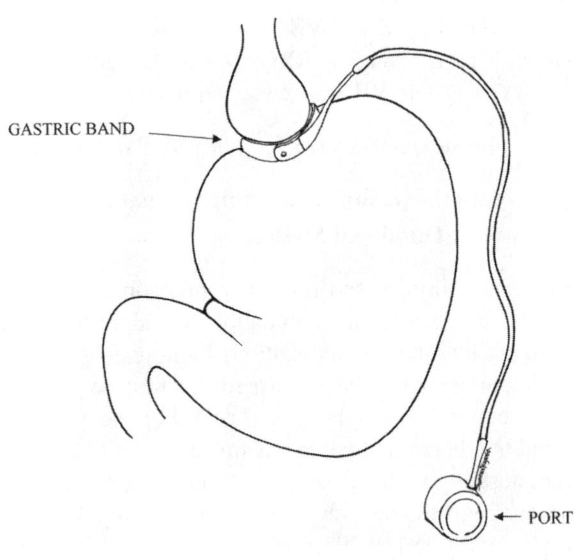

FIGURE 7.2 Adjustable gastric band. (Sherman Bigornia, Boston University School of Medicine.)

done almost exclusively laparoscopically (laparoscopic adjustable gastric banding [LAGB]) and has the previously mentioned advantage of no staple- and incision-related risks but can be fraught with device-related problems [11]. The evolution of the band technique, commonly called the pars flaccida approach, seems to have reduced the frequency of gastric herniation and prolapse [15].

Weight loss with a laparoscopically placed band tends to take more time than does weight loss resulting from procedures with a malabsorptive component. Some surgeons have reported excellent success, with an average of 44.3% of their patients' excess body weight (EBW) lost at 1 yr; however, less than 25% of patients who had undergone this procedure were seen at the 1-yr follow-up visit [16]. A recent literature review presented by Australian bariatric surgeons reported follow-up of up to 4 yr for patients who had undergone weight loss surgery with laparoscopic banding. In the first year of follow-up, a wide range of weight loss was reported — from 20% EBW loss to as high as 71% EBW loss, with an average loss of 40 to 50%. The few studies with 4-yr follow-up showed a loss of 44 to 68% EBW [17]. Typically, most patients were able to maintain 5 to 15% body weight loss in the long term [18].

Nutritional complications following purely restrictive procedures are rare. However, there have been case reports of patients with inadequate intake of phosphorus; iron; zinc; copper; iodine; and vitamins A, C, D, E, K, B1, and B6, despite the patients receiving postoperative vitamin supplementation. During rapid weight loss, protein-calorie malnutrition has also been reported. This usually responds to supplemental enteral nutrition or stoma enlargement. Two main reasons are believed to cause these deficiencies: (1) excessive prolonged vomiting and (2) the "soft calorie" syndrome, in which the patient favors high-calorie and high-carbohydrate foods over more nutritional choices [11]. In one systematic review, which compared restrictive procedures (i.e., LAGB and VBG) with combined malabsorptive/restrictive procedures (Roux-en-Y gastric banding [RYGB]), nutrient deficiency was not observed in LAGB patients, vs. 0.34% in VBG patients, and 6.01% in RYGB patients [17].

7.3.3 Combined Malabsorptive and Restrictive Procedures

7.3.3.1 Biliopancreatic Diversion and Biliopancreatic Diversion with Duodenal Switch

Although separate malabsorptive and restrictive procedures were being developed independently, many surgeons felt a combination procedure would optimize weight loss while minimizing long-term complications by adjusting the length of bypass. In 1979, Nicola Scopinaro of Italy performed the first combined malabsorptive and restrictive procedure for weight loss. The biliopancreatic diversion (BPD) originally consisted of a horizontal partial gastrectomy with closure of the duodenal stump, a gastrojejunostomy with a 250 cm alimentary limb, and anastomosis of the long biliopancreatic limb to the ileum at a distance of 50 cm proximal to the ileocecal valve (Figure 7.3) [19,20]. This was modified almost 15 yr later by Marcia et al. who used a greater curvature gastric tube ("sleeve gastrectomy"), thus preserving the pylorus, anastomosing the enteric limb to the proximal duodenum, and cross-stapling (but not dividing) the distal duodenum [11]. In 1998,

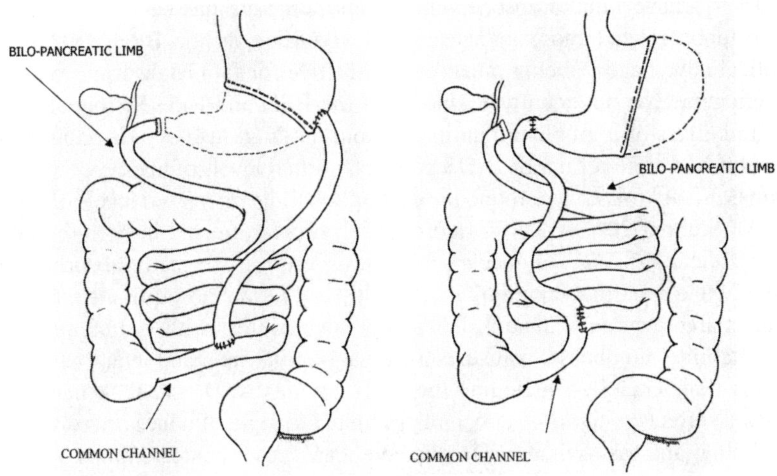

FIGURE 7.3 BPD (distal gastrectomy; sleeve gastrectomy, and duodenal switch). (Sherman Bigornia, Boston University School of Medicine.)

Hess and Hess further modified the BPD by completely dividing the duodenum, as many staple-line disruptions were noted in previous procedures (Figure 7.4) [21]. This procedure — the BPD with duodenal switch (BPD-DS) — is currently performed both laparoscopically and robotically [22].

Weight loss after a BPD-DS is substantial. Some report an initial weight loss of up to 73% of EBW. It should be noted that a typical weight regain in the long term in the patient population who reported this was approximately 7 kg per patient [19].

Nutritional deficiencies are more severe after any bypass procedure compared to a purely restrictive procedure, and the pattern of deficiencies varies depending on how distal the bypass is. These deficiencies include those of protein, calcium, vitamins A, B12, D, and E, and iron, and anemia. In the bypass procedures that cause steatorrea, namely BPD and BPD-DS, all of the fat-soluble vitamins — K, A,

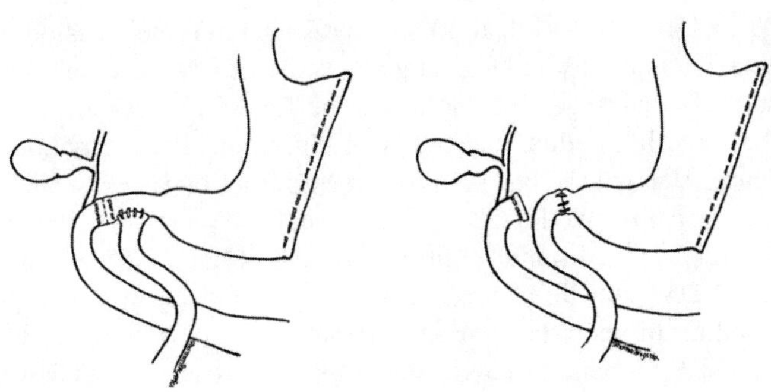

FIGURE 7.4 BPD/DS — two surgical techniques. (Sherman Bigornia, Boston University School of Medicine.)

D, and E — have limited absorption. Hypoproteinemia has been reported, but it appears to be related more to nausea and vomiting, as the BPD-DS offers the theoretical advantage of being much more selective for fat malabsorption. Vitamin-B12 deficiency has not been well studied in the BPD and BPD-DS population but seems to be less of a problem than in the Roux-en-Y gastric bypass population. In an unpublished series of lap BPD-DS patients, normal levels of hemoglobin, ferritin, vitamin B12, and folate were found in addition to mildly decreased levels of vitamins A and D in about 20% at 1 yr. Calcium absorption is affected in both the original BPD and the BPD-DS. This occurs because calcium is normally absorbed in the duodenum and proximal jejunum, and, in addition, fat malabsorption contributes to calcium malabsorption. Calcium deficiency can manifest with symptoms of bone pain, irritability, numbness, parasthesias, myalgia, diarrhea, and tetany [11].

Other deficiencies — including those of vitamins A, D, and E — can produce typical side effects; vitamin-A deficiency is linked to night blindness, xerophthalmia, photophobia, and rash; vitamin-D deficiency can cause muscle cramps and rarely, tetany; and vitamin-E deficiency sometimes manifests as weakness, phlebitis, and hypercoagulability. It is, therefore, essential for routine (at least annual) monitoring of vitamin as well as protein levels in patients post weight loss surgery. Routine postoperative follow-up is also imperative, so that the health care provider can monitor potential signs and symptoms of early deficiencies. There have been case reports of night blindness from vitamin-A deficiency in patients who were noncompliant with follow-up and with vitamin/mineral supplementation [23]. It has recently been shown that as many as 69% of patients 4 yr out from a BPD-DS can be vitamin-A deficient. In this same study, 68% of post-BPD-DS patients were vitamin-K deficient and 63% were vitamin-D deficient. Calcium homeostasis was also severely affected in 3% of patients who had evidence of bone resorption [24].

7.3.3.2 Roux-en-Y Gastric Bypass

The gastric bypass in the traditional sense was first developed by Mason and Ito in 1969. This was not the standard procedure performed today, but consisted of a horizontally divided stomach and a loop gastrojejunostomy between the proximal gastric pouch and proximal jejunum. Early modifications of the procedure decreased the pouch size from 100 to 150 cc to less than 50 cc. The Roux-en-Y modification, not a new procedure in the realm of gastric-ulcer surgery, was used first for weight loss in 1977 by Griffen et al. The advantage of this procedure for weight loss includes reducing tension on the loop, bile reflux, and marginal ulceration. Later variations included vertically oriented staple lines, band reinforcement, distal bypasses, smaller pouches, and, in 1994, the laparoscopic RYGB by Wittgrove, Clark, and Tremblay [11,25].

Resulting weight loss from a traditional RYGB (Figure 7.5) is comparable to that of the BPD-DS, and differences between open and laparoscopic procedures seem unsubstantial. In one report, at approximately 12 mo follow-up, weight loss averaged 68% EBW for patients having undergone laparoscopic RYGB versus 62% loss by patients with an open procedure. The difference in percent of EBW loss between these groups was not statistically significant [26].

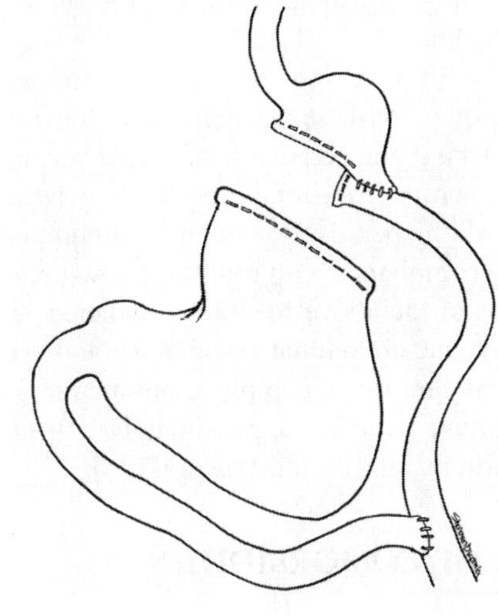

FIGURE 7.5 Long-limb gastric procedure. (Sherman Bigornia, Boston University School of Medicine.)

Late outcomes of RYGB were examined by MacLean et al [27] with a more than 90% follow-up rate and an average of 5.5 yr follow up, 60% of the obese and superobese subgroups had excellent results (BMI < 30), 33% results were considered good (BMI 30–35), and 7% experienced failure (BMI > 35). When compared to the BPD-DS, it would seem that RYGB has a similar maximum average BMI loss (BMI < 35), with some centers reporting a high of 81% EBW for the BPD-DS group and 79% EBW for the RYGB group [19,27].

Nutritional deficiencies are a normal consequence of bypassing the duodenum, as well as excluding part or all of the stomach. Primary potential deficiencies of an RYGB include those of iron, vitamin B12, and folate [27]. In some series, up to 82% of patients had some deficiency: 47% iron deficiency, 37% vitamin-B12 deficiency, 35% folate deficiency, and 54% iron deficiency anemia. Dietary B12 is protein bound and must be enzymatically cleaved before absorption can occur. The absence of gastric acid (hydrochloride [HCl]) and pepsin in a small stomach pouch, as well as the exclusion of the duodenum, where other pancreatic enzymes are released, are most likely responsible for B12 deficiency in weight loss surgery patients. Normally, oral supplementation of B12 and folate are sufficient; however, some patients need additional supplementation because of their noncompliance and dietary habits. Iron deficiency is also common after an RYGB. Not only is red meat — a primary source of iron — difficult to consume after RYGB but its primary site of absorption is the duodenum and proximal jejunum. Also, absorption is aided by gastric acid, which is minimized after bypass. In addition, up to 20% of menstruating women have low or no iron reserves, which adds to their risk for iron deficiency. Folate deficiency can be caused by both decreased intake and lack of gastric acid. Some investigators suggest that folate levels increase further out from bypass as bacteria in the proximal small bowel begin to synthesize the nutrient as a response to achlorhydria [11].

Not surprisingly, patient noncompliance with vitamin and mineral supplementation is primarily responsible for these deficiencies. In some reports, only one third of patients were routinely taking preoperatively mandated supplementation. Routinely, a complete blood count, serum iron, total iron-binding capacity, and vitamin-B12 levels should be checked preoperatively and, at minimum, on an annual basis. This also depends on patient compliance with routine follow-up. As in BPD-DS patients, long-term consequences of the above-mentioned deficiencies may include anemia, neurological sequelae, vague abdominal complaints, and even glossitis [11]. It has been observed that overall nutritional complications are rare in the compliant patient. In one study of compliant patients, approximately 1% of patients after RYGB developed protein-calorie malnutrition or anemia [26].

7.4 RESOLUTION OF COMORBIDITIES

Weight loss after successful bariatric surgery has contributed greatly to the reduction of preoperative comorbidities. Several studies with BPD-DS patients have shown moderate reduction in lipid concentrations [19,21], which is apparent as early as 3 mo postoperatively [21], and resolution of diabetes in nearly all patients [19]. Some studies even report patients with type 2 diabetes leaving the hospital postoperatively without requiring any oral hypoglycemic agents [21].

RYGB patients have shown similar results. Substantial sustained improvement or resolution of diabetes, hypertension, degenerative joint disease, reflux, sleep apnea, and venous stasis disease are consistently reported [11,26,28]. A 5-yr follow-up study of open VBG or open gastric bypass was associated with a significant reduction in the risk of developing cancer, cardiovascular disease, endocrine disorders, infectious diseases, musculoskeletal problems, and respiratory disorders [29]. Findings from a 10-yr follow-up study include a reduction of significance in hypertryglyceridemia, diabetes, hyperuricemia, and hypertension in surgical patients undergoing fixed banding, VBG, or gastric bypass [30].

The overall mortality at 15 yr in obese subjects treated with surgery compared to without surgery was lower. Flum et al. reported a 16.3% mortality rate in non-operated patients compared to 11.8% in the surgical arm. However, that study did show a 2% risk of death in the first 30 postoperative days, which may be correlated with surgeon experience [31].

On comparing laparoscopic gastric bypass and LAGB, Biertho et al. also showed sustained weight loss, in the LAGB patients, of 58% estimated weight loss (EWL) at 4 yr [29,32]. At 18-month follow-up, the results from laparoscopic gastric bypass were superior, with 74.6% EWL, compared to 40.4% EWL with the LAGB.

7.5 SURGICAL COMPLICATIONS

Surgical complications are classified as early and late complications. Early complications occur less than 30 d after surgery, and late complications occur 30 d or more after surgery.

7.5.1 Early Complications

Although risk may be minimized by optimal preoperative, intraoperative, and postoperative preparation and attention, complications are not always avoidable. Older patients tend to have more pre- and postoperative comorbidities as a result of atherosclerotic heart disease [28] and less physiologic reserve to tolerate complications. The complication rate is higher in the morbidly obese. Complications may include renal derangements from fluid and electrolyte imbalance; pulmonary problems including atelectasis, pneumonia, or those resulting from sleep apnea; deep vein thrombosis and pulmonary embolism; leaks; obstructions; and wound infections that are potentially reduced through laparoscopic procedures [26]. Early mobilization and pulmonary toilet are essential. It is recommended that activity be resumed the evening of surgery.

Early anastomotic leaks are possible whenever a hollow viscus is stapled or sutured. Several steps can reduce but not eliminate the chance of leaks from these surgically created weaknesses and anastomoses. Treatment depends on the severity and location of the leak, timing in reference to surgery, and the patient's condition. Intraoperatively, the surgeon may test for leaks in several ways. The first method is intraoperative endoscopy, which can be used to examine the patency of the gastrojejunal anastomosis, as well as to gently test the suture or staple line by insufflating air past the anastomosis. At the same time, the anastomosis is submerged in the operative field, so the surgeon can look for air bubbles. The physician can also evaluate an anastomosis by instilling diluted methylene blue through an orogastric tube to observe staple and suture lines for blue discoloration as the contrast passes the anastomosis or surgically altered viscus. These techniques allow the surgeon to address any potential weak areas immediately — during the original operation. A second method is a limited upper gastrointestinal series with gastrograffin, possibly followed by barium in the absence of leaks, on postoperative days 1 or 2, prior to the patient's initiating oral intake. A leak may manifest as extraluminal extravisation of contrast.

Treatment of leaks depends on timing postsurgery, patient condition, and extent of the leak. Controlled leaks (in which a drain is present at the anastomosis or minimal extravasation) may be treated with bowel rest, parenteral nutrition, and intravenous antibiotics. Inpatients with clinical signs of sepsis, reoperation is often necessary. The frequency of leaks is approximately 1 to 2% of patients undergoing bypass surgery. Marceau's series of BPD-DS had a leak rate of approximately 1% [19]. A similar population of RYGB patients had similar leak rates [26].

Bowel obstruction can also occur in the early postoperative period following bariatric surgery. This is often caused by edema at the proximal anastomosis, which is common in this location, second to the narrow stoma formed purposely to curb intake of nutrients. However, this bowel obstruction is rare and is found in less than 1% of patients [26]. Bowel obstructions are self-limiting but, in more persistent cases, may require reoperation.

Thromboembolic complications are more common in obese patients. As a prophylactic measure, early ambulation should be encouraged. Many also use sequential compression devices routinely, as well as low-dose heparin injections from the time of surgery through discharge. Some high-risk patients even require preoperative vena cava filter placement. The incidence of pulmonary complications, including pulmonary embolism, has been reported in as many as 9% of postbariatric patients, and many of these were fatal [26].

7.5.2 Late Complications

Patients undergoing bariatric surgery should receive lifelong follow-up. This is essential to follow any nutritional deficiencies and to identify early any potential surgical complications that may develop.

In the RYGB as well as the BPD-DS, stenosis can occur at the proximal anastomosis (gastrojejunostomy or duodenojejunostomy, respectively). This often manifests as nausea and vomiting, usually postprandially. Although an upper gastrointestinal series may be helpful, an upper endoscopy may be both diagnostic and therapeutic, as balloon dilatation may be employed to widen the outlet. This procedure is successful in most patients; however, some may require multiple dilations and a few cases may require surgical revision to enlarge the opening.

In rare cases, a patient may present with gastrointestinal hemorrhage after weight loss surgery because of marginal ulceration at the proximal anastomosis. This is more often seen on the jejunal side in RYGB patients. It is most easily diagnosed endoscopically and responds most frequently to conservative therapy of H-2 blockers or proton pump inhibitors. A few cases will require surgical revision [11,19,26].

Adhesions or internal hernias can form after many abdominal surgeries, and patients who undergo bariatric procedures can also develop these complications. Partial or complete small bowel obstructions are more commonly seen after RYGB and BPD-DS, than after purely restrictive procedures, as the potential for internal hernias increases with rerouting of bowel and mesenteries. Internal hernias are potential spaces that are created, usually in mesenteric defects, during surgery. They serve as potential sites of obstruction, which has led many surgeons to close these defects with sutures during the original surgery. Adhesions may act similarly, although they occur less frequently since the advent of laparoscopic techniques. Patients may present with abdominal pain, nausea, and/or vomiting. An upper gastrointestinal series or computed tomography scan may aid in diagnosis. Some partial obstructions will respond to conservative management; however, many require reoperation [11,26].

Some late sequelae of bariatric surgery are related more to the rapid weight loss and known physiologic side effects of bypass. Up to 32% of patients after RYGB will develop gallstones from rapid weight loss. Not all will become symptomatic. Bile acid binders may help decrease this risk preoperatively. Sugerman has found that a daily dose of 600 mg of ursodiol, beginning within 10 d after gastric bypass in patients without preexisting stone disease, reduced the rate of gallstone formation from 32% to 2% [28]. Those who have diagnosed gallstones preoperatively will often have concomitant cholecystectomy at the time of bypass to prevent future problems. Almost all patients undergoing a BPD-DS will have a cholecystectomy at the time of their bypass. Some bypass patients will also experience what has been termed "dumping syndrome," which follows a hyperosmolar oral sugar load and may manifest as nausea, vomiting, diarrhea, or diaphoresis. It is a self-limited phenomenon and serves to reinforce dietary changes that are recommended preoperatively. Most RYGB patients will no longer experience dumping after 1 yr postsurgery, except possibly after consuming dairy products [16,27].

Banding procedures (LAGB) have their own potential complications; device-related problems make them unique as compared to malabsorptive procedures. In addition to nausea and vomiting, gastroesophageal reflux disease (GERD) is experienced by as many as 15% of patients during the first postoperative year. These symptoms may simply be related to maladaptive eating behaviors, postbanding; however, they may lead to or indicate band-related problems. Overeating with an appropriately tight or an overtightened band may manifest with nausea and vomiting. It may also improve as the esophagus dilates proximal to the band and serves as a food reservoir — a state that, if not discovered early — can result in permanent esophageal dysfunction and increased risk of aspiration. Treatment early in the course consists of deflation of the band at the expense of weight loss. Vomiting whether from overeating or other illness can cause band slippage. Slippage may be a misnomer as the stomach actually herniates above the band and thus causes the band position to change, acting as more of a prolapse. This may lead to outlet obstruction or incarceration. Deflating the band often enables the stomach to return to its initial position, but often surgery is required. Maladaptive eating behaviors can also force the band caudad, which creates obstructive type symptoms. Again, sometimes, this can be solved by deflation of the band; however, in some circumstances, it may require surgery. Slippage has been reported in approximately 1.6% of LAGB cases in systematic reviews [11,17].

7.6 EXPERIMENTAL PROCEDURES

There is much interest in novel surgical approaches for weight loss. Investigators are currently evaluating the theory that appetite control can be stimulated or suppressed with manipulation of the gastric tonicity through electrical stimulation. In limited series, several investigators have attempted to induce gastric paresis or vagally induced satiety, and some researchers postulate that this can be accomplished through gastric pacing; stimulating the stomach from proximal to distal, or vice versa, could affect gastric emptying. Early studies conducted in a porcine model demonstrated approximately a 10% weight loss with higher frequency stimulation. In early human studies, at 35 mo, mean weight loss was approximately 19.1 kg in patients with an initial BMI > 40. Weight gain occurred with battery end-of-life or lead malfunction. Further studies are under way. Most frequently cited complications associated with early gastric electrical stimulation lead placement were gastric perforation at implant, complete lead dislodgement, and abdominal discomfort [6,11].

7.7 REOPERATIVE SURGERY

The field of bariatric surgery has evolved tremendously over the last 50 yr. Now, more than ever, outcome measurements, procedure modification, and multidisciplinary team approaches have necessitated replacement of earlier surgical approaches for obesity, which lacked scientific evidence, acceptable malabsorptive complications, or adequate patient selection and education. As a result, there is renewed interest in revisional bariatric surgery for both anatomically intact and anatomically failed procedures. It is imperative that expectations of revisions are clear to both the surgeon and the patient as both may have entirely different notions of the rationale for the revision. Revisions may be undertaken for excessive weight loss and, more frequently, for inadequate weight loss.

7.7.1 Failures of the Surgical Procedure

Given the multitude of bariatric procedures that have evolved over the past five decades, it is easy to see how procedures have evolved, secondary to lessons learned from those performed early on in the field's development. It is not within the scope of this chapter to discuss all potential surgical failures; however, the evolution of bariatric surgery has reduced these numbers by further refining techniques.

Many advances in restrictive and malabsorptive procedures have minimized or eliminated the most serious of complications. For example, the JIB, although effective for weight loss, because of its severe malabsorption, often leads to severe nutritional sequelae as well as potentially life-threatening liver disease. Many of these procedures had to be reversed, as a result. Even today, the RYGB and BPD-DS are reversed occasionally because the patient experiences excessive weight loss and severe protein malnutrition. More often, the procedures are revised to make the bypass less severe to increase nutrient absorption or to surgically (or nonsurgically) place enteral feeding tubes to increase the patient's caloric intake.

Early gastric restrictive procedures with fixed outlet size failed to allow the patient adequate long-term weight loss. Gastrogastric fistula from staple-line breakdown in nondivided stomachs have led to techniques that utilized complete separation of the stomach pouch to decrease oral food capacity, as well as absorption of nutrients not bypassing the biliopancreatic or Roux limbs [13]. Early on, high gastric fistula rates (12 to 50%) were reported for stapled but nondivided stomachs [33–36]. Also, stomal ulceration was found to be higher in patients with gastrogastric fistulas [35]. Fistula rates for completely divided stomachs (now the procedure of choice) have ranged anywhere from 0 to 6% [33,34].

Regardless of the improvements they may provide, all revisionary surgical procedures are associated with increased risk. Risk is increased in malnourished individuals or those who are still obese. Any decision to revise a bariatric procedure should be made on an individual basis.

7.7.2 Failures of the Patient

Some bariatric patients fail to maintain adequate weight loss or to achieve an acceptable BMI despite anatomically intact procedures, because of their failure to alter their lifestyles as directed by the multidisciplinary team and as required by the surgical procedure. Some purely restrictive procedures that lack a malabsorption component can be easily overcome by the intake of liquid calories and grazing behaviors. In fact, most bariatric procedures can result in inadequate weight loss or inadequate weight maintenance if the patient is noncompliant with dietary advice.

Current definitions of success for bariatric surgery are not all encompassing and do not necessarily equate to a BMI of 25. Successful and maintained weight loss is considered by many to be a loss of more than 50% of the patient's EBW. This amount can vary dramatically, depending on the patient's starting BMI. For example, a patient with an initial BMI of 70 may lose 200 lb, well above the 50% loss of EBW, but still have a BMI > 40, which is defined as "morbidly obese." In reality, this patient may still have had resolution of his or her comorbidities — diabetes, stress incontinence, back pain, etc. — and now be able to participate in activity that was impossible before weight loss. In this example, resolution of comorbidities must be taken into account and considered as success.

Each patient who has "failed" an intact surgical procedure should be reviewed individually. Early in bariatric surgical experience, patients did not undergo extensive preoperative evaluation and may not have been educated on the importance of lifelong dietary and exercise requirements. Lack of follow-up, in general, may have been a problem. Maladaptive eating patterns and psychological disorders may not have been identified preoperatively. This is often the case even today, despite more extensive screening tools.

In addition, individuals who underwent long-limb bypasses and restricted gastric pouches have few, if any, surgical options remaining. Other patients may attain mild to moderate weight loss with revisional surgery, with further limitation of the gastric pouch or with increased severity of the bypass.

Ultimately, any patient undergoing a surgical revision of a previous bariatric procedure for additional weight loss needs a full evaluation, which should include the identification of the original procedure and the use of a variety of tools to arrive at a reasonable plan. Some patients may simply not be candidates for any revision despite a BMI that places them in the obese category. Others need to have realistic expectations of further surgical weight loss, with an emphasis placed on diet, exercise, and lifelong follow-up. There also needs to be a clear understanding of their surgical risk, which will vary with the patient.

7.8 SUMMARY

The evolution of surgical procedures for weight loss has changed dramatically during the last 50 yr and most specifically in the last 10 yr. Increasing experience, refinement of technique, and public awareness of surgical options, with the current epidemic of obesity in the U.S., have made surgery an attractive alternative. Surgical weight loss has helped many patients improve or resolve medical problems that were obesity related and endangering their lives. It has even been recommended by the World Health Organization as the most effective way of reducing weight and maintaining weight loss in the severely and morbidly obese, as well as the least expensive treatment after 4 yr on a kg/weight-loss basis [37].

Surgery, however, requires a long-term commitment. It brings potential lifelong problems, including those commonly related to surgery and nutritional deficiencies. The process must include a patient's commitment to dietary and lifestyle modification and the commitment of a dedicated team of health care professionals, e.g., surgeons, primary care physicians, dietitians, psychotherapists, and exercise physiologists, for long-term success. An intact social support system is also extremely advantageous.

The ultimate success of weight loss surgery is dependent on all these factors, as well as the patient's desire and effort toward success.

REFERENCES

1. Flegal KM, Carroll MD, Ogden CL, Johnson CL. Prevalence and trends in obesity among US adults, 1999–2000. *JAMA*. 2002; 288(14):1723–1727.
2. Brody F. Minimally invasive surgery for morbid obesity. *Cleve Clin J Med.* 2004; 71(4):289,293,296–298.
3. Steinbrook R. Surgery for severe obesity. *N Engl J Med.* 2004; 350(11):1075–1079.
4. NIH conference. Gastrointestinal surgery for severe obesity. Consensus Development Conference Panel. *Ann Intern Med.* 1991; 115(12):956–961.
5. Kremen AJ, Linner JH, Nelson CH. An experimental evaluation of the nutritional importance of proximal and distal small intestine. *Ann Surg.* 1954; 140(3):439–448.
6. Buchwald H, Buchwald JN. Evolution of operative procedures for the management of morbid obesity 1950–2000. *Obes Surg.* 2002; 12:705–717.
7. Lambert DM, Sudan R, Forse AR. Choice of bariatric procedures. In Farraye FA, Forse RA, eds. *Bariatric Surgery: A Primer for Your Medical Practice*. Thorofare, NJ: 2005.
8. Matts JP, Buchwald H, Fitch LL, et al. Subgroup analyses of the major clinical endpoints in the Program on the Surgical Control of the Hyperlipidemias (POSCH): overall mortality, atherosclerotic coronary heart disease (ACHD) mortality, and ACHD mortality or myocardial infarction. *J Clin Epidemiol.* 1995; 48(3):389–405.
9. Requarth JA, Burchard KW, Colacchio TA, Stukel TA, Mott LA, Greenberg ER, Weismann RE. Long-term morbidity following jejunoileal bypass. The continuing potential need for surgical reversal. *Arch Surg.* 1995; 130(3):318–325.
10. Sylvan A, Sjolund B, Janunger K. Favorable long-term results with the end-to-side jejunoileal bypass. *Obes Surg.* 1995; 5(4):357–363.
11. Martin LF. The evolution of surgery for morbid obesity. In: Martin LF, ed. *Obesity Surgery.* McGraw-Hill, New York, NY: 2004:15–47.
12. MacLean LD, Rhode BM, Forse RA. Late results of vertical banded gastroplasty for morbid and super obesity. *Surgery.* 1990; 107(1):20–27.
13. Maclean LD, Rhode BM, Forse RA. A gastroplasty that avoids stapling in continuity. *Surgery.* 1993; 113(4):380–388.
14. Moreno P, Alastrue A, Rull M, et al. Band erosion in patients who have undergone vertical banded gastroplasty: incidence and technical solutions. *Arch Surg.* 1998; 133(2):189–193.
15. Fielding GA, Allen JW. A step-by-step guide to placement of the LAP-BAND adjustable gastric banding system. *Am J Surg.* 2002; 184(6B):26S–30S.
16. Ren CJ, Weiner M, Allen JW. Favorable early results of gastric banding for morbid obesity: the American experience. *Surg Endosc.* 2004; 18:543–546.
17. Chapman AE, Kiroff G, Game P, et al. Laparoscopic adjustable gastric banding in the treatment of obesity: a systematic literature review. *Surgery.* 2004; 135(3):326–351.
18. Inabnet W, Demaria W, Ikramuddin S. *Nonsurgical Means of Weight Loss in Laparoscopic Bariatric Surgery.* Lippincott, Williams & Wilkins, Philadelphia, PA: 2005, 13–19.
19. Marceau P, Hould FS, Simard S, et al. Biliopancreatic diversion with duodenal switch. *World J Surg.* 1998; 22:947–954.
20. Scopinaro N, Adami GF, Marinari GM, et al. Biliopancreatic diversion. *World J Surg.* 1998; 22(9):936–946.
21. Hess DW, Hess DS. Biliopancreatic diversion with a duodenal switch. *Obes Surg.* 1998; 8:267–282.

22. Sudan R, Sudan D. Development of a totally intracorporeal robotic assisted biliary pancreatic diversion with duodenal switch. Video presentation. The 19th Annual Meeting of the American Society for Bariatric Surgery, June 2002.
23. Hatzifotis M. Symptomatic vitamin A deficiency following biliopancreatic diversion. *Obes Surg.* 2003; 13:655–657.
24. Slater GH, Ren CJ, Seigel N, et al. Serum fat-soluble vitamin deficiency and abnormal calcium metabolism after malabsorptive bariatric surgery. *J Gastrointest Surg.* 2004; 8(1):48–55.
25. Wittgrove AC, Clark GW, Tremblay LJ. Laparoscopic gastric bypass, Roux-en-Y: preliminary report of five cases. *Obes Surg.* 1994; 4:353–357.
26. Nguyen NT, Goldman C, Rosenquist CJ, et al. Laparoscopic versus open gastric bypass: a randomized study of outcomes, quality of life, and costs. *Ann Surg.* 2001; 234(3):279–289.
27. MacLean LD, Rhode BM, Nohr CW. Late outcome of isolated gastric bypass. *Ann Surg.* 2000; 231(4):524–528.
28. Sugerman HJ, DeMaria EJ, Kellum JM, Sugerman EL, Meador JG, Wolfe LG. Effects of bariatric surgery in older patients. *Ann Surg.* 2004; 240(2):243–247.
29. Christou NV, Sampalis JS, Liberman M, et al. Surgery decreases long-term mortality, morbidity, and health care use in morbidly obese patients. *Ann Surg.* 2004; 240(3): 416–424.
30. Sjostrom L, Lindroos AK, Peltonen M, et al. Lifestyle, diabetes, and cardiovascular risk factors 10 years after bariatric surgery. *N Engl J Med.* 2004; 351(26):2683–2704.
31. Flum DR, Dellinger EP. Impact of gastric bypass operation on survival: a population-based analysis. *J Am Coll Surg.* 2004; 199(4):543–551.
32. Biertho L, Steffen R, Ricklin T, et al. Laparoscopic gastric bypass versus laparoscopic adjustable gastric banding: a comparative study of 1,200 cases. *J Am Coll Surg.* 2003; 197(4):536–545.
33. Cucchi SG, Pories WJ, MacDonald KF, Morgan EJ. Gastrogastric fistulas. A complication of divided gastric bypass surgery. *Ann Surg.* 1995; 221(4):387–391.
34. Capella JF, Capella RF. Gastro-gastric fistulas and marginal ulcers in gastric bypass procedures for weight reductions. *Obes Surg.* 1999; 9(1):22–27.
35. MacLean LD, Rhode BM, Nohr C, Katz S, McLean AP. Stomas ulcer after gastric bypass. *J Am Coll Surg.* 1997; 185(1):87–88.
36. Fobi MA, Lee H, Igwe D Jr, Stanczyk M, Tambi JN. Prospective comparative evaluation of stapled versus transected silastic ring gastric bypass: 6-year follow-up. *Obes Surg.* 2001; 11(1),18–24.
37. Obesity: Preventing and managing the global epidemic. Report of a WHO Consultation on Obesity, 3–5 June 1997, Geneva, WHO/NUT/NCD/98.1. <http://64.233.187.104/search?q = cache:lcvai8y30rIJ:www.who.int/nut/documents/obesity_executive_summary.pdf+report+of+WHO+consultation+on+obesity+geneva&hl=en&client=safari>. Accessed Nov 11, 2005.

8 Gastrointestinal Complications of Bariatric Surgery

Christopher S. Huang and Francis A. Farraye

CONTENTS

8.1 INTRODUCTION

Bariatric surgery, in particular the Roux-en-Y gastric bypass (RYGBP) operation, has been shown to have several significant benefits, including long-term excess weight loss, improvement in quality of life, and amelioration or resolution of obesity-related comorbidities [1–3]. Recent studies have also demonstrated that many gastrointestinal (GI) symptoms, such as abdominal pain and heartburn/acid reflux, significantly improve after laparoscopic RYGBP [4,5]. While the majority of patients achieve successful outcomes following bariatric surgery, a small but significant proportion develop GI complications at some point during their postoperative course. With the dramatic escalation in the number of bariatric surgeries now being performed, these GI complications have become an important cause of morbidity. Therefore, primary care providers must become familiar with these complications and play an active role in their appropriate long-term management [6].

Gastrointestinal complications of bariatric surgery can be categorized into four main categories (Table 8.1): 1) adverse GI symptoms, which occur as an expected result of the alteration in the upper GI tract anatomy, 2) structural complications associated with the operation, 3) hepatobiliary complications and 4) nutritional complications. The purpose of this chapter is to review the most common GI complications of bariatric surgery and provide management recommendations for primary care providers regarding the care of patients with these complications.

8.2 ADVERSE GASTROINTESTINAL SYMPTOMS

Certain adverse GI symptoms are to be expected in patients who undergo bariatric surgery, and they occur as a result of the alteration in the upper GI anatomy and physiology. These symptoms tend to improve over time through patient education and intestinal adaptation.

TABLE 8.1
Gastrointestinal Complications of Bariatric Surgery

Adverse Gastrointestinal Symptoms	Structural Complications	Hepatobiliary Complications	Nutritional Complications
Nausea and vomiting	Marginal ulcer	Cholelithiasis	Iron deficiency
Diarrhea	Stomal stenosis	Liver disease	Vitamin B12 deficiency
Dumping syndrome	Staple line dehiscence		Folate deficiency
Gastroesophageal reflux	Band erosion		Thiamine deficiency
	Small bowel obstruction		Vitamin D and calcium deficiency

TABLE 8.2
Appropriate Eating Habits after Restrictive Bariatric Surgery

Eat slowly and undisturbed
Chew meticulously
Stop eating before onset of discomfort
Do not drink liquid during meals; wait at least 2 h after ingestion of solids before drinking
Avoid high-caloric, high-osmolar foods and drinks

8.2.1 Nausea and Vomiting

Nausea and vomiting are perhaps the most common complaints after bariatric surgery and are typically due to dietary indiscretion or noncompliance with the "gastroplasty diet" [7]. The restrictive bariatric operations, such as the RYGBP, vertical banded gastroplasty (VBG), and laparoscopic adjustable silicone gastric banding (LASGB), result in a small gastric "pouch" that is designed to markedly limit the amount of food that can be ingested during a meal. Successful outcomes of these operations depend on strict patient compliance with dietary recommendations and appropriate eating habits (Table 8.2).

Patients who have persistent nausea and vomiting despite dietary compliance should undergo diagnostic investigation for structural complications, such as marginal ulcers, stomal stenosis, and small bowel obstruction (Table 8.3). Marginal ulcers, with or without stomal stenosis, are a common cause of nausea and vomiting in patients after RYGBP and should be strongly suspected in patients who present within the first six postoperative months with these symptoms [8]. Sudden onset of nausea and vomiting in a patient previously tolerating a proper diet suggests acute stomal obstruction, commonly due to bezoar or food impaction at the gastrojejunal anastomosis [9]. Vomiting accompanied by abdominal pain should raise the suspicion for complications such as biliary colic or small bowel obstruction (due to adhesions or internal hernias). These complications are discussed separately in greater detail below. Finally, RYGBP patients may suffer from the "Roux stasis

TABLE 8.3
Differential Diagnosis of Nausea and Vomiting after Bariatric Surgery

Inappropriate eating behavior/dietary noncompliance
Stomal obstruction due to stenosis, food impaction, or bezoar formation
Marginal ulcer
Small bowel obstruction due to internal hernia, adhesions
Roux stasis syndrome
Symptomatic gallstone disease
Food intolerance
Gastroesophageal reflux
Dumping syndrome

TABLE 8.4
Differential Diagnosis of Diarrhea after Bariatric Surgery

Dumping syndrome
Surgically induced malabsorption
Lactose intolerance
Food sensitivity
Bacterial overgrowth/blind loop syndrome
Gastrointestinal infection
Underlying gastrointestinal disorders not unique to bariatric patients (inflammatory bowel disease, celiac disease and other malabsorptive disorders, irritable bowel syndrome, etc.)
Medication-induced

syndrome," characterized by abdominal pain, nausea, vomiting, and bloating made worse by eating. This syndrome is caused, in part, by a motility disorder of the Roux limb that occurs as a result of transecting the jejunum from the natural small intestinal pacemaker located in the duodenum [10]; this results in a functional obstruction in the Roux limb.

8.2.2 Diarrhea

Diarrhea after bariatric surgery has many different potential causes (Table 8.4). These include dumping syndrome (see below), lactose intolerance, food sensitivity, bacterial overgrowth, malabsorption, and infection [9]. Diarrhea is a "necessary evil" following the malabsorptive bariatric operations, such as the jejunoileal bypass and biliopancreatic diversion [11,12], occurring primarily as a result of the truncated absorptive stream and diminished reabsorption of bile acids. In these situations, diarrhea is typically nonbloody and foul smelling, varies directly with fat intake, and subsides with fasting. There is a general tendency for diarrhea to diminish with time, as the segment of small intestine remaining in the absorptive stream undergoes adaptation, enhancing its absorptive capacity.

Significant diarrhea after RYGBP or the restrictive operations is uncommon. It is important to consider other causes of diarrhea in these patients, which may be unrelated to their bariatric operation, such as inflammatory bowel disease, bacterial or parasitic infections, celiac disease, etc. The presence of systemic symptoms (e.g., fever, malaise), abdominal pain, bloody stools, or greater-than-expected weight loss should alert the physician to the possibility of a separate underlying disease process.

8.2.3 Dumping Syndrome

Dumping syndrome is characterized by early postprandial GI (diarrhea, cramping, nausea, vomiting) and vasomotor symptoms (hypotension, palpitations, flushing, lightheadedness, syncope), resulting from osmotic fluid shifts and release of vasoactive mediators [13]. These mediators induce postprandial peripheral and splanchnic vasodilatation, resulting in relative hypovolemia. Late dumping symptoms are believed to arise as a consequence of reactive hypoglycemia, which is caused by an exaggerated release of insulin and glucagon-like peptide-1 [14]. This syndrome is precipitated by the rapid entry of food and liquids into the small bowel, as can occur after RYGBP or biliopancreatic diversion. Patients who are noncompliant with their diets or who ingest foods with high sugar content are at increased risk for developing dumping syndrome. Prevention includes consumption of small meals, avoidance of foods with high sugar content, and drinking liquids between (not during) meals.

While dumping syndrome is considered an adverse side effect of bariatric surgery, it actually serves to condition patients to avoid high-caloric, high-osmolar foods. Severe symptoms occur very rarely, and in most patients, dumping symptoms are short-lived and disappear as they adapt to their bypass anatomy [6].

8.2.4 Gastroesophageal Reflux

The effects of bariatric surgery on gastroesophageal reflux (GER) are controversial. In particular, studies on the effect of gastric banding on GER have reported conflicting results [15,16]. One key factor that determines how GER is affected by gastric banding is the presence and size of the gastric pouch proximal to the band: reflux and esophagitis appear to be worsened when a large gastric pouch is present (as can occur with band slippage), but improved when the band is placed at or just below the gastroesophageal junction, thereby augmenting the effect of the lower esophageal sphincter [17].

Vertical banded gastroplasty appears to have no significant effect on GER, whereas RYGBP typically reduces GER [5,18]. An increase in reflux symptoms after RYGBP may indicate the development of staple line dehiscence with gastrogastric fistulization, which allows acid from the bypassed stomach to enter the pouch and reflux into the esophagus.

8.3 STRUCTURAL COMPLICATIONS

Structural complications of bariatric surgery can occur at any point in time during the postoperative course. Early/immediate postoperative complications, such as anastomotic leak or acute gastric distension after RYGBP, are typically managed by surgeons. This section, therefore, focuses on the late GI complications that primary care providers may encounter while caring for bariatric surgical patients.

8.3.1 Marginal Ulcer

Marginal ulcers (i.e., ulcers located at the gastrojejunal anastomosis) develop in up to 16% of patients following RYGBP [19–22], usually within the first two to four postoperative months [9]. Their etiology remains unclear, but potential contributory factors include gastric acidity (especially in the presence of a staple line dehiscence and gastrogastric fistula), nonsteroidal anti-inflammatory drug (NSAID) use, *Helicobacter pylori* infection, and local ischemia and tension at the anastomosis [21,23–26].

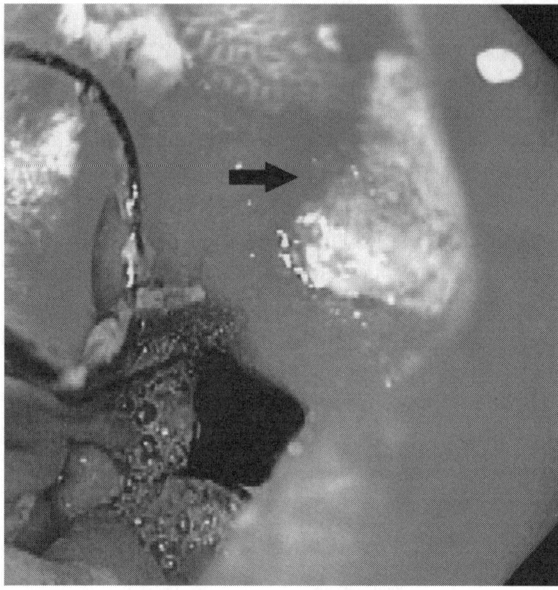

FIGURE 8.1 Endoscopic appearance of a clean-based marginal ulcer (arrow).

Marginal ulcers are often accompanied by some degree of stomal stenosis and commonly present with epigastric abdominal pain, nausea, and vomiting [8]. Marginal ulcers are also a common cause of upper GI hemorrhage occurring in the late postoperative period [27].

Upper endoscopy is the diagnostic test of choice for detecting marginal ulcers (Figure 8.1). Treatment is largely empirical, but may include antisecretory therapy with a proton pump inhibitor, sucralfate, and avoidance of NSAIDs. Standard antibiotic regimens for *H. pylori* infection should also be administered if there is histologic or serologic evidence of infection. Whether *H. pylori* actually has a role in the formation of these ulcers is not known, although there is uncontrolled data suggesting that preoperative treatment of *H. pylori* reduces the incidence of postoperative marginal ulcers [25].

Occasionally, marginal ulcers can be refractory to medical therapy; such ulcers may be due to ischemia at the gastrojejunal anastomosis [28]. Other causes of peptic ulcer disease, such as Zollinger–Ellison syndrome or Crohn's disease, should be considered in the appropriate clinical context. Ultimately, surgical revision may be required to treat refractory ulcers, especially when they are associated with chronic stomal stenosis.

8.3.2 Stomal Stenosis

Stomal stenosis is a relatively common complication of RYGBP and VBG, and typically presents within the first six postoperative months [22,29–34]. Symptoms of this complication include postprandial epigastric pain, vomiting, and dysphagia.

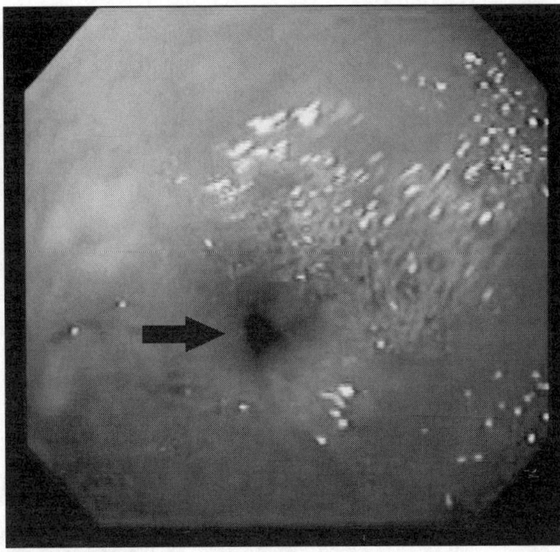

FIGURE 8.2 Endoscopic appearance of significant stomal stenosis (stoma indicated by arrow).

Patients with stomal stenosis may also present with food impaction at the gastrojejunal anastomosis.

Stomal stenosis can be diagnosed on upper GI barium studies, but endoscopy is the preferred test due to its greater accuracy in determining stomal diameter and the ability to perform therapeutic intervention at the time of diagnosis (Figure 8.2). Endoscopic dilation of stomal stenosis has been shown to be safe, durable, and effective, essentially obviating the need for surgical revision except in rare cases [29,30].

8.3.3 Staple Line Dehiscence

Staple line dehiscence is a potential complication of RYGBP and VBG, resulting in a gastrogastric fistula between the pouch and bypassed stomach. This complication is less common today because of improvements in surgical techniques that reinforce and isolate the staple lines. Small dehiscences are typically asymptomatic, whereas large dehiscences may present with weight gain due to reduced satiety from meals and normal absorption of nutrients in the previously bypassed small bowel. Staple line dehiscences may also present with GER or marginal ulcers, presumably as a result of acid refluxing from the bypassed stomach into the gastric pouch [19,20,26].

Upper GI barium studies can readily detect the presence of staple line dehiscence and should be obtained as the first diagnostic test when this complication is suspected (Figure 8.3). Endoscopy may be warranted to exclude the presence of a concomitant marginal ulcer in symptomatic patients. The standard treatment for clinically significant staple line dehiscences is surgical revision, although small studies have reported successful endoscopic therapy using a variety of techniques [35,36].

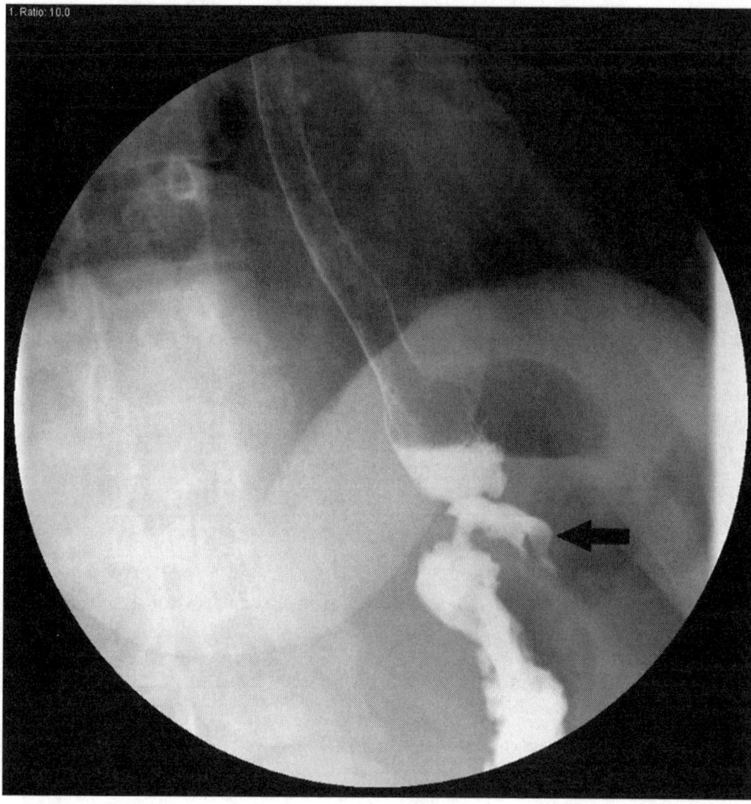

FIGURE 8.3 Staple line dehiscence with a gastrogastric fistula (arrow) demonstrated on barium study.

8.3.4 Band Erosion

Band erosion is a relatively uncommon complication of VBG and LASGB, occurring in approximately 1 to 2% of VBG patients and 1 to 11% of LASGB patients [37–39]. In VBG patients, band erosion may cause pain, but more often presents with weight gain due to reduced restriction in food intake. Band erosion is a potentially serious complication after LASGB and can result in pain, vomiting, bleeding, intraabdominal abscess, or fistula formation [9]. Band erosion after LASGB can also present with sudden weight gain, and, in many cases, the first sign of band erosion is infection at the subcutaneous access port site [38]. The diagnosis of band erosion is made by endoscopy. Endoscopic removal of eroded bands has been described [40,41], but surgical removal is generally recommended, as patients will typically require a redo bariatric operation.

8.3.5 Small Bowel Obstruction

Small bowel obstruction (SBO) occurs in approximately 1 to 4% of patients after laparoscopic RYGBP [42–45]. Early SBO is commonly due to internal hernias, narrowing of the jejunojejunostomy, and obstruction of the Roux limb at the level of the transverse mesocolon. Obstructions that occur later in the postoperative course are typically caused by internal hernias or adhesions [45]. Intussusception and superior mesenteric artery syndrome have also been described as potential causes of SBO several months after RYGBP [46–48].

Patients in whom an SBO is suspected should be evaluated radiographically, with an upper GI series and/or abdominal computed tomography (CT) scan [49]. Surgical exploration is necessary for definitive treatment in most cases.

8.4 HEPATOBILIARY COMPLICATIONS

8.4.1 Cholelithiasis

Rapid weight loss is a recognized risk factor for the development of cholesterol gallstones. It is therefore not surprising that approximately 30% of patients develop gallstones within six months after RYGBP, 40% of whom will experience symptomatic disease [50]. While some surgeons advocate for routine cholecystectomy at the time of the bariatric operation [51], this remains a matter of controversy because of the increased time of operation and postoperative hospitalization, as well as all the potential complications of cholecystectomy [52,53]. Furthermore, cholecystectomy is technically easier to perform after weight loss occurs. One potential alternative to cholecystectomy is medical dissolution therapy. Controlled trials have demonstrated the efficacy of ursodiol therapy in decreasing the incidence of gallstone formation [54,55]. Ursodiol therapy is safe and generally well tolerated, but the costs of long-term use may be prohibitive.

Patients with suspected symptomatic or complicated gallstone disease should undergo abdominal ultrasonography as the initial diagnostic test. Radionuclide cholescintigraphy and abdominal CT scan can be useful when the diagnosis is uncertain or when severe intraabdominal complications are suspected.

8.4.2 Liver Disease

Cirrhosis develops in approximately 7 to 8% of patients following jejunoileal bypass (JIB) [11,56], a procedure that is no longer performed due to the numerous complications associated with it. However, as one of the first major bariatric procedures, the JIB was very popular in the 1970s; so primary care providers must still be able to recognize and manage the long-term consequences such as chronic liver disease. Unfortunately, significant liver disease can develop with little or no clinical evidence and may become evident only when the patient develops ascites, variceal hemorrhage, and hepatic encephalopathy [56]. Reversal of the JIB can improve hepatic inflammation and fibrosis if performed early enough, but once advanced cirrhosis has developed, JIB reversal carries a high perioperative mortality rate, and liver transplantation may be the only effective therapy [56,57].

8.5 NUTRITIONAL COMPLICATIONS

Following bariatric surgery, patients are at risk for a number of nutritional complications. Restriction of dietary intake, intolerance of certain foods, and diversion of food from the stomach and proximal small bowel impair absorption of several important micronutrients, which can potentially result in significant hematologic, neurologic, and metabolic disorders.

8.5.1 Iron Deficiency

Iron deficiency is a common complication of RYGBP and biliopancreatic diversion, developing in 20 to 49% of patients [58–60]. Premenopausal women are particularly at risk, due to menstrual losses. The etiology of iron deficiency in these patients is multifactorial and includes both malabsorption and maldigestion [61]. The primary site of iron absorption is the duodenum, which is bypassed and totally excluded from digestive continuity in RYGBP. Also, the relatively achlorhydric state in the gastric pouch after RYGBP impairs the essential step for iron bioavailability in which ferric iron in food is reduced to the ferrous state in the presence of gastric acid. Finally, postoperative changes in eating habits and food preferences may lead to reduced intake of iron-rich foods, particularly red meat. Studies have shown that prophylactic iron supplementation can prevent iron deficiency and that the concomitant use of vitamin C can improve iron absorption in RYGBP patients [61,62].

8.5.2 Vitamin B12 Deficiency

Vitamin B12 deficiency is common after bariatric surgery, occurring in 25 to 75% of RYGBP patients [60,63–65]. Mechanisms of vitamin B12 deficiency in these patients include achlorhydria (preventing cleavage of B12 from foods), decreased B12 intake due to intolerance of meats and milk, and inadequate secretion of intrinsic factor following surgery. Symptomatic B12 deficiency is uncommon, but significant deficiency can lead to megaloblastic anemia, thrombocytopenia, leukopenia, and glossitis. Persistent deficiency can ultimately lead to subacute combined degeneration of the dorsal and lateral spinal cord columns. Therefore, supplementation with either intramuscular injection (1000 μg/month) or oral crystalline B12 (at least 350 μg/d) is generally recommended.

8.5.3 Folate Deficiency

Folate deficiency after RYGBP occurs as a result of decreased folate consumption, achlorhydria, and bypass of the proximal small intestine. In addition, vitamin B12 deficiency may lead to folate deficiency, as B12 acts as a coenzyme in the metabolism of folate. As with B12 deficiency, symptomatic folate deficiency is uncommon and is easily corrected with the use of a daily multivitamin [66].

8.5.4 Thiamine Deficiency

Thiamine deficiency following bariatric surgery can occur as a result of inadequate intake (often due to protracted vomiting) and/or malabsorption, secondary to surgical bypass of the proximal small bowel. Several cases of Wernicke's encephalopathy have been reported [67–70], highlighting the importance of prevention, early recognition, and immediate treatment of thiamine deficiency.

8.5.5 Vitamin D and Calcium Deficiency

In highly malabsorptive procedures, such as biliopancreatic diversion, fat-soluble vitamin deficiency, including vitamin D deficiency, can occur [71]. Calcium deficiency occurs as a result of surgical bypass of the primary site of active absorption (duodenum) and inadequate intake. As a result, metabolic bone disease is recognized as a potential complication of bariatric surgery [72–76]. It is therefore recommended that all bariatric patients undergo routine measurements of 25-hydroxy vitamin D and calcium levels, and receive lifelong supplemental calcium (1200 to 1500 mg/d of calcium citrate) with vitamin D.

8.6 MANAGEMENT RECOMMENDATIONS

8.6.1 General Guidelines

Primary care providers should become involved in the care of bariatric surgical patients soon after the operation, in conjunction with the patient's surgeon and bariatric team. Regular follow-up is recommended to allow for early identification of long-term complications, including nutritional deficiencies as well as the GI complications discussed in this chapter.

When patients present with GI symptoms after bariatric surgery, the first step is to assess their compliance with appropriate dietary recommendations and eating habits. As mentioned above, many symptoms such as nausea, vomiting, and diarrhea can be ascribed to dietary noncompliance alone. However, when symptoms persist despite dietary compliance, or when symptoms are accompanied by alarm features, such as dehydration, gastrointestinal bleeding, unanticipated weight loss, or severe abdominal pain, further diagnostic testing is recommended.

8.6.2 Diagnostic Testing

The evaluation of GI symptoms typically involves a combination of endoscopic and/or radiographic tests, depending on the suspected site of pathology. Patients in whom a stomal complication is suspected (e.g., marginal ulcer, stomal stenosis) should be referred to a gastroenterologist for upper endoscopy. Band erosion after VBG or LASGB is also best diagnosed by upper endoscopy. Finally, overt or occult GI bleeding deserves endoscopic evaluation, which, depending on the patient's age and presentation, may involve colonoscopy, enteroscopy, and even examination of the bypassed stomach in RYGBP patients.

The three most useful radiologic tests are the barium upper GI series, CT scan, and ultrasonography. Barium upper GI series are most useful for the detection of staple line dehiscence, gastrogastric fistula, and stenosis of the jejunojejunostomy, and for the evaluation of small bowel obstruction. Abdominal CT scans can provide important complementary information in patients with small bowel obstruction, such as the site and cause of obstruction, as well as exclude other extralumenal disease processes. Ultrasonography is the diagnostic test of choice for patients with suspected gallstone disease.

8.7 SUMMARY

Gastrointestinal complications after bariatric surgery have become an important cause of morbidity, owing to the rapid escalation in the performance of RYGBP and other bariatric operations. Primary care providers involved in the long-term care of these patients must become familiar with the common adverse GI symptoms that are "expected" after surgery, as well as the true structural and hepatobiliary complications that can develop. Patients who have persistent symptoms despite dietary compliance, and those with symptoms accompanied by alarm features, should be evaluated for structural complications and underlying disease processes.

SELECTED INTERNET RESOURCES FOR PATIENTS

1. www.collagevideo.com: Collage Video sells exercise videos and includes detailed information and reviews to assist in selecting videos on the basis of preferences and physical limitations.
2. www.eatright.org: The American Dietetic Association offers information on nutrition, healthy lifestyle, and how to find a registered dietitian.
3. www.fitday.com: FitDay.com gives nutrition analysis of calories, fat, protein, carbohydrates, and fiber in table and graph form, as well as offering journals and goal-setting and activity-tracking tools.
4. www.healthetech.com: Healthetech offers information on its Palm or Windows software program for personalized weight management.
5. www.nal.usda.gov/about/oei/index.htm: National Heart, Lung, and Blood Institute Obesity Education Initiative offers information on selecting a weight loss program, menu planning, food label reading, and BMI calculation and interpretation.
6. www.niddk.nih.gov/health/nutrit/win.htm: Weight Control Information Network has weight loss articles from the National Institutes of Health.
7. www.diet.com: Diet.com offers a subscription-based online program based on personal identification of eating, exercise, and coping lifestyle patterns. Coaching is available by a physician and registered dietitian. Includes interactive boards, chat rooms, recipes, and trackers.
8. www.eDiets.com: eDiets.com offers a subscription-based online diet, fitness, and counseling network providing a personal profile. Management team consists of licensed dietitians and psychologists.

9. www.Cyberdiet.com: Cyberdiet.com provides free planning for meals and an exercise profile designed by a registered dietitian.
10. www.Calorieking.com: Calorieking.com is a searchable database of over 40,000 foods and a diet and food tracker.
11. www.efit.com: efit.com is a free e-newsletter on nutrition tips. Also offers weight loss counseling services by a registered dietitian.
12. www.WebMD.com: WebMD.com offers an eating plan based on small changes to current reported eating behaviors, food preferences, and lifestyle. Staff includes a registered dietitian and exercise physiologists.
13. www.obesityhelp.com: Obesityhelp.com offers information for and by gastric bypass patients, and individuals considering weight loss surgery. All aspects of the surgical process are discussed, including insurance issues, as well as chat rooms and message boards.

REFERENCES

1. Choban, P.S., et al., A health status assessment of the impact of weight loss following Roux-en-Y gastric bypass for clinically severe obesity, *J Am Coll Surg,* 188, 491, 1999.
2. Buchwald, H., et al., Bariatric surgery: a systematic review and meta-analysis, *JAMA*, 292, 1724, 2004.
3. Sjostrom, L., et al., Lifestyle, diabetes, and cardiovascular risk factors 10 years after bariatric surgery, *N Engl J Med*, 351, 2683, 2004.
4. Clements, R.H., et al., Gastrointestinal symptoms are more intense in morbidly obese patients and are improved with laparoscopic Roux-en-Y gastric bypass, *Obes Surg*, 13, 610, 2003.
5. Foster, A., et al., Gastrointestinal symptomatic outcome after laparoscopic Roux-en-Y gastric bypass, *J Gastrointest Surg*, 7, 750, 2003.
6. Presutti, R.J., Gorman, R.S., and Swain, J.M., Primary care perspective on bariatric surgery, *Mayo Clin Proc*, 79, 1158, 2004.
7. Pandolfino, J.E., Krishnamoorthy, B., and Lee, T.J., Gastrointestinal complications of obesity surgery, *MedGenMed*, 6, 15, 2004.
8. Huang, C.S., et al., Endoscopic findings and their clinical correlations in patients with symptoms after gastric bypass surgery, *Gastrointest Endosc*, 58, 859, 2003.
9. Ukleja, A. and Stone, R.L., Medical and gastroenterologic management of the post-bariatric surgery patient, *J Clin Gastroenterol*, 38, 312, 2004.
10. Tu, B.N. and Kelly, K.A., Motility disorders after Roux-en-Y gastrojejunostomy, *Obes Surg*, 4, 219, 1994.
11. Hocking, M.P., et al., Jejunoileal bypass for morbid obesity. Late follow-up in 100 cases, *N Engl J Med*, 308, 995, 1983.
12. Hocking, M.P., et al., Long-term consequences after jejunoileal bypass for morbid obesity, *Dig Dis Sci*, 43, 2493, 1998.
13. Hasler, W.L., Dumping syndrome, *Curr Treat Options Gastroenterol*, 5, 139, 2002.
14. Vecht, J., Masclee, A.A., and Lamers, C.B., The dumping syndrome. Current insights into pathophysiology, diagnosis and treatment, *Scand J Gastroenterol Suppl*, 223, 21, 1997.
15. Ovrebo, K.K., et al., Gastroesophageal reflux in morbidly obese patients treated with gastric banding or vertical banded gastroplasty, *Ann Surg*, 228, 51, 1998.

16. Lundell, L., Ruth, M., and Olbe, L., Vertical banded gastroplasty or gastric banding for morbid obesity: effects on gastro-oesophageal reflux, *Eur J Surg*, 163, 525, 1997.
17. de Jong, J.R., et al., The influence of laparoscopic adjustable gastric banding on gastroesophageal reflux, *Obes Surg*, 14, 399, 2004.
18. Ortega, J., et al., Outcome of esophageal function and 24-hour esophageal pH monitoring after vertical banded gastroplasty and Roux-en-Y gastric bypass, *Obes Surg*, 14, 1086, 2004.
19. Capella, J.F. and Capella, R.F., Staple disruption and marginal ulceration in gastric bypass procedures for weight reduction, *Obes Surg*, 6, 44, 1996.
20. Capella, J.F. and Capella, R.F., Gastro-gastric fistulas and marginal ulcers in gastric bypass procedures for weight reduction, *Obes Surg*, 9, 22, 1999.
21. MacLean, L.D., et al., Stomal ulcer after gastric bypass, *J Am Coll Surg*, 185, 1, 1997.
22. Sanyal, A.J., et al., Stomal complications of gastric bypass: incidence and outcome of therapy, *Am J Gastroenterol*, 87, 1165, 1992.
23. Sapala, J.A., et al., Marginal ulcer after gastric bypass: a prospective 3-year study of 173 patients, *Obes Surg*, 8, 505, 1998.
24. Pope, G.D., et al., Peptic ulcer/stricture after gastric bypass: a comparison of technique and acid suppression variables, *Obes Surg*, 12, 30, 2002.
25. Schirmer, B., Erenoglu, C., and Miller, A., Flexible endoscopy in the management of patients undergoing Roux-en-Y gastric bypass, *Obes Surg*, 12, 634, 2002.
26. Jordan, J.H., et al., Marginal ulcer following gastric bypass for morbid obesity, *Am Surg*, 57, 286, 1991.
27. Braley, S.C., Nguyen, N.T., and Wolfe, B.M., Late gastrointestinal hemorrhage after gastric bypass, *Obes Surg*, 12, 404, 2002.
28. Byrne, T.K., Complications of surgery for obesity, *Surg Clin North Am*, 81, 1181, 2001.
29. Ahmad, J., et al., Endoscopic balloon dilation of gastroenteric anastomotic stricture after laparoscopic gastric bypass, *Endoscopy*, 35, 725, 2003.
30. Barba, C.A., et al., Endoscopic dilation of gastroesophageal anastomosis stricture after gastric bypass, *Surg Endosc*, 17, 416, 2003.
31. Sataloff, D.M., Lieber, C.P., and Seinige, U.L., Strictures following gastric stapling for morbid obesity. Results of endoscopic dilatation, *Am Surg*, 56, 167, 1990.
32. Kretzschmar, C.S., et al., Balloon dilation for the treatment of stomal stenosis complicating gastric surgery for morbid obesity, *Surgery*, 102, 443, 1987.
33. Blachar, A. and Federle, M.P., Gastrointestinal complications of laparoscopic Roux-en-Y gastric bypass surgery in patients who are morbidly obese: findings on radiography and CT, *AJR Am J Roentgenol*, 179, 1437, 2002.
34. Matthews, B.D., et al., Initial results with a stapled gastrojejunostomy for the laparoscopic isolated Roux-en-Y gastric bypass, *Am J Surg*, 179, 476, 2000.
35. Thompson, C.C., et al., Peroral endoscopic repair of staple-line dehiscence in Roux-en-Y gastric bypass: a less invasive approach [abstract], *Gastroenterology*, 126 (Suppl. 2), A, 2004.
36. Catalano, M.F., et al., Weight gain following bariatric surgery secondary to staple line disruption and stomal dilation: endotherapy using sodium morrhuate to induce stomal stenosis prevents need for surgical revision [abstract], *Gastrointest Endosc*, 59, AB149, 2004.
37. Greve, J.W., Surgical treatment of morbid obesity: role of the gastroenterologist, *Scand J Gastroenterol Suppl*, 60, 2000.
38. Abu-Abeid, S., et al., The clinical spectrum of band erosion following laparoscopic adjustable silicone gastric banding for morbid obesity, *Surg Endosc*, 17, 861, 2003.

39. Westling, A., et al., Silicone-adjustable gastric banding: disappointing results, *Obes Surg*, 8, 467, 1998.
40. Weiss, H., et al., Gastroscopic band removal after intragastric migration of adjustable gastric band: a new minimal invasive technique, *Obes Surg*, 10, 167, 2000.
41. Chaptini, L., et al., Successful endoscopic management of band erosion complicating gastric bypass surgery, *J Clin Gastroenterol*, 38, 914, 2004.
42. Felsher, J., Brodsky, J., and Brody, F., Small bowel obstruction after laparoscopic Roux-en-Y gastric bypass, *Surgery*, 134, 501, 2003.
43. Champion, J.K. and Williams, M., Small bowel obstruction and internal hernias after laparoscopic Roux-en-Y gastric bypass, *Obes Surg*, 13, 596, 2003.
44. Higa, K.D., Ho, T., and Boone, K.B., Internal hernias after laparoscopic Roux-en-Y gastric bypass: incidence, treatment and prevention, *Obes Surg*, 13, 350, 2003.
45. Nguyen, N.T., et al., Bowel obstruction after laparoscopic Roux-en-Y gastric bypass, *Obes Surg*, 14, 190, 2004.
46. Goitein, D., et al., Superior mesenteric artery syndrome after laparoscopic Roux-en-Y gastric bypass for morbid obesity, *Obes Surg*, 14, 1008, 2004.
47. Bocker, J., et al., Intussusception: an uncommon cause of postoperative small bowel obstruction after gastric bypass, *Obes Surg*, 14, 116, 2004.
48. Duane, T.M., Wohlgemuth, S., and Ruffin, K., Intussusception after Roux-en-Y gastric bypass, *Am Surg*, 66, 82, 2000.
49. Merkle, E.M., et al., Roux-en-Y gastric bypass for clinically severe obesity: normal appearance and spectrum of complications at imaging, *Radiology*, 2005.
50. Shiffman, M.L., et al., Gallstone formation after rapid weight loss: a prospective study in patients undergoing gastric bypass surgery for treatment of morbid obesity, *Am J Gastroenterol*, 86, 1000, 1991.
51. Fobi, M., et al., Prophylactic cholecystectomy with gastric bypass operation: incidence of gallbladder disease, *Obes Surg*, 12, 350, 2002.
52. Hamad, G.G., et al., Elective cholecystectomy during laparoscopic Roux-en-Y gastric bypass: is it worth the wait?, *Obes Surg*, 13, 76, 2003.
53. Sreenarasimhaiah, J., Prevention or surgical treatment of gallstones in patients undergoing gastric bypass surgery for obesity, *Curr Treat Options Gastroenterol*, 7, 99, 2004.
54. Miller, K., et al., Gallstone formation prophylaxis after gastric restrictive procedures for weight loss: a randomized double-blind placebo-controlled trial, *Ann Surg*, 238, 697, 2003.
55. Sugerman, H.J., et al., A multicenter, placebo-controlled, randomized, double-blind, prospective trial of prophylactic ursodiol for the prevention of gallstone formation following gastric-bypass-induced rapid weight loss, *Am J Surg*, 169, 91, 1995.
56. Requarth, J.A., et al., Long-term morbidity following jejunoileal bypass. The continuing potential need for surgical reversal, *Arch Surg*, 130, 318, 1995.
57. Markowitz, J.S., et al., Liver transplantation for decompensated cirrhosis after jejunoileal bypass: a strategy for management, *Transplantation*, 65, 570, 1998.
58. Avinoah, E., Ovnat, A., and Charuzi, I., Nutritional status seven years after Roux-en-Y gastric bypass surgery, *Surgery*, 111, 137, 1992.
59. Brolin, R.E., et al., Multivitamin prophylaxis in prevention of post-gastric bypass vitamin and mineral deficiencies, *Int J Obes*, 15, 661, 1991.
60. Halverson, J.D., Micronutrient deficiencies after gastric bypass for morbid obesity, *Am Surg*, 52, 594, 1986.
61. Brolin, R.E., et al., Prophylactic iron supplementation after Roux-en-Y gastric bypass: a prospective, double-blind, randomized study, *Arch Surg*, 133, 740, 1998.

62. Rhode, B.M., et al., Iron absorption and therapy after gastric bypass, *Obes Surg*, 9, 17, 1999.
63. Rhode, B.M., et al., Vitamin B-12 deficiency after gastric surgery for obesity, *Am J Clin Nutr*, 63, 103, 1996.
64. Schilling, R.F., Gohdes, P.N., and Hardie, G.H., Vitamin B12 deficiency after gastric bypass surgery for obesity, *Ann Intern Med*, 101, 501, 1984.
65. Simon, S.R., et al., Hematologic complications of gastric bypass for morbid obesity, *South Med J*, 82, 1108, 1989.
66. Brolin, R.E., et al., Are vitamin B12 and folate deficiency clinically important after Roux-en-Y gastric bypass?, *J Gastrointest Surg*, 2, 436, 1998.
67. Mason, M.E., Jalagani, H., and Vinik, A.I., Metabolic complications of bariatric surgery: diagnosis and management issues, *Gastroenterol Clin North Am*, 34, 25, 2005.
68. Angstadt, J.D. and Bodziner, R.A., Peripheral polyneuropathy from thiamine deficiency following laparoscopic Roux-en-Y gastric bypass, *Obes Surg*, 15, 890, 2005.
69. Nautiyal, A., Singh, S., and Alaimo, D.J., Wernicke encephalopathy — an emerging trend after bariatric surgery, *Am J Med*, 117, 804, 2004.
70. Salas-Salvado, J., et al., Wernicke's syndrome after bariatric surgery, *Clin Nutr*, 19, 371, 2000.
71. Slater, G.H., et al., Serum fat-soluble vitamin deficiency and abnormal calcium metabolism after malabsorptive bariatric surgery, *J Gastrointest Surg*, 8, 48, 2004.
72. Coates, P.S., et al., Gastric bypass surgery for morbid obesity leads to an increase in bone turnover and a decrease in bone mass, *J Clin Endocrinol Metab*, 89, 1061, 2004.
73. Collazo-Clavell, M.L., et al., Osteomalacia after Roux-en-Y gastric bypass, *Endocr Pract*, 10, 195, 2004.
74. Goode, L.R., et al., Bone and gastric bypass surgery: effects of dietary calcium and vitamin D, *Obes Res*, 12, 40, 2004.
75. Goldner, W.S., et al., Severe metabolic bone disease as a long-term complication of obesity surgery, *Obes Surg*, 12, 685, 2002.
76. Shaker, J.L., et al., Secondary hyperparathyroidism and osteopenia in women following gastric exclusion surgery for obesity, *Osteoporos Int*, 1, 177, 1991.

9 Follow-Up Strategies for the Treatment of Obesity in Primary Care Settings

Valerie H. Myers and Donna H. Ryan

CONTENTS

9.1 THE KEY ROLE OF PRIMARY CARE PROVIDERS IN OBESITY MANAGEMENT

Primary care providers and allied health care professionals play an important role in addressing behavioral risk factors, prevention, and chronic disease management in the general population [1] and are a critical source of health risk advice for most individuals [2,3]. Specifically, survey data suggest that over 80% of adults between the ages of 18 and 64 report having a usual source of care when they are sick or are in need of health advice [4], and greater than 40% of adults over the age of 40 have had the same physician for longer than five years [5]. Most adults visit a physician more than twice per year [6,7]. Estimates suggest that primary care physicians treat over 11% of the U.S. population each month [8], and obesity is one of the most common presenting chronic conditions to these clinics [9]. Notably, one study found that obesity-related physician visits have increased by over 80% in the past few years alone [10].

Most patients report valuing the advice and guidance that their physician provides, and advice from a health care provider is a powerful predictor of patient behavior change [11,12]. However, despite the frequency of attendance of individuals seeking treatment from their primary care physician and the significant influence that physician advice has on many patients, it remains uncommon for physicians to advise overweight patients to lose weight [13]. Specifically, several studies have found that estimates of patient self-report for their physician advising them to lose weight remains low (e.g., 5 to 42%) [14–17], and most physicians do not counsel on diet or exercise [13,18]. Thus, it is not currently the norm for primary care providers to initiate weight loss, much less be concerned with sustaining the weight loss effort or achieving rescue from relapse to weight gain.

Because obesity-related health expenditures are approximately 6% of total health care costs in the U.S. [19] and primary care clinics offer a logical and conventional setting to implement primary and secondary obesity prevention interventions, there has been a recent push in public health policy to recognize the importance that primary care settings have in combating the obesity epidemic. As a result, there has been an increase in calls for action for physician-delivered weight loss interventions by the American Medical Association, the American Academy of Family Physicians, and the Surgeon General [9,20,21].

9.2 PHYSICIAN-DELIVERED OBESITY-COUNSELING STUDIES: EVIDENCE FOR SUCCESS

The use of the primary care setting to monitor patients' weight, give educational materials and referrals, and manage weight-related comorbidities has been the focus of several systematic studies [22]. The results of these physician-delivered obesity-counseling studies are promising. For example, studies have demonstrated that weight management interventions delivered by the physician alone [23,24], or in combination with specific dietary interventions, can produce weight losses [25–27]. Concise educational materials and interactive instructional methods (e.g., modeling, role-playing) have demonstrated improvement in physician weight-counseling skills [28]. After receiving behavior training, physicians have reported improved patient response to weight counseling, increased physician self-confidence, and improved quality and frequency of weight management recommendations [9,29,30].

There are a number of studies documenting the effectiveness of nutritional counseling for weight loss in primary care settings [31]. However, the majority of these studies have not utilized the primary care physician solely. Rather, most of these studies have used a combination of health educators, nurses, or dietitians. Traditionally, registered dietitians have been the primary source of nutritional counseling, and only a few studies have compared the effectiveness of physicians and other health care providers to dietitians in weight loss counseling. In one clinical study, Ashley and colleagues [32] reported a 26-session dietitian-led group counseling intervention, which was compared with the dietitian-led counseling or physicians' sessions with meal replacements. Notably, this trial revealed that shortened counseling sessions with a health care provider (10 to 15 min duration) combined with meal replacements led to similar degrees of weight loss as the hour-long dietitian-led group sessions. Both were superior to dietitian-led counseling alone. This suggests that health care providers can be effective, especially if teamed with effective tools such as meal replacements. It also demonstrates that physicians and other allied health care professionals can be trained effectively in weight loss counseling. We are optimistic that in the future, primary care providers will routinely engage in office-based obesity prevention and weight loss management for overweight and obese individuals.

9.3 STRATEGIES FOR FOLLOW-UP: THE CHRONIC CARE MODEL

Two issues require discussion in any review of follow-up strategies. The first is the issue of follow-up of those who are undergoing a weight loss effort, and the second is the issue of follow-up of those individuals who are seeking to maintain weight following a successful weight loss effort. Both of these discussions relate to understanding obesity as a chronic disease and its treatment as a chronic care model.

9.3.1 "Chronic Care" Model and the Five As of Counseling

One strategy for treating obesity is to view it as a chronic disease [33]. Obesity is similar to other chronic conditions in its course. Therefore, treatment approaches that focus on preventing and/or managing obesity rather than "curing" it may be more effective [34]. This would require implementing strategies that have been successful with other chronic diseases, such as frequent assessment, continuity of care, and long-term access to viable treatments [34]. For example, the U.S. Preventative Services Task Force (USPSTF) Counseling and Behavioral Interventions Work Group recently recommended the adoption of the "5A's" as a conceptual framework for evaluating and describing health behavioral counseling in primary care [35]. The 5A's framework is derived from the "4A's" approach used successfully in the smoking cessation literature. The 5A's consists of the following elements: Assess, Advise, Agree, Assist, and Arrange (see Table 9.1). "Assess" refers to assessment of patients' behaviors including their knowledge, attitudes, and beliefs. This step identifies who may be in need of

TABLE 9.1
The Five A's of Counseling

Assess: assessment of patients' behaviors, including their knowledge, attitudes, and beliefs	Providers should assess their patients' risk of obesity-related conditions and identify obesity-related comorbidities and risk factors for cardiovascular disease (CVD)
Advise: provider advice should be personalized, supportive, and relevant to the patient's symptoms and concerns	Providers should advise patients on how to design a weight loss program individually tailored to their needs. For those patients who are not ready to initiate a weight loss program, providers should counsel on maintaining weight, and preventing more weight gain
Agree: emphasizes collaboration between provider and patient; weight management goals and outcomes to measure target goals should be established	Providers and patients should mutually agree on the course of the treatment program including medically appropriate and realistic weight loss goals
Assist: behavioral counseling for a target behavior, problem-solving, barriers to success, and increasing self-efficacy in the patient	Providers should assist patients in implementing appropriate lifestyle modification interventions, such as dietary reduction and physical activity promotion, as well as continually monitoring levels of motivation to continue weight loss efforts; during this step, the provider may be inclined to refer to other health professionals who may be specialists in other health domains
Arrange: establishing the frequency and duration of subsequent contacts with the primary care team	Providers should arrange for regular follow-up and continually monitor progress of target goals; providers and patients should develop weight maintenance plans and relapse prevention programs; providers should also continue to reinforce patient efforts and offer long-term support

Source: Adapted from Whitlock et al., *Am. J. Prev. Med.,*22, 267, 2002; Serdula et al., *JAMA,*289, 1747, 2003.

behavioral counseling and will allow tailoring of treatment. "Advise" is supported by the literature in that the provider has a powerful impact on his/her patient. In this step, provider advice should be personalized, supportive, and relevant to the patient's symptoms and concerns. "Agree" is the conceptual step that emphasizes collaboration between provider and patient. In this step, both patient and physician identify target weight management goals and establish measures to define the outcomes of the target goals. The "Assist" step incorporates behavioral counseling for a target behavior, problem-solving, barriers to success, and increasing self-efficacy in the patient. During this step, the provider may be inclined to refer to other health professionals who may be specialists in a certain domain (e.g., nutritional counseling, behavior change). Finally, the "Arrange" step involves establishing the frequency and duration of subsequent contacts with the primary care team. This step can include follow-up visits in multiple formats, including face-to-face, telephone, or Internet interventions [1].

9.3.2 Follow-Up Care: A Three-Stage Approach

After an initial evaluation and assessment of health risk and need for weight loss, the physician should follow a three-stage approach to a weight management program (see Table 9.2) [21]. In stage one, the provider should discuss the prevention of further weight gain with the patient. This stage is helpful for the patient with lower health risk, or the patient who may be prepared to only attempt a minor lifestyle change at the present time. The second stage is utilized with those patients who are ready to attempt a weight loss intervention. This stage involves multiple components and is the core of a weight loss program. Overall goals in this stage are to establish weight goals and provide dietary and physical activity management. The third stage is the weight maintenance stage. This stage is reached after the patient has attained the goal weight. This stage consists of continued lifestyle change for long-term weight maintenance.

TABLE 9.2
Three-Stage Approach to Weight Management

Stage	Target Population	Overview
1: Prevention of weight gain	Patients with lower health risk or patients committed to only making minor lifestyle changes	Discuss the benefits and importance of prevention of future weight gain; prevention requires the use of lifestyle modification; patients may feel less threatened if focused on making small steps toward improved health, rather than focusing on specific weight loss goals
2: Active weight loss	Patients who are low to moderate risk and are ready to attempt active weight loss	Encourage a 5 to 10% reduction in weight; establish specific weight goals and dietary and physical activity management approaches; incorporate behavioral techniques, such as self-monitoring, stimulus control, goal setting, cognitive restructuring, and problem solving
3: Weight loss maintenance	Patients who have successfully met weight loss goals	Encourage continued long-term maintenance of behavior change through use of ongoing lifestyle interventions; focus on continued monitoring of diet and physical activity; provide ongoing encouragement and support even after weight goals have been met

Source: Adapted from American Medical Association, *Assessment and Management of Adult Obesity: A Primer for Physicians,* American Medical Association, Atlanta, 2003.

9.4 FOLLOW-UP DURING THE WEIGHT LOSS EFFORT

Patients who have initiated a weight loss regimen should be seen for an office visit within 2 to 4 weeks of initiating treatment, in order to monitor the treatment side effects and effectiveness [36]. Monthly visits are appropriate for the first 3 mo after beginning treatment, provided weight loss is favorable and there are few side effects [36]. More frequent visits are based on the medical judgment of the physician, particularly in cases where the patient has comorbidities that may be adversely affected by weight loss. This is especially true in the case of diabetes, where medications must be actively managed (reduced) to prevent hypoglycemia during negative energy balance. Each visit should include a weigh-in and measurement of blood pressure and pulse. Height is measured only annually. Waist circumference and blood lipids should be reevaluated much less frequently. Results of these measures can be motivating for patients. Visits should incorporate monitoring compliance with food and exercise diaries, setting new goals, and providing support and encouragement.

There are no well-established guidelines for the frequency of visits and for duration of behavior change programs in the primary care setting. However, previous studies of physician-directed change programs [30] and optimal time recommendations for dietary therapy [33] suggest that at least 6 mo of regular follow-up may prove helpful. This corresponds well with the literature on the effectiveness of behavioral weight loss programs over the past three decades. Specifically, in the 1970s, behavioral treatment for weight loss typically lasted 8 to 10 weeks and resulted in 8 to 9 lb losses. In the 1980s, there was an increased focus on improving weight loss results. Treatment was lengthened to 13 to 16 sessions and results improved to 15 to 22 lb losses [37]. In a review of the literature, Foreyt and Goodrick [38] found that the average duration of the behavioral program was 18 weeks, with weight losses of 9.9 kg (0.5 kg per week) and an attrition rate of less than 15%. In a review by Williamson and Perrin [39], length of treatment increased to 20 weeks and follow-up to 43 weeks between the years 1991 and 1995; however, weight loss remained fairly stable. In another review, behavioral programs lasted typically 15 to 24 weeks, and were delivered in a group format with an average weight loss of 8.5 kg [40]. In a recent review by Wadden and colleagues [41], the authors noted that between the early 1970s and more recent studies (1996 to 2002), three decades later, the amount of weight loss reported in behavioral programs has nearly tripled. This review revealed that treatments in 1974 lasted 8.4 weeks, with a mean weight loss of 3.8 kg. Behavioral treatment studies between 1996 and 2002 lasted an average of 31.6 weeks and produced an average weight loss of 10.7 kg. Notably, this increase in weight loss corresponds to a nearly threefold increase in the duration of treatment. The authors concluded that the most parsimonious explanation for the observed improvement in weight loss is the longer duration of treatment. Comparisons of studies with individual and group treatment modalities suggest that group therapy produces greater weight loss than individual therapy [42]. Other studies have suggested that the intensity of the medical and behavioral approaches can influence the amount of weight loss (see Table 9.3) [43–46]. More recently, the focus of behavior therapy in weight loss has been on long-term maintenance and improving the effects of other weight loss strategies, such as low-calorie diets (LCD)

TABLE 9.3
Effectiveness of Weight Loss Approaches

Treatment	Effectiveness	Annual Cost Estimates
Commercial (Weight Watchers)	6% at 6 mo	$12/week; $624/yr
Behavioral programs	8–10% at 6 mo	$800/yr group; $1700/yr individual
Meal replacement (SlimFast)	8% at 3 mo	$12/week; $624/yr
Medically supervised liquid diet	15–25% at 4 mo	$3000/6 mo; $6000/yr
Pharmacotherapy (sibutramine/orlistat)	7–10% at 6 mo	$1100–$1350/yr
Combined behavior programs/medication	16% at 6 mo	$1900–$3000/yr
Gastric surgery	25–30% at 6–12 mo	$25,000 surgery + $1200/yr for the next 6 yr

Source: Adapted from data based on Wolf A.M. et al., *Obesity: Mechanisms and Clinical Management*, Eckel, R.H., Ed., Lippincott Williams & Wilkins, Philadelphia, 523–549, 2003; Agren, G., et al., *Int. J. Obes.*, 26, 184–192, 2002; NHLBI, *The Practical Guide to the Identification, Evaluation, and Treatment of Overweight and Obesity in Adults.* Bethesda, MD: National Institutes of Health; NIH Publication No. 00-4084, 2000; Wadden, T.A. and Osei, S., in *Handbook of Obesity Treatment*, Wadden, T.A. and Stunkard, A.J., Eds., The Guilford Press, New York, 242, 2002.

and medication. For example, intensive medical approaches using combined elements, such as group and individual behavior therapy, very-low-calorie and structured diets, increased physical activity, and medications have been shown to produce weight loss exceeding 16% [47,48].

9.5 FOLLOW-UP DURING MAINTENANCE FOLLOWING WEIGHT LOSS

Most active weight loss occurs in the initial 6 mo of treatment [49]. However, maintaining weight loss remains a challenge. In one review of the treatment literature, weight regain can consume as much as 35 to 40% of initial loss [49]. Most opinion leaders argue that exercise or regular physical activity is the most critical factor during the maintenance period [50,51]. Specifically, individuals who are more physically active are more likely to maintain weight loss. The amount of physical activity optimal for weight loss maintenance is more than the 30 min three times a week, recommended for cardiovascular health. Findings suggest that either alone or in combination with other treatment modalities, physical activity that expends 1500 to 2000 kcal/week is necessary to maintain weight loss [51]. In one study, individuals who engaged in an average of 280 min of exercise per week had more weight maintenance [52].

There are several studies of short- and long-term follow-up that suggest the benefits of continued physical activity during weight maintenance. One study with five-year follow-up data on patients losing 12 kg during an acute weight loss period found that 89% of patients maintained their weight loss through increased exercise and dietary attention [50]. Fifty to sixty percent success rates for maintenance of weight loss over a two-year period have been found when caloric restriction and increased physical activity were utilized [53]. A meta-analysis by Miller and colleagues [54] replicated that diet, in combination with exercise, tended to be the superior approach to weight maintenance, compared to diet or exercise alone (8.6 kg, 6.6 kg, 6.1 kg, respectively) at one-year follow-up [54]. Additionally, another review investigating long-term maintenance effects of dietary restriction and exercise demonstrated consistency among all studies, where maintenance of weight loss occurred in conditions that promoted physical activity [55]. Another review of randomized clinical trials with at least one-year follow-up data concluded that exercise, in combination with diet, was more effective for weight loss than diet alone [56]. Furthermore, it was concluded that light exercise (e.g., calisthenics, stretching) may be as effective as moderate exercise, albeit without the cardiorespiratory benefits of moderate exercise. The evidence is thus strong, supporting exercise in combination with caloric restriction as more effective than exercise or diet alone. However, studies to determine the ideal duration, intensity, and regularity of exercise need further exploration.

The National Weight Control Registry (NWCR) is a database of people who have self-reported a weight loss of 30 lb or more and kept it off for at least a year. The average NWCR participant has lost about 60 lb and kept it off for about five years. This self-identified sample recruited from health and weight magazines has been studied to identify parameters associated with successful weight loss. Specifically, NWCR registrants exhibit far greater activity than the general population and report burning an average of 2800 cal a week through exercise [57].

Given the fact that NWCR participants with long-term weight loss success appear to engage in two significant changes: (1) reduction in dietary intake primarily related to dietary fat, and (2) physical activity enough to expend >2500 cal/day [58], the health care provider should actively encourage continuing dietary modification and physical activity promotion during the weight maintenance period, and the focus should be strong for the first 6 mo after the 6-mo visit. The physician should develop a plan, in collaboration with the patient, whereby the patient will weigh frequently, and if weight regain occurs (5 lb), the patient should return for active intervention. Long-term monitoring from the provider can prolong the maintenance of effects and improve chances of long-term success.

9.6 OVERVIEW OF BEHAVIORAL TECHNIQUES OF IMPORTANCE IN FOLLOW-UP SESSIONS

If health care providers are to be effective agents of change in counseling for weight management, they must be knowledgeable in behavioral techniques. Provided below is a brief review of the key behavioral strategies (see Table 9.4) [41,59,60].

TABLE 9.4
Behavioral Strategies for Weight Loss and Maintenance

Behavioral Strategy	Overview
Goal setting	Set specific goals for diet, exercise, and other targeted behaviors; goals should be realistic, attainable, and measurable; establish realistic short-term and long-term goals; goals for weight maintenance include losing small amounts of weight as small increases in weight occur and increasing overall levels of physical activity
Self-monitoring	The "cornerstone" of behavioral treatment: helps to increase awareness and identify unhelpful eating and physical activity patterns, and involves monitoring of all eating and physical activity behaviors on a daily basis (i.e., food and fitness diaries); regular weighing should also be recommended; the physician should review the records regularly to assist with problem-solving and to spot pitfalls
Stimulus control	Stimulus control techniques target environmental antecedents that influence eating or exercise patterns; these techniques are helpful in avoiding and modifying high-risk situations that may initiate relapse or prompt maladaptive eating or sedentary behavior; strategies can include eating three meals a day, eating at the same time or place, or changing serving and food storage
Modification of eating and activity patterns/nutrition	Goal is to alter maladaptive eating and activity behaviors that may lead to excessive eating or reduced physical activity; strategies exist for both eating behavior (i.e., slowing down the pace of eating, portion control, etc) and sedentary behavior (i.e., encouraging more physical activity into daily routine)
Contingency management	Encourage positive reinforcement for adaptive weight management behaviors and recommend the elimination of food rewards early on in the weight loss phase; behavioral contracting with the physician may also be used to gain social reinforcements; replace tangible rewards for weight loss with intangible or internal rewards prior to beginning maintenance
Cognitive behavioral strategies	A combination of traditional behavioral techniques and examination of thinking patterns associated with eating and physical activity patterns; goal is to improve mood, alter irrational beliefs/standards, and correct negative self-evaluations that may be affecting eating and activity behaviors; the physician should continually monitor the patient for high levels of self-criticism and negative thinking, which may act as a trigger for relapse
Stress management	Goal of stress management is to reduce arousal and provide distraction from stressful events; strategies include progressive muscle relaxation, diaphragmatic breathing, and meditation

Source: Adapted from American Medical Association, *Assessment and Management of Adult Obesity: A Primer for Physicians,* American Medical Association, Atlanta, 2003.; Wadden, T.A. et al., *Obes. Res.,* 12, 151S, 2004.; Wadden, T.A., *Baillieres Best Pract. Res. Clin. Endocrinol. Metab.,* 13, 93, 1999. and Foreyt, J.P. and Poston, W.S.C., *Obes. Res.,* 6, 18S, 1998.

9.6.1 Goal Setting

Patients should set goals for diet (i.e., calories, fat), exercise, and other targeted behaviors, which will be beneficial to preventing weight regain. Principles of behavior theory suggest that goals should be realistic, attainable, and objectively measured. Therefore, realistic short-term and long-term goals should be discussed in order to maintain behavior change. Goals for weight maintenance include losing small amounts of weight, as small increases in weight occur, and increasing overall levels of physical activity.

9.6.2 Self-Monitoring

This technique is considered the "cornerstone" of behavioral treatment and involves monitoring of all eating and physical activity behaviors on a daily basis. We recommend weighing weekly during the active weight loss phase, and daily during maintenance. Self-monitoring is utilized to increase awareness of behavior patterns and to identify unhelpful eating and physical activity patterns. Food and activity diaries are the cornerstone of weight loss efforts and can be reinitiated if weight regain occurs. Patients should be encouraged to write down as much information as possible, including recording date, time, and place of eating and activity behaviors, any antecedents to the behavior, and quantity of eating and activity behaviors. The health care providers should review the records to spot pitfalls. The provider should emphasize the importance of self-monitoring during times of weight regain or increased stress, during holidays or periods when maintaining the lifestyle changes are particularly difficult, or when patients are feeling less control over their newly acquired healthful behaviors.

9.6.3 Stimulus Control

Many people are unaware of the impact that their environment has on their behaviors. Stimulus control techniques are used to amend environmental antecedents that influence eating or exercise patterns. The goal of stimulus control is to restrict everyday life circumstances that prompt maladaptive eating or sedentary behavior. Stimulus control strategies can include eating three meals a day, eating at the same time or place, changing serving, and food storage. The goal of weight maintenance is mastery. Therefore, during weight maintenance, the patient should be encouraged to learn to eat troublesome foods in a controlled manner and encouraged to create new, healthier food choices. Stimulus control techniques are helpful in avoiding and modifying high-risk situations that may induce relapse.

9.6.4 Modification of Eating and Activity Patterns/Nutrition

The goal of these techniques is to alter maladaptive eating and activity behaviors that may lead to excessive eating or reduced physical activity. Common strategies include slowing down the pace of eating, portion control, leaving food on plate, measuring food quantity, improving food choices, and eliminating second servings. Additionally, nutrition education on healthy eating is provided. Sedentary behaviors are targeted by increasing efforts to incorporate more physical activity into daily routine (i.e., taking stairs, parking car further out, walking rather than driving) and by increasing programmed/regular exercise. Patients should be encouraged to continue to use modified eating and activity patterns until the newly acquired adaptive behaviors are mastered.

9.6.5 Contingency Management

Positive reinforcement is used to acquire and stabilize new weight management behaviors. Strategies focus on providing positive reinforcing consequences for the development or implementation of targeted behavior changes. Patients are encouraged to eliminate all food rewards and develop other sources of motivation. Behavioral contracting with the physician or other health provider may also be used to gain social reinforcements. Contracting is beneficial, because it (1) makes the patient involved in his/her treatment, (2) reduces forgetfulness and disagreement on goals, and (3) provides information on how rewards are to be earned on the basis of successful completion of a targeted goal. Weight loss is greatly reinforcing and many patients will receive encouragement and accolades during their acute weight loss period. Often times, maintenance of the weight lost can be less reinforcing (e.g., fewer compliments from spouse, friends, or coworkers). Therefore, it is critical to begin replacing tangible rewards for weight loss (e.g., buying yourself something special, monetary reward) with intangible or internal rewards prior to beginning maintenance. Intangible rewards are longer lasting, because they become more internally focused (e.g., feeling good about yourself and what you are doing, the benefits of what you are doing, etc.).

9.6.6 Cognitive Behavioral Strategies

Cognitive behavioral strategies are a combination of traditional behavioral techniques and examination of thinking patterns associated with eating and physical activity patterns. The goal of this strategy is to improve mood, alter irrational beliefs/standards, and correct negative self-evaluations that may be affecting eating and activity behaviors by systematically questioning and improving negative thought statements. These techniques may also include stress management and assertiveness training to improve resilience to high-risk situations. During weight maintenance, the provider should continually monitor for high levels of self-criticism and negative thinking on the part of the patient, which may act as a trigger for relapse.

9.6.7 Stress Management

The goal of stress management is to reduce arousal and provide distraction from stressful events. Strategies include progressive muscle relaxation, diaphragmatic breathing, and meditation. Stress management is a critical tool with regards to relapse prevention. Therefore, the provider should continue to encourage these skills during maintenance in order to reduce triggers and high-risk situations that may provoke relapse.

9.7 THE TOOLBOX APPROACH

In our experience, the best follow-up strategy is to avoid a rigid treatment protocol, but rather to adopt a "toolbox approach," where a variety of different treatment schemes are available and may be implemented on the basis of provider and patient preferences. We employ a variety of dietary strategies, behavioral strategies, physical activity strategies, and referral to commercial programs, depending on our patients' needs and desires.

9.7.1 Dietary Strategies

The general goal for dietary modification is overall reduction of calories. Traditionally, the recommended diet for weight loss has been a low-fat diet (less than 30% fat) [61,62], and traditional dietary counseling has promoted moderate reduction of calories (e.g., daily caloric deficit of 500 to 1000 kcal) to achieve a steady weight loss of 1 to 2 lb per week. Caloric needs are generally different for men and women. Therefore, our practice is to encourage women to consume between 1200 to 1500 kcal/day in order to produce a 1 lb-per-week weight loss, whereas we advise men to consume between 1500 and 1800 kcal/day [45]. The traditional strategy includes teaching about calorie content of different foods, food composition (i.e., fats, carbohydrates, and proteins), reading nutrition labels, types of foods to buy, and how to prepare foods.

Traditional dietary recommendations are useful and effective; however, we believe it is acceptable for health care providers to utilize other pragmatic dietary approaches in order to assist in recharging weight loss efforts. For example, portion control strategies (e.g., meal replacements) have documented success in weight loss. Meal replacements are portion- and calorie-controlled foods typically in the form of drinks or bars that are intended to replace a meal. Meal replacements have grown in public popularity for a number of reasons, including their effectiveness, taste, simplicity, and ease of obtaining, preparing, and transporting. A meta-analysis of meal replacement in weight management found that participants prescribed either meal replacement or calorie-reduced diet lost significant amounts of weight at 3 mo and 1 yr follow-up compared to controls [63]. Notably, those receiving meal replacement lost significantly more weight compared to those on a reduced calorie diet. Meal replacement participants lost 7 to 8% of body weight compared to 3 to 7% lost by the reduced calorie group. Other studies have also found significant weight losses. Heber [64] found weight losses of approximately 17 lb at 12 to 24 weeks (males and females respectively), which was maintained for up to 2 yr. Another study found meal replacement participants lost 16 lb at 12 weeks, while those prescribed a calorie-restricted diet lost 3 lb [65].

Compliance has been shown to play a major role in weight loss success through meal replacement [64,65]. Simplified meal plans can decrease meal planning, reduce delays in preparing food, and do not rely on restriction of foods [66]. Therefore, meal replacements can act as a valuable stimulus control and technique for relapse prevention. Meal replacements are an easy alternative to skipping meals, are nutritionally balanced, and appear to be a promising tool for weight loss and maintenance.

Portion control diets are flexible and malleable, given the needs and goals of the patient. Providers can determine the extent of the portion-controlled diet required during the acute weight loss phase (e.g., two meal replacements and portion-controlled snacks, and one structured meal), and then encourage meal replacement as needed in the maintenance phase (e.g., single meal replacement daily).

Another pragmatic approach to weight loss is the use of alternative diets. Our patients frequently express an interest in such popular alternative diets such as the low-carbohydrate, high-protein diets. Health care providers must stay abreast of all the popular diets. We keep an open mind about these approaches and generally tolerate them as acceptable approaches to "recharging" weight loss efforts, as long as we consider them safe. Studies have shown that when calories are maintained in a constant manner, fat loss is identical, regardless of the macronutrient composition [67]. Low-carbohydrate, high-fat diets limit food choices, which may account for their success. It appears that the macronutrient focus may help patients alter the food environment and they seem to help some people consume fewer calories in an environment that promotes overconsumption.

Also to consider is emerging evidence that the low-carbohydrate approach may not be so harmful and may be modestly effective. One study evaluated obese men and women over the course of a year, comparing a low-carbohydrate, high-protein diet to a conventional high-carbohydrate, low-fat diet [68]. Results demonstrated greater weight loss for the high-protein, low-carbohydrate diet at months 3 and 6 (7% vs. 3.2%), but the difference was not significant at year 1. Notably, lipid improvements were found with the low-carbohydrate diet. Six-month results from another study revealed that the low-carbohydrate/high-fat diet group had greater weight loss (5.6 kg vs. 1.9 kg) and greater reduction in insulin and triglycerides than the high-carbohydrate/low-fat diet [69]. Other studies have found similar results in obese women [70] and adolescents [71]. Although these studies draw attention to the lack of detrimental changes in lipids on a low-carbohydrate/high-fat diet, another study has completed a more sophisticated evaluation of lipids [72]. This study suggests that for individuals with atherosclerotic cardiovascular disease, a low-carbohydrate/high-saturated-fat diet resulted in a significant decrease in body weight and triglycerides, and an increase in HDL and LDL particle size. More sophisticated testing has shown that *de novo* lipogenesis was less on a low-carbohydrate/high-fat diet compared to a high-carbohydrate/low-fat diet [73].

In sum, alternative dietary strategies may be beneficial for certain patients. Therefore, the health care provider is encouraged to evaluate the benefits and costs of introducing an alternative dietary approach for the patient. We consider some of the popular diets to be tools, just as meal replacements are, and we implement these alternative strategies on a case-by-case basis.

9.7.2 Commercial Weight Loss Programs

Commercial weight loss programs are a popular choice for many individuals attempting to lose weight, and we do refer patients to some of these. Weight Watchers International is the largest commercial weight loss program and its efficacy is supported by published data [74]. Successful participants have been studied, and results from one study suggest that 37% of these individuals have maintained their goal weight for 5 yr [75]. An additional study demonstrated that 19.4% of "lifetime members" were within 5 lb of their goal weight, 5 yr posttreatment [76]. A 2-yr multicenter randomized clinical trial compared a structured Weight Watchers program to a self-help group condition consisting of two brief nutritional counseling sessions and self-help materials [77]. After 1 yr, participants in the Weight Watchers condition had lost significantly more weight than those in the self-help group, 4.3 and 1.3 kg, respectively. At 2 yr follow-up, the commercial weight loss participants' weight loss was significantly greater than in the self-help group, 2.9 kg and 0.2 kg, respectively [77]. Weight Watchers is popular because it is economical, provides social support, and is effective, if followed.

In a recent meta-analysis, Tsai and Wadden [78] reviewed randomized trials of 12-week duration, which included a commercial weight loss component. In addition to the Weight Watchers data, these authors evaluated medically supervised, very-low-calorie diet programs and found that patients who completed treatment lost approximately 15 to 25% of their initial weight. However, these programs were associated with high costs, high attrition, and high weight regain. Still, commercial programs may be a promising alternative for some patients and are a "tool" to consider.

9.7.3 Self-Monitoring Tools

Food diaries are useful tools and have demonstrated weight loss facilitation [79]. They assist patients by helping them learn more about their nutrition and dietary habits (e.g., "what, when and why" they eat). Patients should be encouraged to write down everything they eat, when they eat, and how much they eat, as soon as they consume something, in order to prevent forgetting. Patients should be reminded to record all food and drink that is consumed, including snacks and soft drinks. Ideally, the physician should introduce the food diary to the patient and model its use with an example of the patient's previous meal. The physician should encourage the patient to use the food diary daily and review the food records at the next scheduled visit. This will assist the physician by providing information on the amounts and types of food consumed, as well as clarifying eating patterns that may be modifiable (i.e., eating while watching television, skipping, meals, etc.) [80].

Physicians should also encourage patients to weigh themselves regularly. Data from the National Weight Control Registry suggest that 75% of successful maintainers of weight loss weighed themselves at least once a week [57].

9.7.4 Physical Activity Tools

When discussing behavioral targets for physical activity with a patient, the physician should target reducing sedentary behavior and increasing lifestyle physical activity. Physicians should educate patients on the benefits of increased physical activity, including improvements in general health and life expectancy, as well as the specific benefits that exercise may promote for the patient's personal health status. Furthermore, physicians should educate patients on the fact that any exercise is better than none [81].

Initially, physicians should encourage patients to document their physical activity levels using self-monitoring techniques (e.g., physical activity diary). Next, the physician should discuss initiating a walking program. Walking is a useful and common form of physical activity [82]. Patients should be instructed to begin with 15 to 30 min a day at a comfortable pace. If this goal is too cumbersome, encourage patients to begin with a 5-min walk at a slower pace, with the goal of gradually progressing to more time and intensity. If the patient reports time constraints, suggest to the patient that he/she attempt a 5-min walk three times a day. After 1 to 2 weeks, review the physical activity record with the patient, and encourage an increase in physical activity time (additional 5 min), and intensity (increased pace, swinging arms, etc.). The physician may want to inquire about social support level (i.e., friends, family) who may be beneficial in encouraging or participating with the patient in exercise. The physician should also emphasize finding additional opportunities for increasing physical activity other than walking. This can include taking the stairs rather than the elevator, parking the car further out in the lot, gardening, substituting a day of walking for another form of fun exercise, playing with children/grandchildren, and making television time an active time (e.g., walking during commercials).

Physical activity can be measured objectively by a pedometer. A pedometer is a device about the size of a pager that is worn around the waist, and can be attached to a belt or waistband. Pedometers record the number of steps taken based on the body's movement, and can be a great motivational tool for many patients. Analog pedometers measure the number of steps taken, whereas digital pedometers can measure distances walked and calories burned. Pedometers are available for a relatively nominal amount, and can be easily obtained through a number of stores and on-line resources. Since a pedometer is an objective measure, it is not subject to the biases associated with self-reported physical activity assessments. However, pedometers are limited in that they only assess physical activity during the time the patient is wearing the device. Therefore, patients should be encouraged to wear and monitor their pedometer daily. All patients should be given instructions on how to properly use a pedometer, how to monitor their daily steps, and encouraged to take 10,000 steps a day [83,84].

In addition to encouraging the use of self-monitoring tools and pedometers for physical activity, we also promote the use of programmed exercise at local health clubs, and the use of professional trainers. Providers may find it useful to have a referral and resource list of local professionals and facilities dedicated to physical activity promotion available for dissemination to patients.

9.7.5 The Office Visit Is a Tool

Anderson and Wadden [81] suggest that providers should evaluate patients every 3 mo to assess changes in physical health, and discuss progress in dietary and activity changes (reiterate goals, establish new goals, document behavior change attempts, etc.). Additionally, they suggest that it may be helpful to set aside a designated block of time each week (e.g., Mondays from 4:00 to 5:00) for 2-min visits for patients who wish to weigh-in and have food and exercise diaries reviewed. It is suggested that these brief visits can provide a continual and helpful contact with patients in a cost-effective manner.

9.7.6 Pharmacotherapy

Medication management is a key element in managing the obese patient. Health care providers must be aware of medications that promote weight gain. Antidepressants (exceptions are venlafaxine and bupropion) are frequent offenders, as are many of the medications used for diabetes management and medications for neuropsychiatric disorders. Health care providers who manage overweight and obese patients should be aware of this complication and prescribe weight-neutral or weight loss-promoting drugs when possible. A recent review provides guidance [85].

Medications to aid weight loss attempts are part of our treatment toolbox. We consider weight loss medications to be biologic reinforcement for behavioral attempts to reduce food intake. We endorse the use of the two FDA-approved drugs for long-term use — orlistat and sibutramine — for selected patients (those with BMI $\geq$ 30 kg/m^2 or 27 kg/m^2 with a comorbidity, no contraindications, and prior attempt at weight loss that was less than successful). These medications and rimonabant, which is expected to reach the market soon, are discussed thoroughly in Chapter 6.

9.7.7 Surgery

Surgery is another tool in our therapeutic toolbox. Surgery should be considered for individuals with a BMI $\geq$ 40 kg/m^2 or 35 kg/m^2 and a serious comorbid condition. It is not unusual for us to see individuals with class III obesity, who have lost >100 lb, only to experience regain. Surgery has been shown to produce sustained weight loss for ten or more years [86]. For highly-motivated patients, who are acceptable candidates for these procedures and who are willing to comply with postsurgical dietary alterations, we recommend consultation with an experienced bariatric surgeon. This topic is thoroughly detailed in Chapter 7.

9.8 CONCLUSION

Health care providers are challenged by a large population of overweight and obese patients. The traditional approach has been to focus on comorbidity management, with the emphasis on prescribing antihypertensives, lipid-lowering medications, and diabetes medications. Primary care providers are in a unique position to impact their patients' health risks through weight management. This will entail more than the traditional advice to "eat less and exercise more;" but providers who engage in the follow-through of weight management will be rewarded by prevention of comorbid diseases and improvement in risk factors.

REFERENCES

1. Goldstein, M.G., Whitlock, E.P., and DePue, J.D., Multiple behavioral risk factor interventions in primary care, *Am. J. Prev. Med.*, 27, 61, 2004.
2. Steptoe, A. et al., Sociodemographic and psychological predictors of changes in dietary fat consumption in adults with high blood cholesterol following counseling in primary care, *Health Psychol.*, 19, 411, 2000.

3. Vogt, T.M. et al., The medical care system and prevention: the need for a new paradigm, *HMO Practice.*, 12, 5, 1998.
4. National Center for Health Statistics., *Health, United States, 2003,* National Center for Health Statistics, Hyattsville, 2003.
5. Davis, D. et al., Room for Improvement: Patients Report on the Quality of Their Health Care, The Commonwealth Fund, New York, 2002.
6. U.S. Bureau of the Census, *Statistical Abstract of the United States: 1998,* 118th ed., Washington, D.C., 1998.
7. Goldberg, R.J. et al., Physicians' attitudes and reported practices toward smoking intervention, *J. Cancer Educ.,* 8, 133, 1993.
8. Green, L.A. et al., The ecology of medical care revisited, *N. Engl. J. Med.*, 344, 2021, 2001.
9. Simkin-Silverman, L.R. and Wing, R.R., Management of obesity in primary care, *Obes. Res.,* 5, 603, 1997.
10. Horgen, K.B. and Brownell, K.D., Policy change as a means for reducing the prevalence and impact of alcoholism, smoking, and obesity, in *Treating Addictive Behaviors,* 2nd ed., Miller, W.R. and Heather, N., Eds., Plenum Press, New York, 105, 1998.
11. Hiddink, G.J. et al., Consumers' expectations about nutrition guidance: the importance of primary care physicians, *Am. J. Clin. Nutr.,* 65, 1974S, 1997.
12. Potter, M.B., Vu, J.D., and Croughan-Minihane. M., Weight management: what patients want from their primary care physicians, *J. Fam. Pract.,* 50, 513, 2001.
13. Simkin-Silverman, L.R. et al., Predictors of weight control advice in primary care practices: patient health and psychosocial characteristics, *Prev. Med.,* 40, 71, 2005.
14. Serdula, M.K., Khan, L.K., and Dietz, W.H., Weight loss counseling revisited, *JAMA,* 289, 1747, 2003.
15. Scott, J.G. et al., Speaking of weight: how patients and primary care clinicians initiate weight loss counseling, *Prev. Med.,* 38, 819, 2004.
16. Huang, J. et al., Physicians' weight loss counseling in two public hospital primary care clinics, *Acad. Med.,* 79, 156, 2004.
17. Stafford, R.S. et al., National patterns of physician activities related to obesity management, *Arch. Fam. Med.,* 9, 631, 2000.
18. Wee, C.C. et al., Physician counseling about exercise, *JAMA,* 282, 1583, 1999.
19. Finkelstein, E.A., Fiebelkorn, I.C., and Wang, G., State-level estimates of annual medical expenditures attributable to obesity, *Obes. Res.,* 12, 18, 2004.
20. U.S. Department of Health and Human Services, *The Surgeon General's Call to Action to Prevent and Decrease Overweight and Obesity,* U.S. Department of Health and Human Services, Public Health Services, Office of the Surgeon General, Rockville, 2001.
21. American Medical Association., *Assessment and Management of Adult Obesity: A Primer for Physicians,* American Medical Association, Atlanta, 2003.
22. Aronne, L.J., Treating obesity: a new target for prevention of coronary heart disease, *Prog. Cardiovasc. Nurs.,* 16, 98, 2001.
23. Cohen, M.D., D'Amico, F.J., and Merenstein, J.H., Weight reduction in obese hypertensive patients, *Fam. Med.,* 23, 25, 1991.
24. Logsdon, D.N., Lazaro, C.M., and Meier, R.V., The feasibility of behavioral risk reduction in primary medical care, *Am. J. Prev. Med.,* 5, 249, 1989.
25. Bowerman, S. et al., Implementation of a primary care physician network obesity management program, *Obes. Res.,* 9, 321S, 2001.
26. Martin, P.D. et al., Weight maintenance and the prevention of weight gain in the primary care setting: the final results of the PCOMO study, *Obes. Res.,* 11, A148, 2003.

27. The Counterweight Project Team, A new evidence-based model for weight management in primary care: the Counterweight Programme, *J. Hum. Nutr. Diet.,* 17, 191, 2004.
28. Kenner, M.M. et al., Primary care providers need a variety of nutrition and wellness patient education materials, *J. Am. Diet. Assoc.,* 99, 462, 1999.
29. Lazarus, K., Nutrition practices of family physicians after education by a physician nutrition specialist, *Am. J. Clin. Nutr.,* 65, 2007S, 1997.
30. Ockene, J.K. et al., Physician training for patient-centered nutrition counseling in a lipid intervention trial, *Prev. Med.,* 24, 563, 1995.
31. Eaton, C.B. et al., Teaching nutrition skills to primary care practitioners, *J. Nutr.,* 133, 563S, 2003.
32. Ashley, J. et al., Weight control in the physician's office, *Arch. Intern. Med.,* 161, 1599, 2001.
33. NHLBI Obesity Education Initiative., *Clinical Guidelines on the Identification, Evaluation, and Treatment of Overweight and Obesity in Adults: The Evidence Report,* NIH Publication No. 98-4083, U.S. Department of Health and Human Services, Public Health Service, National Institutes of Health, National Heart, Lung, and Blood Institute, Bethesda, 1998.
34. Logue, E. et al., Obesity management in primary care: assessment of readiness to change among 284 family practice patients, *J. Am. Board Fam. Pract.,* 13, 164, 2000.
35. Whitlock, E.P. et al., Evaluating primary care behavioral counseling interventions: an evidence-based approach, *Am. J. Prev. Med.,* 22, 267, 2002.
36. Aronne, L.J. Treatment of obesity in the primary care setting, in *Handbook of Obesity Treatment,* Wadden, T.A. and Stunkard A.J., Eds., The Guilford Press, New York, 2002.
37. Brownell, K.D. and Jeffery, R.W., Improving long-term weight loss: pushing the limits of treatment, *Behav. Ther.,* 18, 353, 1987.
38. Foreyt, J.P. and Goodrick, G.K., Evidence for success of behavior modification in weight loss and control, *Ann. Intern. Med.,* 119, 698, 1993.
39. Williamson, D.A. and Perrin, L.A., Behavioral therapy for obesity, *Endocrinol. Metab. Clin. North Am.,* 25, 943, 1996.
40. Perri, M.G., Obese populations, in *Compliance in Healthcare and Research,* Burke, L.E. and Ockene, I.S., Eds., Futura Publishing Company, Armonk, 219, 2001.
41. Wadden, T.A., Butryn, M.L., and Byrne, K.J., Efficacy of lifestyle modification for long-term weight control, *Obes. Res.,* 12, 151S, 2004.
42. Renjilian, D.A. et al., Individual versus group therapy for obesity: effects of matching participants to their treatment preferences, *J. Consult. Clin. Psychol.,* 69, 717, 2001.
43. Wolf, A.M., Manson, J.E., Colditz, G.A. The economic impact of overweight, obesity, and weight loss. In *Obesity: Mechanisms and Clinical Management*, Eckel, R.H., Ed., Lippincott Williams & Wilkins, Philadelphia, 523–549, 2003.
44. Agren, G., Narbro, K., Naslund, I., Sjostrom, L., Peltonen, M. Long-term effects of weight loss on pharmaceutical costs in obese subjects. A report from the SOS intervention study. *Int. J. Obes.,* 26, 184–192, 2002.
45. National Heart Lung and Blood Institute (NHLBI), North American Association for the Study of Obesity (NAASO). *The Practical Guide to the Identification, Evaluation, and Treatment of Overweight and Obesity in Adults.* Bethesda, MD: National Institutes of Health; NIH Publication No. 00-4084, 2000.
46. Wadden, T.A. and Osei, S., Behavioral assessment of the obese patient, in *Handbook of Obesity Treatment*, Wadden, T.A. and Stunkard, A.J., Eds., The Guilford Press, New York, 242, 2002.

47. Apfelbaum, M. et al., Long-term maintenance of weight loss after a very-low calorie diet: a randomized blinded trial of the efficacy and tolerability of sibutramine, *Am. J. Med.,* 106, 179, 1999.
48. Wadden, T.A. et al., Benefits of lifestyle modification in pharmacologic treatment of obesity, *Arch. Int. Med.,* 161, 218, 2001.
49. Wing, R. Behavioral weight control, in *Handbook of Obesity Treatment*, Wadden, T.A. and Stunkard, A.J., Eds., The Guilford Press, New York, 301, 2002.
50. Klem, M.L., A descriptive study of individuals successful at long-term maintenance of substantial weight loss, *Am. J. Clin. Nutr.,* 66, 239, 1997.
51. Rippe, J.M. and Hess, S., The role of physical activity in the prevention and management of obesity, *J. Am. Diet. Assoc.,* 10, S31, 1998.
52. Jackicic, J. et al., Relationship between presence of exercise equipment in the home and physical activity level, *Am. J. Health Promot.,* 11, 363, 1997.
53. Safer, D.J., Diet, behavior modification, and exercise: a review of obesity treatments from a long-term perspective, *South. Med. J.*, 84, 1470, 1991.
54. Miller, W.C., Koceja, D.M., and Hamilton, E.J., A meta-analysis of the past 25 years of weight loss research using diet, exercise or diet plus exercise intervention, *Int. J. Obes.,* 21, 941, 1997.
55. Cowburn, G., Hillsdon, M., and Hankey, C.R., Obesity management by lifestyle strategies, *Br. Med. Bull.,* 53, 389, 1997.
56. NHS Centre for Reviews and Dissemination., The prevention and treatment of obesity, *Eff. Health Care,* 3, 1, 1997.
57. Wing, R.R. and Hill, J.O., Successful weight loss maintenance, *Ann. Rev. Nutr.,* 21, 323, 2001.
58. Klem, M.L. et al., Psychological symptoms in individuals successful at long-term maintenance of weight loss, *Health Psychol.,* 17, 336, 1998.
59. Wadden, T.A., Sarwer, D.B., and Berkowitz, R.I., Behavioural treatment of the overweight patient, *Baillieres Best Pract. Res. Clin. Endocrinol. Metab.,* 13, 93, 1999.
60. Foreyt, J.P. and Poston, W.S.C., What is the role of cognitive-behavior therapy in patient management?, *Obes. Res.,* 6, 18S, 1998.
61. Melanson, K. and Dwyer, J., Popular diets for treatment of overweight and obesity, in *Handbook of Obesity Treatment*, Wadden, T.A. and Stunkard, A.J., Eds., The Guilford Press, New York, 249, 2002.
62. Luepker, R.V. et al., Outcomes of a field trial to improve children's dietary patterns and physical activity. The Child and Adolescent Trial for Cardiovascular Health, CATCH collaborative group, *JAMA,* 275, 768, 1996.
63. Heymsfield, S.B. et al., Weight management using a meal replacement strategy: meta and pooling analysis from six studies, *Int. J. Obes.,* 27, 537, 2003.
64. Heber, D. Meal replacements in the treatment of obesity, in *Eating Disorders and Obesity: A Comprehensive Handbook,* 2nd ed., Fairburn, C.G. and Brownell, K.D., Eds., The Guilford Press, New York, 529, 2002.
65. Ditschuneit, H.H. et al., Metabolic and weight-loss effects of a long-term dietary intervention in obese patients, *Am. J. Clin. Nutr.,* 69, 198, 1999.
66. Barnard, N.D., Akhtar, A., and Nicholson, A., Factors that facilitate compliance to lower fat intake, *Arch. Fam. Med.,* 4, 153, 1995.
67. Lewis, S.B. et al., Effect of diet composition on metabolic adaptations to hypocaloric nutrition: comparison of high carbohydrate and high fat isocaloric diets, *Am. J. Clin. Nutr.,* 30, 160, 1977.
68. Foster, G.D. et al., A randomized trial of a low-carbohydrate diet for obesity, *N. Engl. J. Med.,* 348, 2082, 2003.

69. Samaha, F.F. et al., A low-carbohydrate as compared with a low-fat diet in severe obesity, *N. Engl. J. Med.,* 348, 2074, 2003.
70. Brehm, B.J. et al., A randomized trial comparing a very low carbohydrate diet and a calorie-restricted low fat diet on body weight and cardiovascular risk factors in healthy women, *J. Clin. Endocrinol. Metab.,* 88, 1617, 2003.
71. Sondike, S.B., Copperman, N., and Jacobson, M.S., Effects of a low-carbohydrate diet on weight loss and cardiovascular risk factor in overweight adolescents, *J. Pediatr.,* 142, 253, 2003.
72. Hays, J.H. et al., Effect of a high saturated fat and no-starch diet on serum lipid subfractions in patients with documented atherosclerotic cardiovascular disease, *Mayo. Clin. Proc.,* 78, 1331, 2003.
73. Schwarz, J.M. et al., Hepatic de novo lipogenesis in normoinsulinemic and hyperinsulinemic subjects consuming high-fat, low-carbohydrate and low-fat, high-carbohydrate isoenergetic diets, *Am. J. Clin. Nutr.,* 77, 43, 2003.
74. Womble, L.G., Wang, S.S., and Wadden, T.A., Commercial and self-help weight loss programs, in *Handbook of Obesity Treatment,* Wadden, T.A. and Stunkard, A.J., Eds., The Guilford Press, New York, 395, 2002.
75. Christakis, G. and Miller-Kovach, K., Maintenance of weight goal among Weight Watchers lifetime members, *Nutr. Today.,* 31, 29, 1996.
76. Lowe, M.R. et al., An initial evaluation of a commercial weight loss program: short-term effects on weight, eating behavior, and mood, *Obes. Res.,* 7, 51, 1999.
77. Heshka, S. et al., Weight loss with self-help compared with a structured commercial program, *JAMA,* 289, 1792, 2003.
78. Tsai, A.G. and Wadden, T.A., Systematic review: an evaluation of major commercial weight loss programs in the United States, *Ann. Intern. Med.,* 142, 56, 2005.
79. Streit, K.J., Food records: a predictor and modifier of weight change in a long-term weight loss program, *J. Am. Diet. Assoc.,* 91, 213, 1991.
80. Hill, J.O. and Wyatt, H., Outpatient management of obesity: a primary care perspective, *Obes. Res.,* 10, 124S, 2002.
81. Anderson, D.A. and Wadden, T.A., Treating the obese patient: suggestions for primary care practice, *Arch. Fam. Med.,* 8, 156, 1999.
82. Siegel, P.Z., Brackbill, R.M., and Heath, G.W., The epidemiology of walking for exercise: implications for promoting activity among sedentary groups, *Am. J. Public Health,* 85, 706, 1995.
83. Swartz, A.M. et al., Increasing daily walking improves glucose tolerance in overweight women, *Prev. Med.,* 37, 356, 2003.
84. Yamanouchi, K. et al., Daily walking combined with diet therapy is a useful means for obese NIDDM patients not only to reduce body weight but also to improve insulin sensitivity, *Diabetes Care,* 18, 775, 1995.
85. Schwartz, T.L. et al., Psychiatric medication-induced obesity: treatment options, *Obes. Res.,* 5, 233, 2004.
86. Sjöström, L. et al., Lifestyle, diabetes, and cardiovascular risk factors 10 years after bariatric surgery, *N. Engl. J. Med.,* 351, 2683, 2004.

10 Maintenance: The Ultimate Goal

Rena R. Wing, Angela Marinilli Pinto, and Heather Niemeier

CONTENTS

10.1 INTRODUCTION

The number one problem in the treatment of obesity is the problem of weight loss maintenance. Most patients who enter weight loss programs are successful initially; however, they typically achieve their maximum weight loss within approximately 6 months and then regain. The purpose of this chapter is to discuss the research on the maintenance of weight loss and to identify those strategies that appear most effective for long-term weight control. Two approaches to understanding maintenance of weight loss will be used. After discussing definitions of weight loss maintenance, this chapter will review randomized clinical trials that have been conducted, evaluating specific treatment strategies and their effect on long-term weight loss maintenance. Then findings from the National Weight Control Registry (NWCR) will be presented which highlight the approaches used by these successful weight losers to achieve long-term maintenance of weight loss.

10.2 PROBLEMS WITH DEFINITIONS OF WEIGHT LOSS MAINTENANCE

It is increasingly clear that weight losses of 5 to 10% of body weight will have marked impact on health [1]. Thus, the goal of treatment is to help patients achieve and maintain weight losses of this magnitude. Despite this consensus, it remains difficult to define "maintenance." In simplest terms, one would think that weight loss maintenance would refer to remaining at the same weight, or losing more weight, after a period of successful weight loss. Thus, individuals who lose 10 lb and regain none would have maintained their weight loss better than individuals who lose 20 lb initially and regain 5. However, in terms of health outcomes, the latter would be expected to produce better results [2]. Consequently, it may be more important to focus on overall long-term weight loss and to worry less about the pattern of weight change. A 250-lb individual who loses 10% of his body weight should be considered successful regardless of whether the person lost 35 lb at 6 mo and then regained 10 lb or lost the 25 lb gradually (with no regain).

This distinction is important because those people who achieve greater initial weight loss are also more likely to experience weight regain, but have the best overall outcome. This paradox is illustrated by data from the Nurses Health Study. Field et al. [3] compared women who lost at least 10% of their body weight from 1989 to 1991 and those who did not lose weight over this period. These investigators found that women

TABLE 10.1
Association between Initial Weight Loss, Subsequent Regain, and Overall Weight Change

Initial Weight	Loss	Regain	Overall
Field et al., 2001 [3]			
Lost <10% or gained	+2.7	+4.1	+6.8
Lost >10%	−14.1	+14.1	0
Jeffery, 1998 [4]			
Smallest weight losses	−6.2 kg	+8.7	+2.5 kg
Middle	−12.5 kg	+10.6	−1.9 kg
Largest weight losses	−18.5 kg	+12.1	−6.4 kg

Source: Adapted from [3] and [4].

who lost >10% body weight initially (1989–1991) regained more weight over the next 4 yr. However, overall (1989–1995), these women had reduced their weight more than those who did not lose weight initially. Table 10.1 shows the patterns of results for women with BMI ≥ 30 kg/m^2, but the same finding was observed in all weight groups.

Similarly, in weight loss programs, those individuals who achieve the largest weight losses initially regain the most over the period of follow-up, but achieve the best long-term outcomes. Jeffery et al. [4] divided patients in a weight loss program into tertiles according to their initial (approximately 6 mo) weight loss. They then followed these participants through 30 mo. Those participants who achieved the largest initial weight losses (18.5 kg) regained the most (12.1 kg) but also were most successful at 30 mo (Table 10.1).

Clinically, it is therefore important to focus on overall weight loss and to recognize that the best way to achieve large overall weight losses is to achieve large initial (6 mo) weight losses.

10.3 BEHAVIORAL APPROACHES AND LONG-TERM WEIGHT LOSS

Behavioral weight loss programs have been shown to provide the most effective approach to long-term weight control. Behavior change strategies were first applied to obesity in the 1970s and have been gradually refined over the last three decades [5]. Behavioral programs are typically offered in a closed group format, with 15 to 20 participants, led by a multidisciplinary team of therapists. The program usually involves weekly meetings for 6 months, followed by biweekly meetings for months 6–12 and then biweekly or monthly meetings for months 12–18. As will be discussed below, the program focuses on changing both diet and physical activity through the use of behavioral strategies such as goal setting, self-monitoring, stimulus control, problem solving, and relapse prevention. In recent studies, the average weight loss was 10.4 kg over the first 6 mo, with an average weight loss of 8.1 kg at 18 months [5]. There is marked variability in outcome, with the standard deviation of weight loss at 18 months almost as large as the average weight loss; thus, some participants will do much better than others. Although the variability is acknowledged, it has proven very difficult to identify baseline variables that allow prediction of who will be successful in the program [6]. Rather, the focus has been on specific treatment components that may improve the average long-term weight loss outcomes. These strategies are discussed in the following sections.

10.3.1 Changing Dietary Intake to Produce Long-Term Weight Loss and Maintenance

Behavioral weight loss programs are designed to produce a 1 to 2 lb/week loss. To accomplish this, participants who weigh less than 200 lb are usually encouraged to consume a 1200 to 1500 kcal/d diet and those weighing more than 200 lb are encouraged to eat 1500 to 1800 kcal/d. Although flexibility is allowed in the specific types of foods selected, participants are encouraged to obtain these calories by following a low-fat diet that conforms to the recommendations of the food guide pyramid.

Studies comparing different dietary strategies for weight loss and weight loss maintenance have typically focused on total calories prescribed, macronutrient distribution of the diet, or ways to simplify the diet. Each of these factors will be described briefly below:

10.3.1.1 Total Calories

In the 1990s, there were several studies that compared balanced low-calorie diets (typically 1200–1500 kcal/d) with very-low-calorie diets (VLCDs) (400 kcal/d, consumed as liquid formula or lean meat, fish, and fowl) [7,8]. Consistently, these studies showed that the VLCD produced greater initial weight losses than the balanced low-calorie regimens, with weight losses on VLCDs averaging 20 kg in 12 weeks; however, these weight losses were not well maintained. Patients prescribed VLCDs regained more weight after the VLCD than those on balanced low-calorie diets; at 12- or 24-mo follow-up, no significant differences were observed in the overall weight loss for the two approaches. Efforts to improve the maintenance of weight loss after VLCDs by providing ongoing therapeutic contact, greater use of behavioral strategies, or periodic reintroduction of the VLCD, were not successful [7,8]. As a result, most programs have moved away from VLCDs, and typically prescribe 1200 or more calories per day.

10.3.1.2 Macronutrient Distribution

Most behavioral weight loss programs use low-calorie, low-fat dietary prescriptions. This is based on several randomized trials that have compared programs that focus on reducing caloric intake only, reducing dietary fat only, or reducing calories plus fat. These studies suggested that restricting both calories and fat intake produces the best overall weight loss [9,10]. Consequently participants in behavioral weight loss programs are given both a daily calorie goal and a fat goal, with the latter prescribed in grams per day and set at a level designed to produce a 20 to 25% fat diet.

There have been several recent studies comparing low-calorie, low-fat diets with low-carbohydrate approaches (e.g., the Atkins diet) [11–13]. These studies have

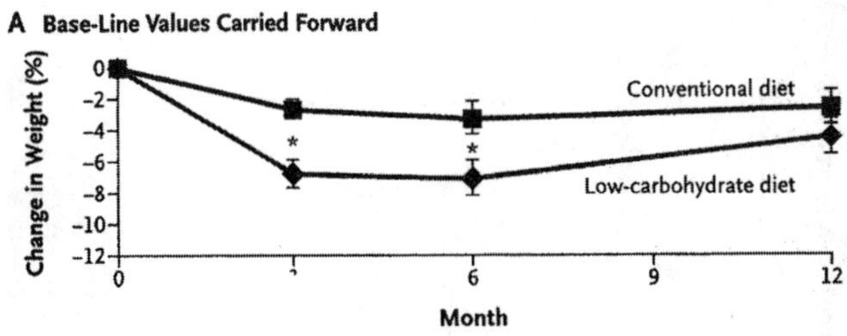

FIGURE 10.1 Mean (± SE) percent change in weight among subjects on the low-carbohydrate diet and those on the conventional (low-calorie, high-carbohydrate) diet, according to an analysis in which baseline values were carried forward in the case of missing values. (Reprinted from Foster, G., H.R. Wyatt, J.O. Hill, B.G. McGuckin, C. Brill, S. Mohammed, P.O. Szapary, D.J. Rader, J.S. Edman, and S. Klein, *N Engl J Med,* 2003. 348(21): p. 2082–2090.)

found that the low-carbohydrate diets produce larger initial weight losses. Foster et al. [11] followed patients through 12 mo and found that compared to those on the low-calorie/low-fat diet, participants who were randomized to the low-carbohydrate diet lost more weight initially, but then regained more weight from 6 to 12 months (Figure 10.1). Consequently, at 12 months, there were no significant differences in weight loss for the two approaches.

Low-carbohydrate diets appear to improve initial weight loss because they help patients adhere to a low-calorie diet. Although low-carbohydrate regimens typically allow participants to eat as much as they want, intake is reduced because many high-calorie items are eliminated from the diet. Patients on low-carbohydrate diets report consuming an average of 1630 kcal/d after 6 months on the diet, representing almost a 500 kcal deficit from baseline [12]. It is also possible that the high-protein, high-fat diets increase feelings of satiety, and thus improve dietary adherence. Over time, however, adherence to these regimens decreases and patients regain their weight.

10.3.1.3 Simplicity or Structure of the Diet

The best diet for long-term weight loss is a diet that helps participants reduce their caloric intake and can be adhered to long term. Adherence may be more strongly associated with the degree of structure of the diet, or its simplicity, rather than the specific macronutrient composition of the diet. This point has been illustrated in several studies. Jeffery, Wing, and colleagues [14,15] randomized weight loss participants to diet programs that were identical in their caloric and macronutrient prescriptions; however, some participants were actually provided with the food they should eat or given meal plans and grocery lists indicating exactly what to eat for each meal. Providing this enhanced structure, through either the foods themselves or the meal plans, improved both short- and long-term results. Participants reported that the structure created a more regular meal pattern and helped them with meal planning and with having appropriate foods available.

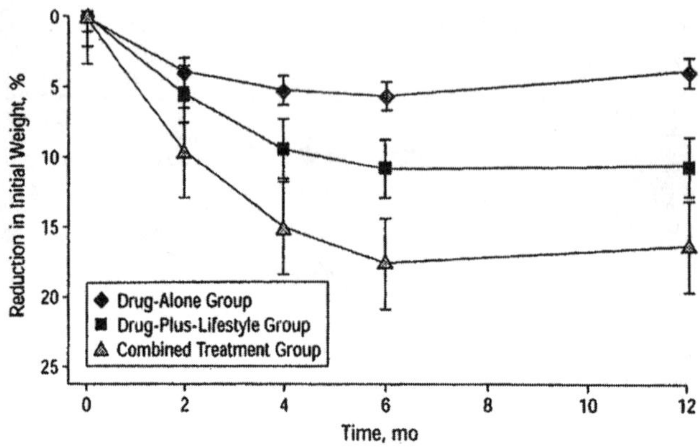

FIGURE 10.2 Percentage reduction in initial body weight for women treated with sibutramine hydrochloride alone (drug-alone), sibutramine plus group lifestyle modification (drug-plus-lifestyle), and sibutramine plus lifestyle modification plus portion-controlled diet (combined treatment), as assessed by a last-observation-carried-forward analysis. (Reprinted from Wadden, T.A., R.I. Berkowitz, D.B. Sarwer, R. Prus-Wisniewski, and C. Steinberg, *Arch Intern Med*, 2001. 161: p. 218–227.)

Another way to simplify the diet is to use portion-controlled foods, such as Slim-Fast, for one to two of the meals each day. Ditschuneit and colleagues [16,17] randomized 100 participants to 1200–1500 kcal/d diets that were either entirely self-selected or comprised two Slim-Fast meal replacements per day, two Slim-Fast snack bars, and a healthy dinner. At the end of 3 months, the Slim-Fast group had lost 7.1 kg, compared to 1.3 kg in the other condition. Subsequently, both groups were encouraged to use one Slim-Fast meal and one snack bar per day, but the difference in weight loss persisted over a full 4 years. Four-year follow-up data on 75% of the original 100 participants indicated a 9.5 kg weight loss in the Slim-Fast group, compared to a 4.1 kg loss in the conventional group. A more recent study by Wadden et al. [18] also supports this suggestion. Wadden et al. randomly assigned participants to weight loss medication (sibutramine), medication plus group behavior modification, or medication plus group behavior modification plus a portion-controlled diet. This diet again included four servings per day of liquid formula and a healthy dinner using regular foods. Results are shown in Figure 10.2.

10.3.2 The Role of Physical Activity in Long-Term Weight Loss Maintenance

The variable that has been most consistently associated with long-term weight loss is physical activity. In correlational studies, those participants who continue to perform the most physical activity are the ones who achieve the largest long-term weight losses [19]. Similarly, comparing weight loss maintainers with regainers, Kayman and colleagues [20] found that 90% of maintainers reported exercising on a regular basis, whereas only 34% of regainers did so.

10.3.2.1 Studies Comparing Diet, Exercise, and the Combination

There have been a number of randomized trials comparing diet only, exercise only, and the combination of diet plus exercise; these studies provide the strongest test of whether exercise improves long-term maintenance of weight loss [21]. Typically in these studies, and in behavioral weight loss programs in general, participants are encouraged to gradually increase their physical activity, using activities that are similar in intensity to brisk walking, until achieving an activity goal of 1000 kcal/week (equivalent to walking 2 miles/d on 5 d/week) or a goal of 150 min per week of activity. Exercise alone has been found to produce a 2 to 4 kg weight loss; diet alone and diet plus physical exercise produce larger weight losses than exercise alone [21]. Most important are the comparisons of diet alone with diet plus exercise. These studies suggest that the combination produces slightly larger initial weight losses than diet alone, but the most significant effect is in terms of the maintenance of weight loss. Almost all studies show better maintenance of weight loss using diet plus exercise.

It should be noted that the effect of diet plus exercise (vs. diet only) on long-term weight loss is not as large as often assumed. Wing [21] noted that only two of six long-term studies found that the diet plus exercise produced *significantly* greater long-term weight losses than diet alone, and a meta-analysis by Miller and colleagues [22] found no difference in weight loss or percent of weight loss retained at 1-yr follow-up for diet only vs. diet plus exercise. The difficulty in seeing an effect of exercise on long-term weight loss probably reflects difficulties in producing long-term adherence to physical activity. In these randomized trials, many participants in the diet plus exercise group stop exercising over time and some in the diet group start to exercise. Moreover, the amount of exercise recommended (often 1000 kcal/week) may not be large enough to produce a significant impact on body weight regulation.

10.3.2.2 Studies Comparing Dose of Exercise

Stronger evidence of the benefits of physical activity for long-term maintenance of weight loss comes from studies prescribing larger doses of exercise. Jeffery, Wing, Sherwood, and Tate [23] recruited 202 overweight men and women and randomly assigned them to a weight control program with a standard or a high exercise prescription. The standard exercise group was instructed to increase their activity to 1000 kcal/week (equivalent to walking 10 miles/week) whereas the high exercise group gradually increased to 2500 kcal/week. As seen in Table 10.2, the exercise manipulation was successful; participants in the high exercise group did significantly more exercise and approached the 2500 kcal/week level. This higher level of activity produced significantly greater weight losses at 12- and 18-month follow-up.

There have been several other studies suggesting that higher amounts of physical activity may help with maintenance of weight loss. In a post hoc analysis of a weight loss intervention, Jakicic and associates [24] divided women into groups according to their self-reported exercise level at 6 and 12 months. As shown in Figure 10.3,

TABLE 10.2
Self-Reported Physical Activity and Weight Loss in a Weight Loss Program with 1000 vs. 2500 kcal/Week Prescriptions for Physical Activity

	Low Exercise (1000 kcal/week)	High Exercise (2500 kcal/week)	
	Self-Reported Physical Activity (kcal/week)		
6 month	1837 ± 1431	2399 ± 1571	$p < 0.01$
12 month	1565 ± 1309	2349 ± 1751	$p < 0.01$
18 month	1629 ± 1483	2317 ± 1854	$p < 0.01$
	Weight Loss (kg)		
6 month	8.1 ± 7.4	9.0 ± 7.1	NS
12 month	6.1 ± 8.8	8.5 ± 7.9	p < 0.07
18 month	4.1 ± 7.3	6.7 ± 8.1	p < 0.04

those women who reported doing at least 200 min of activity at 6 and 12 months had the largest initial and 12-month weight losses. These findings, and data from the NWCR which will be presented later in the chapter, suggest that higher levels of exercise may be needed to maintain weight loss. Consequently many programs are now encouraging over 200 min/week of activity or 2000 to 2500 kcal/week.

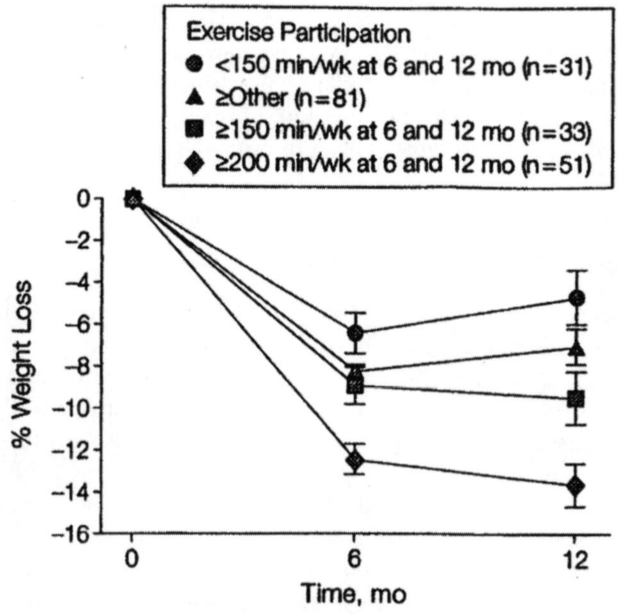

FIGURE 10.3 Percent change in weight loss based on exercise duration (n = 196). (Reprinted from Jakicic, J., B.H. Marcus, K.I. Gallagher, M. Napolitano, and W. Lang, *JAMA*, 2003. 290(10): p. 1323–1330.)

10.3.2.3 Improving Adherence to Physical Activity

As described above in discussing dietary prescriptions, the primary question related to physical activity is how to produce long-term adherence to this behavior. Researchers have shown that adherence can be improved by encouraging patients to divide their physical activity into multiple short (10 min) bouts [25], by providing home exercise equipment [26] and by providing small incentives/reinforcers for activity [27]. Many participants enjoy using pedometers to record their activity, but whether this source of feedback and reinforcement improves long-term adherence has not been studied.

10.3.3 Behavioral Strategies for Improving Long-Term Maintenance

In addition to strengthening the dietary and physical activity components of behavioral weight loss interventions, long-term weight loss maintenance can be improved by increasing support for behavior change and teaching participants specific strategies for problem solving and preventing relapse. These approaches are described below.

10.3.3.1 Extended Contact

One of the most effective strategies for improving long-term weight loss maintenance has been extending the duration of treatment contact. By extending contact, patients are helped to increase their adherence to behavior change and made accountable for their progress. In a series of studies, Perri and colleagues have demonstrated the impact of continued therapeutic contact. For example, Perri et al. [28] compared 20- and 40-week treatment programs that were identical in content and found that weight losses did not differ after 20 weeks, but after 40 weeks, participants in the extended treatment condition had lost more weight than those in the standard program (13.6 vs. 6.4 kg). Although participants in both conditions regained weight between weeks 40 and 72, the extended treatment condition continued to show better overall weight loss at the 72-week follow-up compared to those in the standard program (9.6 vs. 4.6 kg). In another study of extended contact, Perri et al. [29] compared a condition receiving no contact between months 6 and 18 to four different extended contact conditions, each receiving biweekly therapist contact and a combination of other interventions (e.g., social influence and aerobic exercise). At the 18-month follow-up, all of the extended contact conditions had lost more weight than the no contact condition with no differences among the types of interventions. Thus, the frequency of contact seemed to be the important component and the content of the treatment had little effect.

Because of the demonstrated effectiveness of extending treatment, several randomized controlled trials have included weekly group treatments for a full year [7,8]. Unfortunately, these attempts have demonstrated significant problems with attendance at treatment sessions. For example, Wing et al. [8] offered weekly treatment sessions for a full year and found that in the first 12 weeks, participants attended an average of 83% of meetings, while in the last 12 weeks of the year, they attended only 42% of meetings. These findings suggest that different methods are needed to maintain frequent treatment contact while decreasing both participant burden and treatment costs. Perri et al. [30] found that continued phone and mail contact by study therapists significantly improved weight loss maintenance for patients receiving behavior therapy and relapse prevention training as compared to those not receiving such contact. However, Wing et al. [31] compared a phone-based maintenance intervention to a control group receiving no additional contact following a 6-month weight loss intervention and found only modest effects of the phone contact on weight regain. In the phone contact condition, participants received weekly phone calls from research assistants asking them to report their weight and diary data (exercise minutes and calorie and fat intake), thereby hoping to improve their adherence to self-monitoring. However, the use of research assistants rather than therapists may have weakened the efficacy of this ongoing contact.

Recent efforts to extend contact with less participant burden and provider costs have used Internet-based maintenance interventions with mixed results. After participants completed a 6-month face-to-face behavioral treatment program, Harvey-Berino et al. [32] randomly assigned groups to an Internet-based biweekly maintenance program, an in-person biweekly program, or a minimal in-person support program. The Internet-based group regained twice as much weight as the in-person groups. However, the fact that the initial treatment had been done face to face may have influenced this result. In contrast, Harvey-Berino et al. [33] found no significant difference in weight regain among participants who had initially completed treatment through an interactive TV approach and then were randomly assigned to an Internet-based maintenance program or two “in-person” maintenance programs. Those in the Internet-based maintenance program maintained a weight loss of 8.2% at 18-mo follow-up while those in the frequent and minimal in-person contact maintenance programs lost 5.6 and 6.0%, respectively. Although the effectiveness of Internet-based programs in improving long-term weight loss maintenance remains to be seen, further study is warranted, given the potential public health impact of the use of the Internet as a maintenance treatment delivery modality.

10.3.3.2 Social Support

Another approach to improving motivation for ongoing weight control efforts has been the use of social support enhancement interventions. Several early studies focused on the inclusion of spouses or significant others in the treatment process with the goal of extending treatment beyond the clinical context. In a meta-analysis of such studies, Black et al. [34] found that the inclusion of a partner modestly, but significantly, improved initial weight loss outcomes with a trend toward improvement in short-term follow-up as well. More recent approaches to enhancing social support have included a study by Wing and Jeffery [35] in which participants were recruited with or without a group of three friends (recruitment method was not randomly assigned). Results showed that those participating with friends had better initial weight losses and better weight loss maintenance than those recruited alone. The study also tested the addition of an experimenter-created social support intervention including activities to increase intragroup cohesion and intergroup competitions and found that the social support intervention also improved weight loss maintenance. Thus, enhancing social support appears to show promise in improving long-term weight loss maintenance.

10.3.3.3 Problem Solving and Relapse Prevention

Two common skills taught in weight loss maintenance programs are problem solving and relapse prevention. Both skills are aimed at helping participants maintain their behavior changes by coping with challenges that may arise over the long term. Formal problem solving skills are taught as a five-step process based on the work of D'Zurilla and Goldfried [36], and participants are encouraged to engage in problem solving as a group and on their own. The five steps as outlined by Perri et al. [37] include 1) adopting a problem solving orientation, 2) detailed specification of the problem, 3) generation of potential solutions through brainstorming, 4) selection of an approach to try, and 5) implementation of the approach and evaluation of its effectiveness.

Relapse prevention is based on the work of Marlatt and Gordon [38,39] and involves teaching participants to anticipate and plan for high-risk situations with the hope of preventing lapses and relapses while also teaching skills to deal with such events should they occur. Participants are taught to identify their own high-risk situations, which often include situational triggers such as vacations, holidays, and social situations, or emotional triggers such as stress, negative affect, and celebrations. They are then assisted in the development of strategies to overcome such challenges, often using the problem solving approach. A key to relapse prevention is the distinction between lapses (i.e., temporary setbacks) and a relapse (i.e., a significant weight regain). Participants are taught that lapses are normal and are encouraged to take immediate steps to prevent lapses from becoming a relapse by resisting the tendency to allow negative thoughts and feelings about the lapse to influence their behavior. Instead, they are encouraged to view the lapse as one episode in the context of their successful weight loss experience and to immediately take steps to return to their healthy eating and exercise habits. In the case of a relapse, participants are encouraged to have a plan in place, which will allow them to return to the behaviors that helped them in their initial weight loss efforts, including self-monitoring, the use of meal replacements or a structured meal plan, and regular physical activity.

Both problem solving and relapse prevention are standard components of most maintenance programs. However, in one study, a purely problem-solving approach was compared to relapse prevention [40], with problem solving shown to be superior. Perri et al. compared a group receiving no follow-up intervention following a 5-month behavioral weight loss program to groups meeting biweekly for five additional months and receiving either a relapse prevention program or a problem-solving model. In the problem-solving program, interventionists solicited eating- and exercise-related difficulties that had been encountered by group members in the previous week and then led participants in group problem solving to generate a solution plan for each participant. Participants in the problem-solving program had the best long-term weight loss outcome with an average loss of 10.8 kg at 17 mo vs. 5.85 kg in relapse prevention and 4.14 kg in the no-treatment control condition.

10.4 THE NATIONAL WEIGHT CONTROL REGISTRY

Another approach to understanding factors associated with maintenance of weight loss is to study those individuals who have succeeded in this feat. The variables found to be characteristic of successful weight loss maintainers confirm the findings described above and suggest the importance of a low-calorie/low-fat diet, physical activity, and ongoing vigilance.

The NWCR was established in 1994 by Drs. James O. Hill and Rena R. Wing. The NWCR is the largest study of individuals who have succeeded in maintaining long-term weight loss and provides important data on characteristics of these individuals and strategies for their success. To be eligible for membership in the NWCR, individuals must have maintained at least a 30 lb weight loss for at least 1 yr. Eligible participants provide informed consent and are asked to complete several self-report questionnaires that assess weight history, comorbid conditions, quality of life, and behavioral strategies used to lose and maintain weight. Additional follow-up questionnaires are completed annually.

Currently, the NWCR has over 4000 members who have maintained an average weight loss of 73 lb for about 5.7 yr [41]. The average age of members is 47 yr; 77% are women and 95% are Caucasian. Individuals in the Registry report a strong family history of obesity, with almost half (46%) reporting overweight or obesity in one parent and over one quarter (27%) identifying both parents as overweight or obese [42]. In addition, 46% of participants report being overweight as children. A history of prior unsuccessful weight loss attempts is very common, occurring in 90% of Registry participants. When asked what distinguished this successful effort from prior unsuccessful weight loss attempts, NWCR members note greater commitment, stricter dieting, and more use of physical activity as part of this effort.

10.4.1 Approaches Used by NWCR Members for Weight Loss

It has been well established that successful weight loss is best achieved through decreasing caloric intake and increasing physical activity. Indeed, the vast majority of participants in the NWCR (89%) lost weight by making changes in dietary intake (e.g., restricting certain types of foods, limiting portions, counting calories) and by engaging in regular physical activity [43]. They describe using different approaches to lose weight, such that 50% report losing weight on their own, 35% reported losing weight with the help of a formal weight loss program (e.g., Weight Watchers, Jenny Craig, Take Off Pounds Sensibly [TOPS]), and 15% report using a liquid formula diet (e.g., Optifast) [44]. Despite variability in methods for *weight loss,* similar behavioral strategies are employed by large numbers of NWCR members for *weight maintenance,* including: eating a low-calorie low-fat diet that includes breakfast, engaging in regular exercise, and frequent self-monitoring.

10.4.2 Approaches Used by NWCR Members for Weight Loss Maintenance

10.4.2.1 Diet

Dietary intake of NWCR members is assessed using the Block Food Frequency questionnaire [45]. Upon entry into the Registry (which is on average almost 6 yr after losing weight), this group of successful weight loss maintainers report eating an average of 1381 kcal/d comprising 24% fat, 19% protein, and 56% carbohydrates [43]. Given that most people underreport their dietary intake by about 30% [46], these participants are most likely eating approximately 1800 kcal/d, but even this would represent a calorie-reduced regimen. Participants use a number of approaches to control dietary intake, including limiting certain foods (92%), controlling portion size (49%), restricting fat (38%), and counting calories (35%). Members report eating an average of five times per day, with very few eating less frequently than twice a day. While the majority of meals are consumed in the home, participants report having approximately two meals a week in non-fast-food restaurants. These data suggest that while participants demonstrate regular use of behavioral strategies to maintain their weight loss success, they are not using extreme measures (e.g., eating only once a day, eating only one or two types of food) and continue to enjoy occasional restaurant dining. In addition to consuming a diet low in calories and fat, Wyatt and colleagues [47] identified regular consumption of breakfast as a common occurrence among Registry members. Specifically, 78% of successful weight loss maintainers report eating breakfast 7 d/week and almost 90% report eating breakfast on 4 or more days of the week.

10.4.2.2 Physical Activity

In the NWCR, physical activity is measured using the Paffenbarger Physical Activity Questionnaire [48]. Participants report high levels of physical activity, expending an average of 2827 kcal/week through exercise [43]. This level of exercise is comparable to 1 hr of moderate intensity activity (e.g., brisk walking) per day, which is much greater than the minimal physical activity recommendation of the American College of Sports Medicine (ACSM). The ACSM [49] recommends that overweight and obese individuals obtain a minimum of 150 min/week of moderate intensity physical activity. For long-term maintenance of weight loss, the ACSM recommends that levels of physical activity be increased to 200 to 300 min/week or a weekly calorie expenditure of 2000 kcal or more. Of NWCR members, 52% met or exceeded the goal of 2000 kcal/week of physical activity. Registry members report engaging in both medium-intensity (e.g., stationary or road cycling, aerobics, walking) and heavy-intensity (e.g., weight lifting, jogging, using stair-stepper) activity. These findings indicate that individuals who are successful at long-term weight loss have routinely incorporated high levels of physical activity into their lifestyle.

10.4.2.3 Self-Monitoring

Self-monitoring of dietary intake and weight is very effective for weight loss and is included as a key component in behavioral treatments [50]. Self-monitoring of weight is a commonly used strategy for successful weight loss maintainers in the NWCR.

TABLE 10.3
Key Weight Loss Maintenance Strategies Used by National Weight Control Registry Members

Self-monitoring	
	Weigh self regularly (at least once/week)
	Count calories
Dietary intake	
	Consume a low-calorie, low-fat diet
	Eat breakfast regularly
	Limit portion sizes
	Limit intake of high fat/high calorie foods
Physical Activity	
	Engage in high levels of physical activity (comparable to one hour of brisk walking each day)

Upon entry into the study, more than 44% of participants report weighing themselves at least once a day and 31% report weighing themselves once a week [43]. Individuals who are working to maintain weight loss benefit from frequent weighing because it allows them to see small increases in body weight and to re-engage in behavioral strategies to reverse weight gain. In addition to monitoring body weight, self-monitoring of dietary intake is an important element in weight loss treatment because it has the effect of making individuals more aware of the type and quantity of foods they consume. In the NWCR, participants were asked to report their level of cognitive restraint, a measure of conscious control exerted over eating. These successful weight loss maintainers demonstrate levels of cognitive restraint that are higher than non-dieting normal-weight individuals and similar to levels of restraint reported by patients who have recently completed weight loss treatment [51]. Overall, these data suggest that continued self-monitoring of eating behavior and weight are important behavioral strategies that promote successful long-term maintenance of weight loss. Key weight loss maintenance strategies used by NWCR members are summarized in Table 10.3.

10.4.3 Predictors of Weight Regain

The longitudinal nature of the NWCR study allows researchers to follow participants over time to examine factors related to long-term weight maintenance. Even in this successful group of weight losers, regain was common. One year after entry into the study, 35% of members regained 5 lb or more, 59% maintained their weight loss, and 6% continued to lose [52]. Several factors assessed at baseline were associated with elevated risk of weight regain at 1-yr follow-up. Specifically, compared to participants who maintained their weight over 1 yr, those who regained reported 1) larger weight losses (loss of 30% or more of maximum lifetime weight vs. less than 30%), 2) more recent weight losses (loss occurred fewer than 2 yr ago vs. 2 or more years ago), 3) more frequent weight cycling, 4) greater depressive symptoms, 5) greater dietary disinhibition, and 6) more frequent binge eating.

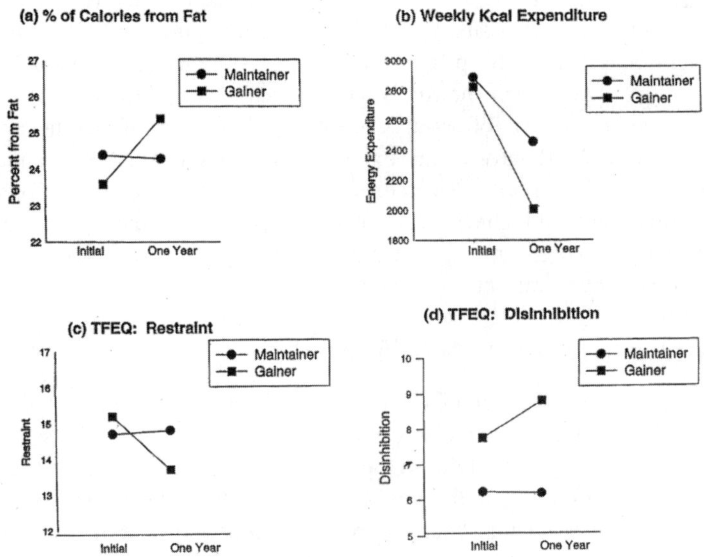

FIGURE 10.4 Changes in (a) percentage of total calories from fat, (b) total energy expenditure, (c) restraint, and (d) dietary disinhibition between initial and 1-year follow-up assessments in weight loss maintainers vs. gainers. *Note:* TFEQ, Three-Factor Eating Questionnaire. (Reprinted from McGuire, M.T., R.R. Wing, M.L. Klem, W. Lang, and J.O. Hill, *J Consult Clin Psychol*, 1999: 67, p. 177–185.)

Although regainers and maintainers reported similar diet and exercise behaviors at baseline, participants who regained weight over 1 yr follow-up reported significant changes in key weight loss behaviors [52]. Compared to maintainers, regainers reported reduced dietary restraint, increased disinhibition, and greater consumption of calories from fat when reassessed at 1-yr (Figure 10.4). While both groups reported decreases in physical activity, participants who regained weight reduced their exercise expenditure by almost twice that of maintainers. These findings suggest that individuals who are more likely to regain weight are those who experience reduced control over eating in conjunction with decreased physical activity, and underscore the importance of continued behavior change for successful long-term weight loss.

Another factor that has been associated with risk for weight regain is lack of dieting consistency. In a study examining consistency of dieting over the course of the week (weekends vs. weekdays), Gorin et al. [53] found that Registry participants who kept consistent dieting habits across days of the week were less likely to regain weight than those who reported stricter dieting on weekdays than on weekends.

To examine the natural course of recovery from weight regain, Phelan et al. followed 2400 participants in the NWCR over a 2-yr period [54]. When assessed at 1-yr follow-up, approximately two thirds of participants had regained some of their weight. Of those individuals, only 11% returned to their initial assessment weight at year 2. Even a relatively small amount of weight regain (e.g., 1 to 3% of initial body weight) was difficult for participants to lose. As expected, individuals with the greatest weight regains over the first year were least likely to return to their initial assessment weight at 2-yr follow-up. Despite the frequency of weight regain, participants in the NWCR have been very successful, with over 96% maintaining a weight loss of 10% or more below their maximum lifetime weight. However, given that few participants were able to recover from even small weight regains, continued focus on methods to prevent weight regain in the first place may be the most effective strategy for continued weight loss maintenance.

10.4.4 Quality of Life in NWCR Members

As described, successful weight loss maintainers must make large and sustained changes in their eating and exercise behaviors to succeed. This has raised questions about whether these individuals experience depression, disordered eating, or impaired quality of life due to their efforts. Findings from the NWCR suggest quite the opposite. NWCR members report levels of depression that are similar to non-depressed community samples, very low levels of binge eating or self-induced vomiting, and marked improvements in their quality of life resulting from their weight loss [43,51].

As noted above, they do, however, continue to be restrained and to consciously work to maintain their new behaviors. A very positive finding is that over time, NWCR members report that maintaining their weight requires less effort and fewer behavioral strategies. Thus, with longer duration of weight loss maintenance, they experience a more positive ratio of pleasure:effort from their success.

10.5 SUMMARY

Data from randomized trials and the NWCR are quite consistent in suggesting approaches that appear to improve long-term maintenance of weight loss. In working with overweight patients, clinicians should emphasize the following strategies from this research:

10.5.1 Goal Setting

Setting a goal of losing 10% of weight is recommended. However, patients should be encouraged to achieve this weight loss within 5 to 6 months. Almost all patients achieve their maximum weight loss in the first 6 months (and then unfortunately regain); so the emphasis should be on increasing initial weight loss success. Larger initial weight losses are associated with larger long-term weight loss.

10.5.2 Targeting Decreased Caloric Intake

The primary approach to weight loss rests on decreasing caloric intake. Typically a calorie goal of 1200 to 1800 kcal/d is prescribed initially, but this goal should be modified as needed to achieve a weight loss of 1 to 2 lb/week. Research suggests that limiting fat intake is an important strategy for reducing overall caloric intake, due to the caloric density of fat. However, other strategies that improve dietary adherence — for example the use of portion-controlled meals — should also be recommended.

10.5.3 Increasing Physical Activity

Increased physical activity is the strongest predictor of maintenance of weight loss. Individuals seeking to lose weight should therefore be encouraged to add physical activity to their daily life. Recent studies suggest that the more physical activity, the better for weight loss maintenance. Thus, aiming for 150 min/week may be a good initial goal, but over time, exercise should be increased to 60 to 90 min/d to increase the probability of long-term weight loss maintenance.

10.5.4 Making Patients Accountable and Vigilant

Changing eating and activity behaviors is clearly difficult. Overweight individuals have been eating in one way for many years and have developed a variety of physical activity habits, social support systems, and environmental structures that maintain these behaviors. Strategies such as self-monitoring of intake and activity, frequent self-weighing, and regular therapist contact are required to provide patients with feedback on their behavior changes and motivate them to continue focusing on these issues.

10.5.5 Teaching Skills Related to Problem Solving and Relapse Prevention

It is helpful to teach participants to anticipate difficult situations related to weight control and to plan strategies to effectively handle these situations. Typical difficult or high-risk situations include positive social events (parties, vacations) and negative affect (depression, anger, boredom). Patients need to realize that despite all their planning, they will at times experience slips or lapses from their healthy eating and exercise behaviors; the important thing is to deal with these lapses quickly and prevent them from leading to relapse.

10.5.6 Helping Patients Realize that Successful Weight Loss Maintenance is Possible

There has been so much negative publicity regarding weight control that many people feel there is no way to ever succeed. This expectation of failure may well set patients up to fail. Hopefully, an important message from the NWCR is that there are many overweight people who have indeed succeeded. They have tried before — unsuccessfully — but this time, they were able to lose significant amounts of weight and keep it off. Although it took work, they found that maintaining their weight loss became less difficult over time and had extremely positive effects on their quality of life. Thus, other overweight patients can indeed be successful at long-term weight loss maintenance.

REFERENCES

1. Diabetes Prevention Program, Research Group, Reduction in the incidence of type 2 diabetes with lifestyle intervention or Metformin. *N Eng J Med*, 2002. 346: p. 393–403.
2. Wing, R.R., R.W. Jeffery, and W.L. Hellerstedt, A prospective study of effects of weight cycling on cardiovascular risk factors. *Arch Int Med*, 1995. 155: p. 1416–1422.
3. Field, A.E., R.R. Wing, J.E. Manson, D.L. Spiegelman, and W.C. Willett, Relationship of a large weight loss to long-term weight change among young and middle-aged US women. *Int J Obes Relat Metab Disord*, 2001. 25(8): p. 1113–1121.
4. Jeffery, R.W., R.R. Wing, and R.R. Mayer, Are smaller weight losses or more achievable weight loss goals better in the long term for obese patients? *J Consult Clin Psychol*, 1998. 66(4): p. 641–645.
5. Wing, R.R., Behavioral approaches to the treatment of obesity, in *Handbook of Obesity: Clinical Applications*, G. Bray and C. Bouchard, Eds., 2004, Marcel Dekker, Inc.: New York.
6. Wing, R.R. and S. Phelan, Behavioral treatment of obesity: strategies to improve outcome and predictors of success, in *Obesity Mechanisms and Clinical Management*, R.H. Eckel, Ed., 2003, Lippincott Williams & Wilkins: Philadelphia.
7. Wadden, T.A., G.D. Foster, and K.A. Letizia, One-year behavioral treatment of obesity: Comparison of moderate and severe caloric restriction and the effects of weight maintenance therapy. *J Consult Clin Psychol*, 1994. 62: p. 165–171.
8. Wing, R.R., E. Blair, M. Marcus, L.H. Epstein, and J. Harvey, Year-long weight loss treatment for obese patients with type II diabetes: Does inclusion of an intermittent very low calorie diet improve outcome? *Am J Med*, 1994. 97: p. 354–362.
9. Schlundt, D.G., J.O. Hill, J. Pope-Cordle, D. Arnold, K.L. Virts, and M. Katahn, Randomized evaluation of a low fat ad libitum carbohydrate diet for weight reduction. *Int J Ob*, 1993. 17: p. 623–629.
10. Pascale, R.W., R.R. Wing, B.A. Butler, M. Mullen, and P. Bononi, Effects of a behavioral weight loss program stressing calorie restriction versus calorie plus fat restriction in obese individuals with NIDDM or a family history of diabetes. *Diabetes Care*, 1995. 18(9): p. 1241–1248.
11. Foster, G., H.R. Wyatt, J.O. Hill, B.G. McGuckin, C. Brill, S. Mohammed, P.O. Szapary, D.J. Rader, J.S. Edman, and S. Klein, A randomized trial of a low-carbohydrate diet for obesity. *N Eng J Med*, 2003. 348(21): p. 2082–2090.
12. Samaha, F.F., N. Iqbal, P. Seshadri, K.L. Chicano, D.A. Daily, J. McGorory, T. Williams, M. Williams, E.J. Gracely, and L. Stern, A low-carbohydrate as compared with a low-fat diet in severe obesity. *N Eng J Med*, 2003. 348(21): p. 2074–2081.
13. Yancy, W.S., M.K. Olsen, J.R. Guyton, R.P. Bakst, and E.C. Westman, A low-carbohydrate, ketogenic diet versus a low-fat diet to treat obesity and hyperlipidemia. *Ann Intern Med*, 2004. 140: p. 769–777.
14. Jeffery, R.W., R.R. Wing, C. Thorson, L.R. Burton, C. Raether, J. Harvey, and M. Mullen, Strengthening behavioral interventions for weight loss: a randomized trial of food provision and monetary incentives. *J Consult Clin Psychol*, 1993. 61(6): p. 1038–1045.
15. Wing, R.R., R.W. Jeffery, L.R. Burton, C. Thorson, K. Sperber Nissinoff, and J.E. Baxter, Food provision vs. structured meal plans in the behavioral treatment of obesity. *Int J Obes Relat Metab Disord*, 1996. 20: p. 56–62.
16. Ditschuneit, H.H., M. Flechtner-Mors, T.D. Johnson, and G. Adler, Metabolic and weight-loss effects of a long-term dietary intervention in obese patients. *Am J Clin Nutr*, 1999. 69: p. 198–204.

17. Flechtner-Mors, M., H.H. Ditschuneit, T.D. Johnson, M.A. Suchard, and G. Adler, Metabolic and weight loss effects of long-term dietary intervention in obese patients: four-year results. *Obes Res*, 2000. 8(5): p. 399–402.
18. Wadden, T.A., R.I. Berkowitz, D.B. Sarwer, R. Prus-Wisniewski, and C. Steinberg, Benefits of lifestyle modification in the pharmacologic treatment of obesity. *Arch Intern Med*, 2001. 161: p. 218–227.
19. Pronk, N.P. and R.R. Wing, Physical activity and long-term maintenance of weight loss. *Obes Res*, 1994. 2: p. 587–599.
20. Kayman, S., W. Bruvold, and J.S. Stern, Maintenance and relapse after weight loss in women: behavioral aspects. *Am J Clin Nutr*, 1990. 52: p. 800–807.
21. Wing, R.R., Physical activity in the treatment of the adulthood overweight and obesity: current evidence and research issues. *Med Sci Sports Exer*, 1999. 31: p. S547–552.
22. Miller, W.C., D.M. Koceja, and E.J. Hamilton, A meta-analysis of the past 25 years of weight loss research using diet, exercise or diet plus exercise intervention. *Int J Obes Relat Metab Disord*, 1997. 21: p. 941–947.
23. Jeffery, R.W., R.R. Wing, N.E. Sherwood, and D.F. Tate, Physical activity and weight loss: does prescribing higher physical activity goals improve outcome? *Am J Clin Nutr*, 2003. 89: p. 684–689.
24. Jakicic, J., B.H. Marcus, K.I. Gallagher, M. Napolitano, and W. Lang, Effect of exercise duration and intensity on weight loss in overweight, sedentary women a randomized trial. *JAMA*, 2003. 290(10): p. 1323–1330.
25. Jakicic, J.M., R.R. Wing, B.A. Butler, and R.J. Robertson, Prescribing exercise in multiple short bouts versus one continuous bout: effects on adherence, cardiorespiratory fitness, and weight loss in overweight women. *Int J Obes Relat Metab Disord*, 1995. 19: p. 893–901.
26. Jakicic, J., R. Wing, and C. Winters, Effects of intermittent exercise and use of home exercise equipment on adherence, weight loss, and fitness in overweight women. *JAMA*, 1999. 282(16): p. 1554–1560.
27. Jeffery, R.W., R.R. Wing, C. Thorson, and L.C. Burton, Use of personal trainers and financial incentives to increase exercise in a behavioral weight-loss program. *J Consult Clin Psychol*, 1998. 66: p. 777–783.
28. Perri, M.G., A.M. Nezu, E.T. Patti, and K.L. McCann, Effect of length of treatment on weight loss. *J Consult Clin Psychol*, 1989. 57(3): p. 450–452.
29. Perri, M.G., D.A. McAllister, J.J. Gange, R.C. Jordan, W.G. McAdoo, and A.M. Nezu, Effects of four maintenance programs on the long-term management of obesity. *J Consult Clin Psychol*, 1988. 56: p. 529–534.
30. Perri, M.G., R.M. Shapiro, W.W. Ludwig, C.T. Twentyman, and W.G. McAdoo, Maintenance strategies for the treatment of obesity: an evaluation of relapse prevention training and posttreatment contact by mail and telephone. *J Consult Clin Psychol*, 1984. 52: p. 404–413.
31. Wing, R.R., R.W. Jeffery, W.L. Hellerstedt, and L.R. Burton, Effect of frequent phone contacts and optional food provision on maintenance of weight loss. *Ann Behav Med*, 1996. 18: p. 172–176.
32. Harvey-Berino, J., S. Pintauro, P. Bulzzell, M. DiGiulio, B. Casey Gold, C. Moldovan, and E. Ramirez, Does using the Internet facilitate the maintenance of weight loss? *Int J Eating Disord*, 2002. 26: p. 1254–1260.
33. Harvey-Berino, J., S. Pintauro, P. Buzzell, and E.C. Gold, Effect of Internet support on the long-term maintenance of weight loss. *Obes Res*, 2004. 12: p. 320–329.
34. Black, D.R., L.J. Gleser, and K.J. Kooyers, A meta-analytic evaluation of couples weight-loss programs. *Health Psychol*, 1990. 9: p. 330–347.

35. Wing, R. and R. Jeffery, Benefits of recruiting participants with friends and increasing social support for weight loss and maintenance. *J Consult Clin Psychol*, 1999. 67(1): p. 132–138.
36. D'Zurilla, T.J. and M.R. Goldfried, Problem solving and behavior modification. *J Abnorm Psychol*, 1971. 78: p. 107–126.
37. Perri, M.G., A.M. Nezu, and B.J. Viegener, Improving the long-term management of obesity, 1992, John Wiley & Sons: New York.
38. Marlatt, G.A. and J.R. Gordon, Determinants of relapse: implications for the maintenance of behavior change, in *Behavioral Medicine: Changing Health Lifestyles*, P.O. Davidson and S.M. Davidson, Eds., 1979, Brunner/Mazel: New York. p. 410–452.
39. Marlatt, G.A. and J.R. Gordon, Relapse prevention: maintenance strategies, in *Addictive Behavior Change*, 1985, Guilford: New York.
40. Perri, M.G., W.F. McKelvey, D.A. Renjilian, A.M. Nezu, R.L. Shermer, and B.J. Viegener, Relapse prevention training and problem-solving therapy in the long-term management of obesity. *J Consult Clin Psychol*, 2001. 69(4): p. 722–726.
41. Wing, R.R. and S. Phelan, Long-term weight loss maintenance. *Am J Clin Nutr*, 2005. In press.
42. Wing, R.R. and J.O. Hill, Successful weight loss maintenance. *Annu Rev Nutr*, 2001. 21: p. 323–341.
43. Klem, M.L., R.R. Wing, M.T. McGuire, H.M. Seagle, and J.O. Hill, A descriptive study of individuals successful at long-term maintenance of substantial weight loss. *Am J Clin Nutr*, 1997. 66: p. 239–246.
44. McGuire, M.T., R.R. Wing, M.L. Klem, and J.O. Hill, Long-term maintenance of weight loss: do people who lose weight through various weight loss methods use different behaviors to maintain their weight? *Int J Obes Relat Metab Disord*, 1998. 22: p. 572–577.
45. Block, G., A.M. Hartman, C.M. Dresser, M.D. Carroll, J. Gannon, and L. Gardner, A data-based approach to diet questionnaire design and testing. *Am J Epidemiol*, 1986. 124: p. 453–469.
46. Hill, R.J. and P.S. Davies, The validity of self-reported energy intake as determined using the doubly labeled water technique. *Br J Nutr*, 2001. 85: p. 415–430.
47. Wyatt, H.R., G.K. Grunwald, C.L. Mosca, M. Klem, R.R. Wing, and J.O. Hill, Long-term weight loss and breakfast in subjectes in the National Weight Control Registry. *Obes Res*, 2002. 10(2): p. 78–82.
48. Paffenbarger, R.S., A.L. Wing, and R.T. Hyde, Physical activity as an index of heart attack risk in college alumni. *Am J Epidemiol*, 1978. 108: p. 161–175.
49. Jakicic, J.M., K. Clark, E. Coleman, J.E. Donnelly, J. Foreyt, E. Melanson, J. Volek, and S.L. Volpe, American College of Sports Medicine position stand. Appropriate intervention strategies for weight loss and prevention of weight regain for adults. *Med Sci Sports Exerc*, 2001. 33(12): p. 2145–56.
50. Wing, R.R., Behavioral weight control, in *Handbook of Obesity Treatment*, T. Wadden and A. Stunkard, Eds., 2002, The Guilford Press: New York. p. 301–316.
51. Klem, M.L., R.R. Wing, M.T. McGuire, H.M. Seagle, and J.O. Hill, Psychological symptoms in individuals successful at long-term maintenance of weight loss. *Health Psychol*, 1998. 17(4): p. 336–345.
52. McGuire, M.T., R.R. Wing, M.L. Klem, W. Lang, and J.O. Hill, What predicts weight regain among a group of successful weight losers? *J Consult Clin Psychol*, 1999. 67: p. 177–185.
53. Gorin, A.A., S. Phelan, R.R. Wing, and J.O. Hill, Promoting long-term weight control: does dietary consistency matter? *Int J Obes Relat Metab Disord*, 2004. 28: p. 278–281.
54. Phelan, S., J.O. Hill, W. Lang, J.R. DiBello, and R.R. Wing, Recovery from relapse among successful weight losers. *Am J Clin Nutr*, 2003. 78: p. 1079–1084.

11 A Clinical Guide to Pediatric Ambulatory Weight Management

Carine M. Lenders, Alan F. Meyers, and Holly Oh

CONTENTS

11.1 INTRODUCTION

Despite a more than threefold increase in the rate of pediatric obesity during the past three decades, there is still a lack of evidence to support current pediatric weight management approaches [1–3]. Nevertheless, the American Academy of Pediatrics (AAP) advises physicians that it is essential to monitor patients throughout their childhood and to counsel parents and caregivers to help prevent obesity in children [4]. As with other chronic conditions, the primary care clinician is responsible for providing patients and their families with information about risk.

Few families realize how serious pediatric obesity is. About half of school-age obese children and 60 to 70% of obese adolescents become obese adults [5], with greater risk of adult morbidity and mortality, independent of adult Body Mass Index (BMI), family history of cardiovascular diseases or cancer, and smoking [6,7].

The racial and socioeconomic disparities in the rates of pediatric obesity are very concerning and should be considered when developing an intervention [7].

While the increase in prevalence of obesity in the general pediatric population is worrisome, the disproportionate effect on minority populations is even more alarming. Over a period of 12 yrs, the prevalence of obesity has increased by 120% among Hispanic and black populations compared to 50% in non-Hispanic white populations [9]; in addition, minority populations are currently increasing rapidly in numbers and are expected to comprise 40% of the U.S. population by the year 2020 [10]. With regard to socioeconomic factors, lacking private health insurance is directly associated with obesity during adolescence [11]. Unfortunately, reimbursement of multidisciplinary weight management programs can be as low as 10% [12]. Thus, treatment strategies taking place in the community should take into account the special needs of minorities and groups from lower socioeconomic backgrounds.

As opposed to medical assessment and monitoring, interventions to modify behavior risk factors can be performed in different settings: group, interpersonal, organizational, and societal level. The importance of behavior modification for the success of interventions has clearly been demonstrated, at least in motivated groups [1]. However, only a small number of families (38%) are ready to change [13]. Although physician counseling has been shown to affect other risk-taking behaviors, no mechanism currently exists to empower primary care clinicians in affecting change in the patient behavior that may lead to obesity.

Attitudes, perception, and barriers to ambulatory pediatric weight management and intervention practices have been evaluated in other settings [14], but no formal curriculum has been designed to train pediatric primary care clinicians in assessing, counseling, and referring patients for weight management. O'Brien et al. have shown that pediatricians in an academic center frequently do not properly diagnose and manage obese children [15]. Additionally, many health care professionals encounter barriers to managing pediatric weight problems and express the need for increased training opportunities related to obesity prevention and treatment [16-18]. Unfortunately, they lack time as shown in one of our Continuous Medical Education (CME) surveys where most clinicians typically had less than 10 min in a session to dedicate to counseling of the patient and their family.

The focus of this chapter is to discuss a practical approach to managing pediatric obesity using evidence-based information or expert opinion when available while taking into account barriers to care. This chapter provides algorithms and tools that were developed for primary care clinicians during a multifaceted intervention intended to increase access to community-based health care and lifestyle resources while optimizing referral to the few multidisciplinary weight management programs available. This intervention had a special focus on primary care providers from Boston HealthNet (Boston Medical Center-partnered health centers) and was based on knowledge updating (lecture format), enabling strategies (workshops, problem-based learning, patient education activities), and reinforcing strategies (reminders, clinical practice guidelines, and primary care clinicians feedback) [19]. This intervention was sponsored in part by the Division of Pediatric Nutrition, the Division of Community Pediatrics at BMC, the New Balance Foundation®, the Physician Nutrition Specialist Award from the American Society for Nutrition, and the Joel and Barbara Alpert Endowment for the Children of the City, and in collaboration with the Massachusetts chapter of the American Academy of Pediatrics.

11.2 DEFINITION

Any definition of obesity is useful only if it predicts morbidity or mortality. Since most complications of obesity are associated with body fat and not muscle mass, measures of obesity represent an attempt to estimate the adipose compartment. At present, there is no precise clinically practical method to measure body fat in children and adolescents. Methods used to define obesity generally measure under- or overweight, not lean or fat. Although imperfect, these measures are inexpensive and practical for use in the clinical setting.

BMI is defined as the weight of the child in kilograms divided by the height in meters squared (kg/m^2) and was established as a useful standard measure of adiposity [20]. Although BMI does not directly measure body fat, it is typically used to evaluate adiposity in adults and has been recognized as a useful predictor of adiposity in children and adolescents and current or future medical complications of obesity [21]. Recognizing that the BMI of children and adolescents tends to predict obesity-related complications in both childhood and adulthood, the Institute of medicine (IOM) recommends that the term obesity rather than overweight be used for children and youth aged 2 to 20 yr who have a BMI at or above the 95th percentile [22].

Thus in this chapter, children and youth with BMI at or above the 85th percentile on the 2000 Centers for Disease Control and Prevention (CDC) growth charts are considered overweight and those at or above the 95th percentile are considered obese (Table 11.1) [23]. Using this definition, nearly 50% of children and youth from minority communities receiving care at BMC ambulatory clinics are overweight or obese ($n = 10{,}991$). There is no definition of obesity on the basis of morbidity or mortality risk in children under the age of 2. Given this limitation and until more evidence becomes available, we will consider that a child is at risk when the weight-for-length is at or above the 95th percentile on the CDC growth charts [23].

11.3 EVALUATION

The evaluation of pediatric obesity requires a comprehensive review of systems, child and family past medical, social and lifestyle history, and physical exam. Given the time constraints of a routine well child visit, the goal of this evaluation would be to identify obesity risk based on growth charts and determine whether a child needs anticipatory guidance [4] or further evaluation, in the form of blood tests coupled with serial follow-up visits. The evaluation for comorbidities allows the primary care pediatrician to decide if the child needs follow-up in their clinic or needs to be referred to a multidisciplinary clinic. This chapter focuses on the medical assessment of pediatric obesity while assessment of nutrition, physical activity, and sedentary behaviors, psychologic risk factors and identification of community resources and barriers are reviewed elsewhere in this book [Chapters 4, 12, 13].

11.3.1 Initial Medical Assessment

11.3.1.1 Identification of Overweight and Obesity

The initial step in the management of pediatric obesity is the identification of overweight and obesity (Table 11.2). Since BMI is calculated using standing but

TABLE 11.1
Obesity Rates (BMI >95th Percentile) by Age, Gender, and Race/Ethnicity in Boston Medical Center Pediatric Ambulatory Care Center Compared to National Rates [24]

	Male			Female		
	Non-Hispanic Black	Hispanic	Non-Hispanic White	Non-Hispanic Black	Hispanic	Non-Hispanic White
2–5 yr old						
NHANES 1999–2000	NA	13.1	6.9	11.7	8.7	10.5
NHANES 2003–2004	9.7	23.2	13.0	16.3	15.1	10.0
BMC 2000–2004	**15.2**	**26.6**	**17.7**	**16.7**	**20.4**	**10.8**
6–11 yr old						
NHANES 1999–2000	17.1	26.7	11.9	22.4	19.8	11.6
NHANES 2003–2004	17.5	25.3	18.5	26.5	19.4	16.9
BMC 2000–2004	**24.9**	**29.6**	**18.6**	**28.8**	**26.8**	**19.6**
12–19 yr old						
NHANES 1999–2000	21.0	27.2	11.8	25.2	19.3	11.0
NHANES 2003–2004	18.5	18.3	19.1	25.4	14.1	15.4
BMC 2000–2004	**24.9**	**28.5**	**19.8**	**26.4**	**22.6**	**23.9**

Note: NHANES: National Health and Nutrition Examination Survey 1999–2000 (n = 4,722) and 2003–2004 with n = 3,958; Boston Medical Center 2000–2004 (n = 10,991)

Source: Adapted based on cross sectional data from Ogden CL, Carroll MD, Curtin LR, McDowell MA, Tabak CJ, Flegal KM. Prevalence of overweight and obesity in the United States, 1999–2004. *JAMA.* 2006;295(13):1549–1555; and data from Wright J, Lee K, Shukla R, Adams W, Lenders C. Prevalence of obesity in an urban pediatric ambulatory center: 2000–2004. *Obesity* 2006; 14(supp):A78, with permission.

not recumbent measurements, children between 2 to 3 yr of age with length measurement are plotted on the weight-for-length rather then the BMI chart. Although weight-for-length is correlated with length and, to a lesser extent, BMI is correlated with height in children but no other practicable measure is available, treatment algorithms proposed in this chapter are based on those parameters. The algorithms should be used after exclusion of children who are failure-to-thrive or undernourished [25]. The provision of anticipatory guidance is based on the percentile on the appropriate growth charts: those children younger than 2 yrs of age who plot below the 95th percentile on the appropriate weight-for-length chart and those 2 yrs of age or older who plot under the 85th percentile on the BMI chart (or gain more than 2 units of BMI yearly). All children who plot at or above the 95th percentile on the weight-for-length chart or above the 85th percentile on the BMI chart would be identified and managed by primary care in conjunction with specific specialists. Children with signs and symptoms of serious and acute

TABLE 11.2A
Proposed Treatment Algorithm for Children Less Than 2 yr Old

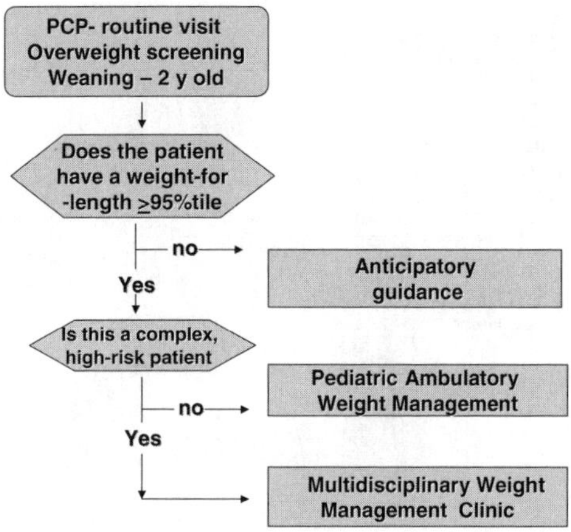

Complex high-risk patient: < 2 y

One or more conditions (acute or serious)

CVD	Moderate/Severe Hypertension
Endocrine/ CNS	CNS = central nervous system (pituitary, hypothalamic, head trauma, high androgens, high cortisol, hypothyroidism)
Genetics	Syndromic
Orthopedic	Blount
Respiratory	Sleep apnea
Psycho-Social	Low socio-economic status (SES) or sleep disorders impending lifestyle changes; psychiatric diagnosis (e.g., mental delay, autism, compulsive eating)

complications would preferably be referred to a more comprehensive multidisciplinary specialty clinic for pediatric weight management when available.

11.3.1.2 Underlying Causes and Complications Related to Obesity

Even though the cause of obesity is typically idiopathic (>95%), the next most important step for the assessment of obesity is the exclusion of potential underlying syndromic and endocrine conditions (Table 11.3).

Screening for short stature (most children with excess weight are average height or tall for their age), developmental delay, dysmorphic features, and abnormal genitalia will help rule out many genetic and endocrine causes of childhood obesity.

TABLE 11.2B
Proposed Treatment Algorithm for Children 2–20 yr

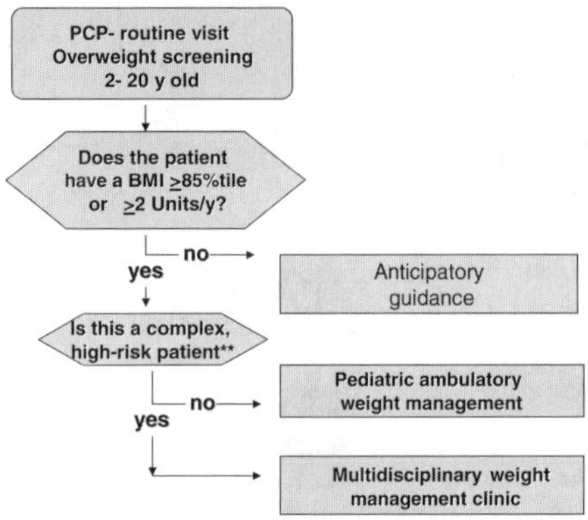

Complex high-risk patient: 2-20 y

** One or more conditions (acute or serious)

CVD	Moderate/severe hypertension, dyslipidemia, heart failure
Endocrine/ CNS	CNS, high androgens, high cortisol, hypothyroidism, Polycystic Ovary Syndrome (PCOS), Pseudotumor cerebri, Type 2 diabetes mellitus (DM)
GI	Encopresis, reflux (GERD), liver disease
Genetics	Syndromic
Orthopedic	Blount, slipped capita femoral epiphysis (SCEFE)
Respiratory	Sleep apnea, hypoventilation syndrome
Psycho-social	Low-self esteem, or sleep d/o, or teasing, or low SES impending lifestyle & school performance; psychiatric diagnosis (e.g. anxiety, compulsive eating, depression)
Lifestyle	Failed several weight treatment attempts for 1 year
Weight gain drugs	Steroids, neuropsychiatric medications

To evaluate the child's stature, the mid-parental height (MPH) potential would be calculated by gender (1 in = 2.5 cm) with an MPH range ± 2.

Boy MPH = (Father's height + [Mother's height + 5"])/2
Girl MPH = ([Father's height − 5"] + Mother's height)/2

TABLE 11.3A
Causes of Obesity

Endogenous (or Organic)	Exogenous (or Idiopathic)
Anatomic or endocrine	Environmental: psychosocial, lifestyle
Syndromic (single gene mutation)	Hereditary

TABLE 11.3B
Causes of Obesity: Typical Assessment

	Endocrine	Syndromic	Exogenous
Bone age	Decreased	Increased	Appropriate
Development delay	No	Yes	No
Dysmorphic features	No	Yes	No
Early obesity onset	No	Yes	No
Hypogonadism	Yes	Yes	No
Kidney condition	No	Yes	No
Muscle strength	Decreased	Normal	Normal
Short stature	Yes	Yes	No
Tone	Normal	Decreased	Normal
Vision/hearing	No	Yes	No

Note: Syndromes may present with tall stature and lack in specific features.

Thus, a child's stature that is not commensurate with his or her MPH potential may invite further investigation into genetic or endocrine causes of childhood obesity (Table 11.3). Furthermore, Mendelian syndromes are distinguishable through their specific features (Table 11.4) and laboratory tests may be performed to confirm the diagnosis, but not as screening tests [26-28]. Although the AAP does not support thyroid function tests in obese children and adolescents [15], parents are always concerned about a "glandular problem," and a negative history and physical exam does not exclude its presence. As syndromes should be identified early, referrals to multidisciplinary pediatric weight management programs before 2 yr of age have been recommended previously by an expert panel on pediatric obesity (Table 11.4) [29].

Complications associated with obesity, which should be identified in children and adolescents have been summarized in Table 11.5 and adapted from several sources [29,42], including the authors' access to their program data. The presence of complications associated with obesity is based on history, physical examination, and laboratory tests. These complications may require a referral to a specialty clinic prior to making community-based lifestyle change recommendations.

Although specific guidelines exist to screen for common comorbid conditions, there may be challenges to implementing these guidelines in the primary setting. For example, specific guidelines to screen for type 2 diabetes mellitus have been developed (Table 11.6) [43–45]. However, these guidelines are controversial as the screening criteria fit a large number of children and youth (more than 2.5 million in the U.S.) and the yield of these tests is relatively low [46].

Specific guidelines to screen for hypercholesterolemia and dyslipidemia have been developed and published by the AAP [47], but are impractical especially given the poor program compliance of challenged populations. The identification of dyslipidemia would require an unacceptable number of visits according to those recommendations. The AAP, in 1992, recommended to screen all children 2 yr of age

TABLE 11.4
Examples of Syndromes Associated with Obesity [30,31]

Syndrome	Chromosome	Clinical Features	Anthropometrics	Cognitive Deficit
Albright (pseudohypo-parathyroidism—type IA)	20q13.2 (recessive)	Bone fibrous dysplasia Hyperpigmentation/vitiligo Neuroendocrine anomalies Polydactily Precocious puberty	Normal or short stature Variable (general) overweight Early onset of overweight	Mild
Alstrom	2p14–p13 (recessive)	Deafness Neuroendocrine anomalies Normal or hypogonadism Retinitis pigmentosa	Normal or short stature Moderate (central) Onset overweight at age 2–5 yr	None
Bardet Biedl	16q21, 15q22–q23	Compulsive behavior Heart anomalies Hypogonadism Hypotonia Polydactyly Renal dysfunction Retinitis	Normal or short stature Moderate (central) overweight Onset overweight at age 1–2 yr	Moderate
Carpenter	Unknown (recessive)	Acrocephaly Flat nasal bridge Heart anomalies High arched palate Hypogonadism Polydactyly Syndactyly	Short stature Central overweight	Mild
Cohen	8q22–q23 (recessive)	Heart anomalies Hypotonia Low hairline Microcephaly Normal or hypogonadism Retinochoroidal dystrophy Short or tall stature Short philtrum	Variable (central) overweight Mid-childhood	Mild
Leptin or leptin receptor	7q31.3 (recessive); 1p31–p32 (recessive)	Hypometabolic rate Hyperphagia Infertility Impaired oral glucose tolerance tests (OGTT) Pubertal delay	Normal stature General overweight Early onset overweight	None

TABLE 11.4 (Continued)
Examples of Syndromes Associated with Obesity [30,31]

Syndrome	Chromosome	Clinical Features	Anthropometrics	Cognitive Deficit
Melacortin 4 (MC4) receptor	18q22 (dominant)	Hyperphagia Increased bone density	Normal stature General overweight Early onset overweight	?
Propiomelano-cortin (POMC)	2p23.3 (recessive)	Adrenocorticotrophic (ACTH) deficiency Hyperphagia Red hair	Normal stature General overweight Early onset overweight	None
Prader–Willi	15q11–q12 (uniparental maternal disomy)	Almond-shaped eyes Compulsive behavior High arched palate Hypogonadism Hypotonia Neuroendocrine anomalies V-shaped mouth	Short stature General moderate/severe overweight Onset overweight at 1–3 yr	Mild to moderate

Source: Adapted from Lenders C and Hoppin A. In: Walker W, Watkins J, Duggan C, Eds. *Nutrition in Pediatrics: Basic Science and Clinical Applications*, 3rd edition. B.C. Decker; ch. 54 2003; 917–934. With permission. For further information, see http://obesity.gene.pbrc.edu

TABLE 11.5
Complications Associated with Obesity in Children and Youth

	Rates (%)	Relevant History and Exam	Diagnostic Tests
Cardiovascular			
Dyslipidemia	17–23	Family Hx; xanthomas	Fasting lipid profile
Hypertension	10–27	Family Hx; 14% children with persistent HBP have LVH	SBP and/or BP >90th percentile
Endocrine			
Impaired OGTT	25	RF of type 2 diabetes mellitus; typically asymptomatic or fatigue	Elevated fasting or 2 hr-OGTT glucose
Type 2 diabetes mellitus	3	High thirst, urination, appetite, fatigue, acanthosis, blurred vision, skin/GU infections, family Hx	Elevated fasting glucose or OGTT
PCOS	?	Amenorrhea, acne, hirsutism, acanthosis (see ACOG, 2005)	Testosterone (total, free), TSH, PRL, 17-OH progesterone

(*continued*)

TABLE 11.5 (Continued)
Complications Associated with Obesity in Children and Youth

	Rates (%)	Relevant History and Exam	Diagnostic Tests
			Optional: ovaries US, LH/FSH
Osteopenia/ osteoporosis	?	May be at increased risk	PTH, 25-OH Vit D, Ca, Mg, Phos
GI/nutrition			
Anemia	5	High HR, pale features, poor growth, fatigue, weakness, cold sensitivity, xs infections	CBC, iron studies, reticulocyte count
Constipation	23	Scybalous, pebble-like, hard stools for a majority of stools; or firm stools two or less times/wk; and no evidence of structural, endocrine, or metabolic disease	Rectal exam, abdominal x-ray
Fecal soiling	15	At least 12 wk: large BM<2X/wk and retentive posturing	Rectal exam, abdominal x-ray
GERD	?	Overfeeding, vomiting, chest pain/burning, asthma	PH probe if treatment trial fails
High ALT (NAFLD)	20	Abdominal pain, nausea, vomiting, asymptomatic	ALT/AST ≥ 3Xnl, repeat liver tests, r/o hepatitis causes
Orthopedic			
Blount's disease	<1	Juvenile; adolescence; one or both knees; deformity; intra-articular instability	X-ray
Flat feet	?	With pain	Ortho
SCFE	<1	Often painless limp; knee pain; flexed hip goes to external rotation	X-ray, MRI, arthroscopy, rapid referral
Neuropsychiatric			
Binge eating (also known as compulsive eating)	?	Large amount of food in discrete time period (2 hr); lack of control, distressed by binging; sneaking/hoarding food; excessive concern with body shape and weight; persists for at least 3 mo, no compensatory behaviors	Eating Attitudes Test—Child Version (chEAT); Eating Disorder Inventory—C (pre-teens and teens); QEWP-A (adolescent version); Eating Disorder Examination (ChEDE)—interview; use ChEDE-Q self-report
Compulsive overeating	6	Characterized by episodic binge eating; may also include uses of purging or restrictive eating; fear of not being able to stop eating; depressed mood; food can become a mood regulator	See above

TABLE 11.5 (Continued)
Complications Associated with Obesity in Children and Youth

	Rates (%)	Relevant History and Exam	Diagnostic Tests
Night eating syndrome	?	Little/no appetite for breakfast; most caloric intake at night; leaves bed to snack at night; anxious; sleep disturbance; persists for at least 2 mo	N/A for children or adolescents, screen for symptoms present
Depression	?	Depressed mood, low self-esteem, ahedoin, irritability, hopelessness, Hx of suicide ideation, sleep disturbance, fatigue, diminished concentration	Child Depression Inventory (CDI)
Anxiety	?	Excessive worry; sleep disturbance; tantrums/crying; obsessive thoughts; fatigue; low self-esteem; avoidance; Hx of trauma; r/o social phobia and separation anxiety	Child Behavior Checklist (CBCL)
Weight teasing (stigmatization, discrimination)	?	Child is target of name-calling, ridicule, put-downs, verbal insults; can occur at home and at school	Teasing and Bullying Survey (TABS-C)—Bodin (2004) (still in research stage)
Pseudotumor cerebrei	<1	Blurred vision; headaches (better with gravity); abnl fundi	Fundi exam, LP
Pulmonary			
Asthma	15	Recurrent episodes of wheezing, chest pain, difficulty breathing; nocturnal cough	Reversible airflow obstruction (peak flow)
Sleep apnea	5–7	Snoring; witnessed apnea; cyanosis; parental concern regarding child's breathing, restless sleep; can lead to heart failure	High RBC; metabolic alkalosis; polysomnography
Dermatologic			
Acanthosis nigricans	81	Elevated skin texture at pressure points	Skin examination
Cutaneous candidiasis	?	Signs of candidiasis	Fasting glucose

Source: Adapted from References [29,42] and data obtained from CL at Children's Hospital of Boston and Boston Medical Center.

and older, with a parent history of premature CAD and/or dyslipidemia [47]. Building on these guidelines, the American Heart Association was less conservative and suggested a fasting lipid profile in all children older than 2 yr and adolescents who smoked, had hypertension, were overweight or obese, or had diabetes (Table 11.7) [48,49].

TABLE 11.6
Assessment of Carbohydrate Metabolism

A. Screening for Type 2 Diabetes Mellitus in Children [43–45]

Definition of body fatness	BMI ≥ 85th percentile
	Wt-for-Ht ≥ 85th percentile
	Wt ≥ 120% ideal body weight
Conditions (two of the three conditions)	Type 2 diabetes mellitus in first- or second-degree relatives
	Race/ethnicty (Native-, African-, Latino-, Asian-American, or Pacific Islander)
	At least acanthosis nigricans, HTN, dyslipidemia, or PCOS
Age and Tanner stage	<10 yr and Tanner stage 2–5
	≥10 yr and Tanner stage 1–5

Source: Copyright 2000. Modified with permission from American Diabetes Association, *Diabetes Care*. 2000; 23(3): 381–389; American Diabetes Association.

B. Tests

Tests (one)	8 hr fast plasma glucose
	OGTT (plasma glucose 2 hr post-challenge)
Frequency	Every 2 yrs if negative

Note: The American Diabetic Association recommends preferentially fasting blood sugar.

C. Reference Values for Children Aged 2 to 20 Yr

	8 hr Fasting Glucose (mg/dL)	2 hr Glucose OGTT (mg/dL)	Random Glucose (mg/dL)	HgbA1c (%)	Fasting Insulin (μU/mL)
Acceptable	<100	<140	<200	5–6	2–15
Borderline	100–125	140–199	NA	6.1–6.9	15.1–19
High	≥126	≥200	≥200	≥7	≥20

Note: HgbA1c is not recommended by the American Academy of Diabetes to diagnose diabetes. However, it is a practical nonfasting predictor. The main concern is that the type of HgbA1C measured and ranges vary somewhat by laboratory. HOMA-IR = (fasting insulin [microU/mL] × fasting glucose [mmol/L])/22.5. Homa-IR is considered a research tool; there is no consensus on a cutoff point in these children.

D. Management: If Fasting Glucose ≥ 100 mg/dL (Possibly Nonfasting HgA1c ≥ 6%)

Weight management with improved diet and exercise (see Chapter 4)
Treat other risk factors (hypertension, dyslipidemia) aggressively to prevent accelerated vascular disease
Refer to endocrinologist
Consider oral agents (e.g., Metformin or glitazones) to improve insulin sensitivity with an endocrinologist

The first line of treatment of dyslipidemia recommended is the Therapeutic Lifestyle Change (TLC, see Chapter 4). The patient is referred to a lipid specialist for further pharmacological evaluation when the nonpharmacologic treatment is unsuccessful or insufficient (Table 11.8).

TABLE 11.7
Dyslipidemia

A. Tests

Non-fasting total cholesterol and HDL_C

10–12-hr fasting lipid profile (total cholesterol, HDL-c, triglycerides); repeat and take average

LDL-c = Total cholesterol –HDL - (triglycerides/5) [if fasting triglycerides <400 mg/dL]

Reference Values for Children Ages 2-19 Years Old [47, 48, 56]

Category	Total cholesterol (TC) (mg/dL)	LDL_C (mg/dL)	HDL_C (mg/dL)	Triglycerides (mg/dL)
Acceptable	<170	<110	≥35–50	≤150–200
Borderline	170–199	110–129	N/A	N/A
High	≥200	≥130	<35–50	>150–200

Note: Definition of dyslipidemia: abnormal cholesterol (TC, LDL-C, or HDL-C) and/or TG concentrations. There is no clear updated consensus since 1992 on the cut off point to be used for abnormal HDL_c and triglycerides among children.

B. Primary Prevention in Children and Youth [48]

Dietary modification: limit foods with

Saturated fast to <10% calories/d

Cholesterol to <300 mg/d

Trans fatty acids

Physical activity

Increase moderate to vigorous ≥60 min/d

Limit sedentary activities ≤2 hr/d

Selective screening

Family history of cardiovascular heart disease

One parent with blood cholesterol >240 mg/dL

No parent history but cardiovascular heart disease risk factors present

≥1 of the following risk factors present: high blood pressure; smoking; sedentary life style; obesity; alcohol intake; use of drugs or diseases associated with dyslipidemia

Source: Reproduced with permission. AHA Scientific Statement, American Heart Association, Managing Abnormal Blood Lipids: A Collaborative Approach © 2005, American Heart Association.

Note: The National Cholesterol Expert Panel (NCEP) and the American Heart Association (AHA) recommend an individualized/high risk approach to identifying dyslipidemia in children, including obese children. A fasting lipid profile in obese children ages 2–20 yrs allows for a comprehensive assessment. The NCEP and AAP recommend to average results of 2 fasting lipids and the AHA recommends to average results of 3 fasting lipid profiles as baseline for guiding treatment.

Finally, guidelines for hypertension have been developed but they are very cumbersome for use in the pediatric office (Table 11.9) [50].

Although the value of screening has been debated [51] and typically has not been recommended before 10 yr of age, it may be useful to determine if there is dyslipidemia and signs of steatosis and glucose intolerance, particularly as new treatments for these conditions are considered [52]. The ideal tests are performed

TABLE 11.8
Treatment of Dyslipidemia

A. Non-Pharmacological Medical Management [47–49]

Borderline LDL	Advise about risk factors for cardiovascular disease Initiate AHA Therapeutic Lifestyle Change (TLC) Diet
High LDL	Evaluate for secondary causes (thyroid, liver, and renal disorders) Evaluate for familial disorders Screen all family members Initiate TLC diet
Low HDL	Counsel regarding smoking, low saturated fat diet, physical activity, and weight management
High triglycerides	Counsel regarding weight management Decrease amount and type of fat and carbohydrates Increase intake of foods rich in fiber Increase consumption of omega-3 fatty acids

Step 1 and 2 diets have been replaced by the American Heart Association TLC diet (Chapter 4)
For further discussion see http://www.emedicine.com/ped/topic2787.htm#target12 (accessed November 11, 2005)

B. Treatment of Dyslipidemia: Indications for Pharmacological Referral [47–49]

Children ≥10 yrs old and after 6–12 m of strict diet therapy

Persistent LDL >190 mg/dL	
Persistent LDL >160 mg/dL	Strong family history of premature CAD (<55 years of age), or ≥2 adult CVD risk factors (low HDL, smoking, high BP, obesity, type 2 diabetes mellitus)

Triglycerides > 400 mg/dL to prevent pancreatitis

Note: Refer to lipid specialist if non-pharmacological management is unsuccessful or if pharmacological management is warranted

C. Pharmacological Agents [47–49]

Bile acid-binding resins or sequestrants (e.g. Choles-teramine)	Documented efficacy
Action: Inhibits bile and thus total cholesterol and LDL-C absorption	Few adverse effects (constipation, nausea/vomiting/diarrhea, higher TG) Apparently safe in children Check TG Supplement with ADEK, folic acid, Fe
Statins–HMG CoA-Reductase Inhibitors	Most effective in lowering LDL (but also TC, ApoB, TG) in adults
(e.g. lovostatin, pravastavin, atorvastatin, simvastatin)	Lowers LDL-C, TC, Apo B in pediatrics
Action: Rate-limiting enzyme in de novo cholesterol synthesis	Safe in children — no liver or muscle damage, no effects on growth or sexual development Check LFTs, CPK

Note: Other agents are not recommended for routine use in children and adolescents except in consultation with a lipid specialist. Prepared by Shirley Huang.

TABLE 11.9
Hypertension

A. Diagnosis and Non-Pharmacological Treatment [50]

	SBP or DBP Percentile*	Frequency of BP Measurement	Therapeutic Lifestyle Changes	Pharmacologic Therapy
Normal	<90th	Recheck at next scheduled physical examination	Encourage healthy diet, sleep, and physical activity	—
Pre-hypertension	90th to <95th or if BP exceeds 120/80 even if <90th percentile up to <95th percentile	Recheck in 6 mo	Weight-management counseling if overweight; introduce physical activity and diet management	None unless compelling indications such as chronic kidney disease, diabetes mellitus, heart failure, or LVH exist
Stage 1 hypertension	95th–99th percentile plus 5 mm Hg	Recheck in 1–2 wk or sooner if the patient is symptomatic; if persistently elevated on 2 additional occasions, evaluate or refer to source of care within 1 mo	Weight-management counseling if overweight; introduce physical activity and diet management	Initiate pharmacological therapy based on indications in Table 11.9.B or if compelling indications exist (as above)
Stage 2 hypertension	>99th percentile plus 5 mm Hg	Evaluate or refer to source of care within 1 wk or immediately if the patient is symptomatic	Weight-management counseling if overweight; introduce physical activity and diet management	Initiate therapy

Source: Reproduced from the National High Blood Pressure Education Program Working Group on High Blood Pressure in Children and Adolescents published in the public domain at http://www.nhlbi.nih.gov/health/prof/heart/hbp/hbp_ped.pdf and also by The American Academy of Pediatrics. *Pediatrics* 2004:114:555–576.

(*continued*)

TABLE 11.9 (Continued)
Hypertension

B. Blood Pressure Measurement Tips

Measure BP at least once in every health care encounter in children >3 years of age

Measure BP in special circumstances in <3 years of age

Blood pressures >90th percentile on oscillometric devices should be repeated by auscultation

Note: Definition of hypertension: SBP and/or DBP ≥95th percentile for age, gender, and height measured on 3 separate readings at rest for at least 5 minutes

C. Hypertension: Systolic and Diastolic Blood Pressure by Age, Gender, and Height

		SPB			DBP		
Age (years)	**BP percentile**	**5-25th percentile for height**	**50th percentile for height**	**75–95th percentile for height**	**5–25th percentile for height**	**50th percentile for height**	**75–95th percentile for height**
1 to 3	90th	94–103	99–105	100–109	49–60	52–61	53–63
	95th	98–107	103–109	104–113	54–64	56–65	57–67
	99th	105–114	110–116	112–120	61–72	64–73	65–75
4 to 6	90th	102–108	107–100	109–113	62–69	65–70	66–72
	95th	106–112	111–114	112–117	66–73	69–74	70–76
	99th	113–119	118–121	120–125	74–81	77–82	78–84
7 to 10	90th	106–114	111–115	113–119	70–74	72–75	73–78
	95th	110–117	115–119	117–123	74–79	76–80	77–82
	99th	117–125	122–127	124–130	82–86	84–88	85–90
11 to 13	90th	113–120	117–122	119–126	74–76	76–77	73–79
	95th	117–124	121–126	123–130	78–80	80–81	81–83
	99th	124–131	129–133	130–137	86–88	88–89	89–91
14 to 17	90th	126–130	125–132	113–136	75–81	78–82	79–84
	95th	124–134	128–136	130–140	80–86	82–87	83–89
	99th	131–141	136–143	138–147	87–93	90–94	91–97

Note: Prepared by Shirley Huang. Categories are collapsed across age and gender to facilitate reading of the table. For precise cutoff points by age, gender, and height, please see source below.

Source: National High Blood Pressure Education Program Working Group on High Blood Pressure in Children and Adolescents published in the public domain at http://www.nhlbi.nih.gov/health/prof/heart/hbp/hbp_ped.pdf and also by The American Academy of Pediatrics. *Pediatrics* 2004:114:555–576.

TABLE 11.10
Pharmacologic Treatment of Hypertension

A. Indications

Symptomatic hypertension
Secondary hypertension
Hypertensive target-organ damage
Diabetes (types 1 and 2)
Persistent hypertension despite non-pharmacologic measures

Source: Reproduced from the National High Blood Pressure Education Program Working Group on High Blood Pressure in Children and Adolescents published in the public domain at http://www.nhlbi.nih.gov/health/prof/heart/hbp/hbp_ped.pdf and also by The American Academy of Pediatrics. *Pediatrics* 2004:114:555–576.

B. Agents

Indications for antihypertensive drug therapy in children include secondary hypertension and insufficient response to lifestyle modifications.

Recent clinical trials have expanded the number of drugs that have pediatric dosing information. Dosing recommendations for many of the newer drugs are provided in the original source document.

Pharmacologic therapy, when indicated, should be initiated with a single drug. Acceptable drug classes for use in children include ACE inhibitors, angiotensin-receptor blockers, b-blockers, calcium channel blockers, and diuretics.

The goal for antihypertensive treatment in children should be reduction of BP to <95th percentile unless concurrent conditions are present, in which case BP should be lowered to <90th percentile.

Severe, symptomatic hypertension should be treated with intravenous antihypertensive drugs.

Source: Reproduced from the National High Blood Pressure Education Program Working Group on High Blood Pressure in Children and Adolescents published in the public domain at http://www.nhlbi.nih.gov/health/prof/heart/hbp/hbp_ped.pdf and also by The American Academy of Pediatrics. *Pediatrics* 2004:114:555–576.

in the fasting state (~12 hr), as most guidelines require fasting laboratory tests for definitive diagnosis. However, in practice, this might be difficult to obtain, especially for clinicians who serve challenged families with multiple barriers to access care. Therefore, blood work should be done in the fasting state if possible, but nonfasting blood work might also be a reasonable alternative for screening (Table 11.11), depending on considerations of adherence. Nonfasting samples showing high thyroid-stimulating hormone (TSH), glucose, hemoglobin A_{1C}, total cholesterol, alanine aminotransferase (ALT), and low HDL-c have been associated with screening of hypothyroidism, diabetes mellitus, dyslipidemia, and nonalcoholic fatty liver disease (NAFL).

Fasting glucose and insulin provide information regarding carbohydrate metabolism and insulin resistance and may predict risk of diabetes mellitus. Measurements of cholesterol may be useful as hypercholesterolemia has been described even in children less than 2 yr of age. The total cholesterol (TC)/HDL-C ratio is another helpful parameter for assessing risk for cardiovascular disease (CVD). The higher

TABLE 11.11
Practicable Blood Tests for Obese Children and Youth

	Initial		Follow-up	
Blood Tests	**Fasting (8–12 hr)**	**Not Fasting**	**Fasting (8–12 hr)**	**Not Fasting**
Total-C (mg/dL)[a]	<170	<170	5 yr or less	5 yr or less
	170–199	170–199	1 yr	1 yr
	200	200	1 yr	1 yr
HDL-C (mg/dL)	≥35–50	≥35–50	5 yr or less	5 yr or less
	<35–50	<35–50	1 yr	1 yr
LDL-C (mg/dL)	<110	—	—	—
	110–129	—	1 yr	—
	130	—	1 yr	—
Triglyceride (mg/dL)	<150–200	—	—	—
	≥150–200	—	1 yr	—
HgBA1c [b] (%)	5–6	5–6	1 yr or loss	1 yr or less
	6.1–6.9	6.1–6.9	Endocrine referral	Endocrine referral
	≥7	≥7	Endocrine referral	Endocrine referral
Glucose (mg/dL)[c]	<100	<200	2 yr or less	2 yr or less
	100–125	NA	Endocrine referral	Endocrine referral
	≥126	≥200	Endocrine referral	Fasting glucose
Insulin[d] (μU/mL)	2–15	—	—	—
	15.1–19	—	—	—
	≥20	—	—	—
ALT/AST	>2–3X nl	>2–3X nl	6 mo[e]	6 mo[e]
Bilirubin T/D	>normal range	>normal range	—	—
BUN/Creatinine	>normal range	>normal range	—	—
TSH	>normal range	>normal range	—	—
CBC	—	—	Per routine	—

Note: We observed that less than 5% of all obese children in a multidisciplinary weight management program had ALT above twice normal range which required gastroenterology referrals (n = 300).

[a] Although based on this guide cholesterol should be checked less frequently when within the normal range [47], levels of cholesterol among obese patients with accelerates weight gain relative to height may need to be checked more frequently.

[b] HgBa1C should be followed every 3 months if the patient has type 2 diabetes mellitus. Although HgBA1C is not recommended as a screening tool for type 2 diabetes mellitus, it might be useful in children with rapid BMI gain. More research is needed.

[c] Follow-up of glucose levels is recommended in overweight and obese children [44] but patients with excessive BMI gain may need more frequent measurements of glucose.

[d] Insulin is not recommended for diabetes screening but may be of utility to document and share with parents the associated risk of insulin resistance. More research is needed.

[e] If liver function tests show persistent elevation of ALT/AST (>2–3X nl) at 6 months, a referral to a gastroenterologist for further investigations should be considered. Further GI workup may include a history of alcohol use, hepatitis B and C virus serology, autoimmune antibody screen, ceruloplasmin, 24-hr urine for copper, lipid profile, fasting glucose, imaging studies, and possibly a liver biopsy.

TABLE 11.12
Useful Tests for Children at Risk for Hypercholesterolemia [47]

TSH
Serum BUN/creatinine
Liver function studies
Lipid panel (TC, HDL-c, LDL-c, and triglycerides)
Pregnancy test

the ratio, the higher the risk of developing CVD. Based on a TC of 150 mg/dL and an HDL-C of 50 mg/dL, the usual TC/HDL-C ratio in children is approximately 3 [53]. In addition, it may be practicable to exclude liver, renal, and thyroid disorders during the same visit when working with challenged populations, as these disorders are associated with hypercholesterolemia (Table 11.12).

Therefore, the tests outlined in Table 11.12 have been included in the practicable tests that may be useful in the assessment of pediatric obesity (Table 11.11). In the same table, a follow-up schedule is proposed, especially for tests that are found to be out of the acceptable range and for children who continue to show excessive relative weight gain as demonstrated on their weight-for-length or BMI charts. Current guidelines do not taken into account the fact that a significant number of patients who are obese continue to show excessive weight gain and thus, waiting 2 or 5 yr for a laboratory follow-up may be too long.

11.3.2 Follow-Up and Monitoring

After obesity risk assessment during a routine visit, the primary care clinician may follow the pediatric ambulatory weight management algorithm and complete the assessment (Table 11.13).

Pertinent points and risks associated with obesity are reviewed with the family based on findings from the growth charts, history, physical exam, and laboratory tests. Further laboratory testing may be necessary in selected cases, but may be expensive or may not be readily available. For example, sleep studies should be performed if there are strong clinical signs of sleep apnea [54] and radiographic evaluation performed when slipped capita femoral epiphysis (SCFE) or Blount disease are suspected. Indirect calorimetry may be used to predict the energy deficit needed for weight loss [55]. This may be very useful when poor program adherence or an eating disorder is suspected and at times may be useful to provide concrete caloric goals to support dietary changes. Bone age may be useful as part of the workup of an endocrinopathy. The child and family readiness to change lifestyles and to follow up in clinic, in either one-on-one or a treatment group program, should be assessed [Chapter 12].

Patients should have their weight, length or height, and weight-for-length or BMI plotted on their growth charts at least at every well child visit in order to prevent obesity and identify excess weight gain relative to linear growth (Table 11.14).

More specifically, children under the age of 2, diagnosed as being at risk for obesity in childhood, should have their weight-for-length plotted and lifestyles reassessed

TABLE 11.13
Algorithm for Pediatric Ambulatory Weight Management

Complex high-risk patient: < 2 y

One or more conditions (acute or serious)

CVD	Moderate/Severe HTN, dyslipidemia
Endocrine/ CNS	CNS (pituitary, hypothalamic, head trauma), high androgens, high cortisol, hypothyroidism)
Genetics	Syndromic
Orthopedic	Blount
Respiratory	Sleep apnea
Psycho-Social	Low SES or sleep d/o impending lifestyle change); psychiatric diagnosis (e.g. mental delay, autism, ADHD, compulsive eating)

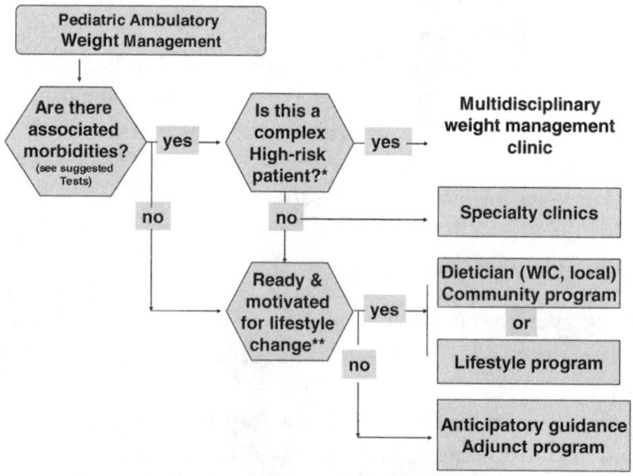

Complex high-risk patient: 2-20 y

One or more conditions (acute or serious)

CVD	Moderate/severe HTN, dyslipidemia, RVH/RVF
Endocrine/ CNS	CNS, high androgens, high cortisol, hypothyroidism, PCOS, Pseudotumor cerebri, Type 2 DM
GI	Encopresis, GERD, liver disease
Genetics	Syndromic
Orthopedic	Blount, SCFE
Respiratory	Sleep apnea, hypoventilation syndrome
Psycho-social	Low-self esteem, or sleep d/o, or teasing, or low SES impending lifestyle & school performance; psychiatric diagnosis (e.g. anxiety, compulsive eating, depression)
Lifestyle	Failed several weight treatment attempts for 1 year
Weight gain drugs	Steroids, neuropsychiatric medications

Note: Practicable follow-up schedule. For the <2-yr-old: followup at scheduled well child visits unless special issues arise. For the 2–20-yr-old: first followup at 1 mo, then based on readiness to change, motivation, comorbidities, and success. See definition on complex righ-risk patient in Table 11.2A and B.

TABLE 11.14
AAP Recommendations for *Prevention* of Obesity in Children and Youth [4]

Identify and track patients at risk by virtue of family history, birth weight, or socioeconomic, ethnic, cultural, or environmental factors
Calculate and plot BMI "once a year" in all children and adolescents
Use change in BMI to identify rate of excessive weight gain relative to linear growth
Encourage, support, and protect breastfeeding
Encourage parents and caregivers to promote healthy eating patterns by offering nutritious snacks, such as vegetables and fruits, low-fat dairy foods, and whole grains; encouraging children's autonomy in self-regulation of food intake and setting appropriate limits on choices; and modeling healthy food choices
Routinely promote physical activity, including unstructured play at home, in school, in child care settings, and throughout the community
Recommend limitation of television and video time to a maximum of 2 hours per day
Recognize and monitor changes in obesity-associated risk factors for adult chronic disease, such as hypertension, dyslipidemia, hyperinsulinemia, impaired glucose tolerance, and symptoms of obstructive sleep apnea syndrome

Source: Adapted with permission from the American Academy of Pediatrics. *Pediatrics*, 2003; 112:424–430.

and readdressed at every well child visit; the 2- to 20-year-olds who are obese would benefit from an initial follow-up at 1 month and frequency, thereafter, determined case-by-case, depending on the readiness to change, comorbid conditions, and lifestyle changes success (Table 11.13). An example of initial and follow-up forms that may be adapted by clinicians to their practices needs is summarized (Table 11.15). Assessment of parent and child for readiness to change is reviewed elsewhere [Chapter 12].

TABLE 11.15
Initial and Followup Ambulatory Pediatric Obesity Triggers for Assessment/Plan and Lifestyle (Example)

A. PCP Obesity Initial Medical Assessment
NAME:
DOB:
DATE OF VISIT:

HPI: Development of Obesity, general health, previous weight loss efforts MEDS and ALTERNATIVE MEDS:
ALLERGIES (food, med):

ROS:

Sleep			**Respiratory**		
Apnea	Y	N	Asthma/SOB?	Y	N
Disturbance	Y	N			

(continued)

TABLE 11.15 (Continued)
Initial and Followup Ambulatory Pediatric Obesity Triggers for Assessment/Plan and Lifestyle (Example)

Central Process			**Musculoskeletal**		
HA/Vision problems?	Y	N	Joint problems?	Y	N
Endocrine			**GI**		
Temperature Intolerance?	Y	N	Constipation/ encopresis	Y	N
Polyuria/polydipsia?	Y	N	Abdominal Pain?	Y	N
Irregular menses?	Y	N	Nausea/Vomiting?	Y	N
Delayed menarche?	Y	N			
Early signs of puberty?	Y	N			
Syndrome			**Other**		
Dysmorphic features?	Y	N			
Dedevelopmental delay?	Y	N			
Short stature?	Y	N			
FAMILY MEDICAL HISTORY					
1st or 2nd Degree Relatives					
Obesity?	Y	N			
Type II DM?	Y	N			
GBD	Y	N			
High cholesterol?	Y	N			
CVD?	Y	N			
HTN?	Y	N			
Stroke?	Y	N			
PSYCHOSOCIAL SCREEN					
Signs of depression?	Y	N			
Teasing?	Y	N			
Overeating	Y	N			
Self-esteem issues?	Y	N			
Anxiety?	Y	N			
Eating disorder?	Y	N			
School performance?					
Who lives at home?					
Stressors at home?					
Food sufficiency problems?					
SEDENTARY AND PHYSICAL ACTIVITIES					
Hours TV/day					
TV in bedroom	Y	N			
Hours computer/day					
Eating in front of TV	Y	N			
Hours video game/day					
Sleeping with TV on	Y	N			

TABLE 11.15 (Continued)
Initial and Followup Ambulatory Pediatric Obesity Triggers for Assessment/Plan and Lifestyle (Example)

Physical activity min/week?
What type of activity?

DIET HISTORY

24 Hour Food Recall	**Food Frequency**
Skip meals?	Dairy
Breakfast	Meat
Snack	Starch
Lunch	Vegetables
Snack	Fruit
Dinner	Fast food (incl school)
Snack	
Juice/Soda: ____oz/day	

PHYSICAL EXAM

Weight
Height
Height %tile
BMI
BMI %ile
BP
Pulse
General Appearance (Moon facies? Dysmorphic features? Hygiene?)
Skin (Acanthosis nigricans, stretch marks, hirsutism)
HEENT (Tonsils size? Thyroid size?)
Chest (Stretch marks? Tanner stage?
CV
Abdomen (Stretch marks? HSM?)
GU (Tanner stage)
Extremities (Edema? Flat feet? Digit issues?)
Neuro

Readiness to change?

Precontemplation: Unaware of the problem, unwilling/discouraged when it comes to changing the problem
Contemplation: Recognizes that a problem exists but is ambivalent regarding making a change
Preparation: Committed to making a change in the near future; on the verge of taking action; trying to gather information
Action: Actively involved in taking steps to change behavior
Maintenance: Working to consolidate gains attained and may be struggling to prevent relapse
Relapse/Recycle: Has returned to problem behavior

(*continued*)

TABLE 11.15 (Continued)
Initial and Followup Ambulatory Pediatric Obesity Triggers for Assessment/Plan and Lifestyle (Example)

IMPRESSION

Plan

1. Medical Risks explained: Type II DM, HTN, CVD, Sleep apnea, Ortho
2. Dietary and/or activity goals (pick 1 or 2)
   a.
   b.
3. Referrals needed:
4. Labs:

Nonfasting □Total Chol/HDL-c □AST/ALT/Bil □BUN/Cr □A1C □Glu □TSH □CBC

Fasting, consider adding: □LDL-C/, □Trg □Insulin

Follow up in ____

Signature

B. PCP Obesity Follow-Up Form

NAME

DOB

DATE OF VISIT

ALLERGIES:

MEDS:

Interval Hx: Recall of goals; successes and barriers; focused ROS

Lifestyle History:

Sedentarity/Physical Activity/Sleep

Hours screen time/day (TV, Video games, computer)?

Minutes/type of physical activity per week?

Sleep time and quality?

Diet History

24-Hour Food Recall:

Skip meals?

Breakfast

Snack

Lunch

Snack

Dinner

Snack

Juice/Soda ___oz day

Food Frequency

Dairy

Meat

Starch

Vegetables

Fruit

Fast Food (incl school)

Physical Exam (Focus)

Weight

Height

BMI

TABLE 11.15 (Continued)
Initial and Followup Ambulatory Pediatric Obesity Triggers for Assessment/Plan and Lifestyle (Example)

	Previous Labs: Fasting or Not Fasting	
BMI %ile	Tchol	Creat
BP	HDL-c	TSH
BP%tile	LDL-c	A1C
General appearance	ALT	Glu
Skin (Acanthosis nigricans? Pedal edema?)	AST	Insulin
Other	Bili	Htc
	BUN	

Impression/Plan

1. Dietary and/or activity goals (repeat or revise previous goals?)
   a.
   b.
2. Referrals needed:
3. Follow up in __________
   Signature

Based on the assessment, the consultations with specialty clinics may include a multidisciplinary pediatric weight management program if the patient has a serious or acute condition, or other pediatric specialties such as sleep disorder, gastroenterology (GI), endocrinology, pulmonary/allergy, otolaryngology (ORL), neurology, genetics and ophthalmology. In addition, children with isolated comorbidities that are neither serious nor acute can certainly be managed in the pediatric ambulatory setting with access to lifestyle interventions in the community and close follow-up, if they are ready to change or become motivated, and with anticipatory guidance, if they are not. However, if these candidates do not show appreciable success in 6 to 12 months of intensive lifestyle modification, referral to a specialty weight management program may be warranted. Involvement in the development of a successful obesity treatment plan may require the expertise of multiple services such as nutrition, exercise physiology, physical therapy, psychology, psychiatry, and social services (Table 11.16).

A variety of drugs may contribute in part to the acceleration of weight gain of some children and youth. These drug treatments are summarized in Table 11.17 and are adapted from a previous review [30]. Finally, herbs are used by some families and may be useful (See Chapter 4).

Tools for anticipatory guidance have been developed most recently by Gerber® in partnership with the American Dietetic Association for children less than 2 yr of age and by WIC (Massachusetts and California) for children age 2 to 5 yr and also for older children. Some interesting web sites for tips on increasing activity, decreasing sedentarity, and nutrition are provided in Table 11.18.

Review of anticipatory guidance for children less than 1 yr (Table 11.19) and 2 to 18 yr are summarized in Table 11.20 [25, 56,57]. Material is readily available for

TABLE 11.16
Potential Referrals

Specialty Clinics	Lifestyle Care Providers	Community Programs	Adjunct Programs
Cardiology	Counselor	After school prog.	WIC
Endocrine	Exercise physiology	Sports club	Food stamps
ORL	Physical therapy	Activity club	Food pantry
GI	Dietician	Relaxation	Social worker
Genetic	Peer leader	Lifestyle	Mentorship
Pulmonary			Transportation
Mental health			Interpreter
Neurology			Support group
Orthopedic			
Sleep			

Note: To locate a nutritionist in your area: http://www.eatright.org/cps/rde/xchg/SID-5303FFEA-531CF821/ada/hs.xsl/home_fanp_consumer_ENU_HTML.htm

To locate a weight-loss program in your area, ask your primary care clinician for a referral or contact your local hospital. For additional general information, contact:
Weight-Control Information Network (WIN)
1 WIN Way
Bethesda, MD 20892-3665
Toll-free: 1-877-9464627
Tel: (202) 828-1025
Fax: (202) 828-1028
E-mail: win@info.niddk.nih.gov
http://www.win.niddk.nih.gov

TABLE 11.17
Drugs Associated with Weight Gain

Drugs with Weight Gain Potential	Alternatives with Less Potential for Weight Gain
Atypical antipsychotics	
Clozapine ++++	Quetiapine
Olanzapine ++++	Ziprasidone
Risperidone ++	—
Mood stabilizers	
Divalproex sodium +++	Lamotrigine (weight neutral)
Lithium +++	Adjunctive topiramate
Tricyclic antidepressants	
Amitriptyline ++	Desipramine
Impramine ++	Nortriptylene
MAO inhibitors	
Phenelzine > isocarboxazide	Tranylcypromine

TABLE 11.17 (Continued)
Drugs Associated with Weight Gain

Drugs with Weight Gain Potential	Alternatives with Less Potential for Weight Gain
SSRIs	
Paroxetine ++	Fluoxetine
Sertraline +	
Atypical antidepressants	
—	Buproprion
Anticonvulsants	
Valproate +++	Zonisamide
Carbamazepine ++	Topiramate
Gabapentin ++	
Antidiabetic agents	
Insulin +++	Metformin
Thiazolidinediones ++	
Steroids	

Source: Adapted with permission from Lenders C and Hoppin A. Management and Treatment of Obesity. In: Walker W, Watkins J, Duggan C, eds. *Nutrition in Pediatrics: Basic Science and Clinical Applications*, 3rd ed. B.C. Decker; 2003: 917–934.

For more details please see Chapter 12.

TABLE 11.18
Helpful Web-Based Tools on BMI, Activity, Sedentarity, Nutrition, and Monitoring

Body mass index calculator and growth charts
- http://www.cdc.gov/nccdphp/dnpa/bmi/bmi-for-age.htm
- http://www.pdacortex.com/STAT_Growth_Charts_Download.htm

Television and the family
- http://www.aap.org/family/tv1.htm

Fitness
- http://www.fitness.gov
- http://www.mja.com.au/public/issues/184_06_200306/bro10547_fm.html
- http://www.brightfutures.org/training/index.html#PA
- http://www.aahperd.org/naspe/pdf_files/brochure.pdf

Nutrition

General
- http://www.cdc.gov/HealthyYouth/nutrition/pdf/facts.pdf
- http://www.healthierus.gov/dietary guidelines
- http://www.calorieking.com/foods/portionwatch
- www.eatright.org
- www.actionforhealthykids.org

(*continued*)

TABLE 11.18 (Continued)
Helpful Web-Based Tools on BMI, Activity, Sedentarity, Nutrition, and Monitoring

http://www.24hourfitness.com/html/24_5/food/exchange/
http://www.diabetes.org/all-about-diabetes/chan_eng/i3/i3p4.htm
http://www.nal.usdwicworksa.gov//Topics/Ethnic.html/

Healthy eating tips for children
http://www.cdc.gov/nccdphp/dnpa/tips/healthy_children.htm
http://www.obesity.org/subs/childhood
http://www.wicworks.ca.gov/education/nutrition/nutritionCards/nutritionCardsIndex.htm
http://www.wicworks.ca.gov/resources/trainManual/Modules/Mod13.pdf

Healthy eating tips for infants
http://www.gerber.com/starthealthy
http://www.wicworks.ca.gov/education/nutrition/nutritionCards/nutritionCardsIndex.htm

Monitoring tool: fitness forward
http://www.fitnessforward.org/

TABLE 11.19
Infant Feeding Guide [25, 56, 57]

Food	0–4 mo	4–6 mo	6–8 mo	8–10 mo	10–12 mo
Br. milk	Short >8 feeds	Short >5 feeds	Demand >5 feeds	Demand	Demand
Formula	6–32 oz; 5–10 feeds	24–40 oz; 4–7 feeds	24–32 oz; 3–4 feeds	16–32 oz; 3–4 feeds	16–32 oz; 3–4 feeds
Cereals and bread	No	No	Infant cereals + H20 2–3 tsp up to 4 Tbsp × 2; **Start slowly at 6 mo**	Cereals; 8–12 Tbsp, Toast, bagel, or cracker taste	Hot/cold not sweet cereals 1/4 cup; Bread, rice, pasta 1/4 cup × 4
Fruit juice	No	No	Optional 4 oz	Optional 4 oz	Optional 4 oz
Vegetable	No	No	Strained, mashed; 1/2–1 jar, avoid corn	Cooked, mashed 1/3–1/2 cup	Cooked, pieces 1/2–3/4 cup
Fruits	None	None	Fresh, cooked, mashed, strained; 4 oz jar or 1/2 cup	Peeled, soft, mashed fruit or wedges; 1/3–1/2 cup	Fresh fruits peeled and seeded; 1/2–1 cup

TABLE 11.19 (Continued)
Infant Feeding Guide

Food	0–4 mo	4–6 mo	6–8 mo	8–10 mo	10–12 mo
Animal	None	None	Yogurt ± soft fresh fruit or apple sauce	Lean meat, chicken, fish strained or small pieces 3–4 tbsp; beans, egg yolk, yogurt, cheese	Meat chicken, fish tender piece 4–5 tbsp; whole egg, yogurt, cooked dried beans

Note: Watch for satiety cues, avoid bottle propping, and use bottle with formula until starts with sip-cup; not juice.
9 mo: wean to cup. If you cannot set limits for juice, do not buy it. No bottles or cup between meals—no bottle to sleep.
Introduce new foods will favor later acceptance; require 10–15 exposures for acceptance of a specific food; no evidence for specific sequence, suggested timing of introduction of new foods two to three per week. The parent decides what the child will eat and the child chooses how much to eat.
No peanut butter, egg white, or cow's milk before 1 yr of age.
New guideline from the AAP—introduction of other food than breast-milk at 6 mo, not earlier.

Source: Adapted with permission from Hendricks, K.M., Weaning: pathophysiology, practice and policy. In: Walker, W., Watkins, J., Duggan, D., Eds., *Nutrition in Pediatrics: Basic Science and Clinical Affiliations,* 3rd ed., B.C. Dekker, 2003; 531-561.

TABLE 11.20
Childhood and Adolescent Feeding Guide (1–18 y)

	1 y	2–3 y	4–8 y	9–13 y	14–18 y
Kilocalories[a]	900	1000			
Female			1200	1600	1800
Male			1400	1800	2200
Fat, % of total kcal	30–40	30–35	25–35	25–35	25–35
Milk/dairy, cups[b]	2[c]	2	2	3	3
Lean meat/beans, oz	1.5	2		5	
Female			3		5
Male			4		6
Fruits, cups[d]	1	1	1.5	1.5	
Female					1.5
Male					2
Vegetables, cups[d]	3/4	1			
Female			1	2	2.5
Male			1.5	2.5	3
Grains, oz[e]	2	3			

(continued)

TABLE 11.20 (Continued)
Childhood and Adolescent Feeding Guide (1–18 y)

	1 y	2–3 y	4–8 y	9–13 y	14–18 y
Female			4	5	6
Male			5	6	7

Note: Calorie estimates are based on a sedentary lifestyle. Increased physical activity will require additional calories by 0-200 kcal/day if moderately physically active and by 200–400 kcal/day if very physically active.

[a] For youth 2 yr and older; adapted from Tables 2 and 3 and Appendix A-2 in US Department of Health and Human Services, US Department of Agriculture. Dietary Guidelines for Americans. 6th ed. Washington, DC: US Government Printing Office; 2005; www.healthierus.gov/dietaryguidelines. Nutrient and energy contributions from each group are calculated according to the nutrient-dense forms of food in each group (eg., lean meats and fat-free milk).
[b] Milk listed is fat-free (except for children under the age of 2 yr). If 1%, 2%, or whole-fat milk is substituted, this will utilize, for each cup, 19, 39, or 63 kcal of discretionary calories and add 2.6, 5.1, or 9.0 g of total fat, of which 1.3, 2.6, or 4.6 g are saturated fat.
[c] For 1-yr-old children, calculations are based on 2% fat milk. If 2 cups of whole milk are substituted, 48 kcal of discretionary calories will be utilized. The American Academy of Pediatrics recommends that low-fat/reduced-fat milk not be started before 2 years of age.
[d] Serving sizes are 1/4 cup for 1 year of age, 1/3 cup for 2 to 3 years of age, and 1/2 cup for ≥4 years of age. A variety of vegetables should be selected from each subgroup over the week.
[e] Half of all grains should be whole grains.

Source: Reproduced with permission. AHA Scientific Statement, American Heart Association, Dietary Recommendations for Children and Adolescents © 2005, American Heart Association.

pediatricians but may need to be adapted to the community served. Tools that may assist the primary care provider in lifestyle monitoring, such as Fitness Forward, have been developed and are readily available on the web (Table 11.18). The American Dietetic Association recommends that primary care clinicians screen for nutrition-related illnesses, prescribe diets, provide preliminary counseling on specific nutritional needs, follow up with patients, and refer patients to appropriate dietetic professionals when necessary [58].

11.4 BENEFITS AND COMPLICATIONS OF WEIGHT LOSS

There is no definition of an optimal BMI following weight loss in children. However, weight loss may improve blood pressure and biologic markers typically associated with the metabolic syndrome (see chapter 2). Weight management in children is viewed mostly as a means to prevent the development of chronic disease such as type 2 diabetes mellitus, hypertension, CVD, certain cancers, and psychosocial consequences of obesity. There are concerns associated with weight loss in children. For example, severe

TABLE 11.21
Goals for Weight Loss and Weight Maintenance

Age (yr)	BMI ≥ 85th and <95th percentile	BMI ≥ 95<95th Percentile	No Associated medical Complications	Associated Medical Complications
2–7	X		Weight maintenance	Weight maintenance
2–7		X	Weight maintenance	Weight loss
>7	X		Weight maintenance	Weight loss
>7		X	Weight loss	Weight loss

Examples of medical complications include hypertension, dyslipidemia, insulin resistance, sleep apnea, genu varum, cutaneous candidiasis.
Weight loss of 1 lb/mo is considered appropriate up to a BMI under the 85th percentile.

Source: Adapted from Barlow and Dietz, *Pediatrics*. 1998;102(3):E29.

caloric restriction may result in linear growth retardation [59] and dieting may possibly result in increased risk of binge eating and mood disturbance [60] and osteoporosis [61].

As a result, The Expert Committee on Childhood Overweight (1998) recommended that the primary goal of a program to manage uncomplicated "overweight" (BMI 85th percentile) be healthy eating and activity, not ideal body weight [29]. However, the committee recommended weight loss for those children aged 7 yr and older, who have a BMI ≥ 85th percentile and have secondary complications, and those who have a BMI ≥ 95th percentile regardless of complications (Table 11.21). Weight loss goals for an obese child or adolescent may need to be tailored to the seriousness or acuteness of other associated conditions. As opposed to adults and adolescents, interventions for younger children typically focus first on weight maintenance and then on weight loss rather than on weight loss and then on weight maintenance [29].

11.5 STRATEGIES TO MAINTAIN OR LOSE WEIGHT

Current lifestyle strategies used for pediatric weight management programs often include family support and developmentally appropriate approaches. These programs typically focus on sedentary behaviors and physical activities, diet and eating behavior, and other behaviors (e.g., socializing, leisure activity). Studies suggest that treatment must take into account family influences on food and activity habits [62] Therefore, it is not surprising that studies suggest that family-based interventions may yield the best long-term results in children [63]. Interventions among obese children are more likely to be effective when they include one or both parents but not the child [64,1], while interventions among obese adolescents are more likely to be effective when they involve parents and adolescents separately [65].

While sedentary behaviors such as TV viewing have been related to increased BMI [66,67], investigators report that 65% of children aged 8 to 18 have a TV in their bedroom [68]. Children who have a TV in their bedroom spend 5 hr or more a week watching TV or videos [69]. As there is a trend toward decreased organized sports and active play among children, incorporating lifestyle physical activities in daily routines (e.g., walking to school) yield greater results in the long term than aerobic activities [70]. Current evidence for physical activity recommendations are reviewed elsewhere [71]. Findings from studies point at the health benefits of such recommendation and activity does not need to be continuous. Thus, decreasing TV viewing and increasing physical activity is important in long-term pediatric weight maintenance (Table 11.22).

TABLE 11.22
Sleep Facts, Sedentary Behavior, and Physical Activity

A. Sleep

During sleep, the brain stores memories and the body recovers and growth
Children and adolescents need a minimum of 9–11 hr of sleep/d
Inadequate sleep in children may result in difficulties to focus, to learn, or to perform daily activities, excessive daytime sleepiness, irritability, easy frustration, and difficulty with impulses and emotions
Sleep deprivation symptoms are often overlooked or erroneously attributed to hyperactivity or behavior disorders
Children with chronic loud snoring or other sleep problems may have a sleep disorder
A study of adolescents found in 1992 that obesity risk increased by 80% for each additional hour of sleep deprivation

Source: Adapted from NHLBI, at http://www.nhlbi.nih.gov/health/public/sleep

B. Sedentary Behavior

Set limits
Plan your child's viewing
Watch TV with your child
Find the right message
Help your child resist commercials
Check the quality of videos and DVDs
Give other options
Set a good example
Express your views

C. Physical Activity

Low	Respiratory and heart rates not increased Able to whistle
Moderate	Respiratory and heart rates slightly increased and light sweating Able to talk but not whistle
Vigorous	Breathing hard and sweating Difficult to talk

Source: Adapted from http://www.mja.com.au/public/issues/184_06_200306/ bro10547_fm. html

The combination of physical activity and diet has been found to be more effective than either one alone [72]. Reduction in total energy intake has been implicated in long-term weight loss and maintenance [73]. One randomized clinical trial using reduction in sugar-sweetened beverages recently showed lower BMI and obesity rates among children [74). Using the Department of Agriculture's 1989–1991 Continuing Survey of Food Intakes by Individuals (CSFII), non-Hispanic white children had the highest intake of grains and dairy and non-Hispanic black children had the highest intake of meat but the lowest of dairy foods, while intake of fruit and dairy foods was directly related to income [75]. While affordability and availability of energy-dense foods has increased among minorities and low socioeconomic groups [76, 77], children are not meeting the recommended servings of five fruits and vegetables a day [78]. As there is no direct evidence that one type of diet is best for the treatment of pediatric obesity [1], combining a moderate energy-reduced diet with current nutrition guidelines can be safely used to treat pediatric obesity. In our clinic, we have learned that the keys to success include improvement in parent–child communication, changes in parenting skills and parent modeling, establishment of a routine including quantity and quality of sleep, as well as not skipping meals, decreasing food items that are high in energy and low in nutrients (e.g., sugary beverages and fast foods) and portion control for foods high in starches and rich in trans fatty acids, as well as saturated fats and cholesterol (see Chapter 4). The methods used to achieve those goals are discussed elsewhere (Chapter 4, 12). Finally, the intensity and quality of physical activity is reviewed elsewhere [71] and in Chapter 5.

Current options for the pharmacologic treatment of obesity are limited, but may have some clinical utility in adults and adolescents [30]. In general, the drugs demonstrate only modest efficacy, minimal adverse effects, and are reviewed elsewhere (Chapter 6). Two drugs have been accepted by the Food and Drug Administration (FDA) for adolescents aged 16 yr and older: orlistat and sibutramine. However, long-term studies are lacking. Metformin is not recommended for weight loss at this point, but several studies are ongoing to evaluate a potential beneficial effect. Lack of adequate data and gaps in knowledge were cited as important reasons for caution in the best practice guidelines for gastric bypass in adolescents developed for Massachusetts (Table 11.23) [78]. Physiological status, comprehensive screening of patients and their families, and required education and counseling were identified as key factors in assessing eligibility for surgery (see Chapter 7).

11.6 CONCLUSIONS

There continues to be a lack of evidence to support current pediatric weight management strategies (summarized in Table 11.24 and Table 11.25) [1,3]. While research updates provide more support in time, there is a need for practical integrated strategies to identify, monitor, treat, and refer pediatric obese patients based on best practice, taking into account barrier to care. To address the pediatric obesity epidemic with greater efficacy at the community and primary care levels, we believe that it is time to train and certify primary care clinicians in pediatric ambulatory weight

TABLE 11.23
Algorithm for Adolescents with Completed Growth (Girls ≥ 13 and Boys ≥ 15 yr) for Referral to a Gastric Bypass Team

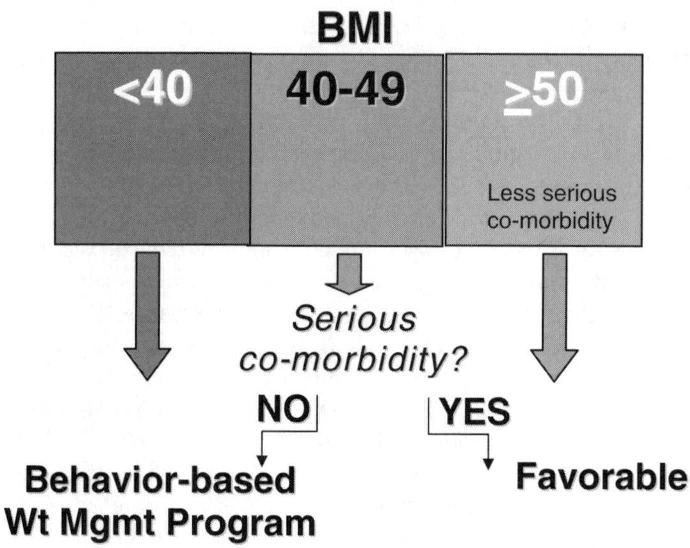

TABLE 11.24
Evidence for Anticipatory Guidance [80]

0–24 mo	2–6 yr	7–12 yr	13–18 yr	Topics
				Nutrition
X				Breast feeding[a]
X				Formula use[c]
X	X			Iron-rich diet[b]
	X	X		Parent role models[c]
	X	X	X	Healthy snacks[c]
	X	X	X	Calcium intake[c]
			X	Folic acid supplements[a]
			X	Limit saturated fat[a]
	X	X	X	5 a day (fruit- and vegetable-rich diet)[c]
			X	Caloric balance/nutrient balance[b]
	X	X	X	**Physical Activity[b]**
				Substance Use/Abuse
X	X	X	X	Tobacco (includes passive exposure)[a]
			X	Problem drinking[a]
			X	Alcohol and other drugs[a]

TABLE 11.24 (Continued)
Evidence for Anticipatory Guidance [80]

0–24 mo	2–6 yr	7–12 yr	13–18 yr	Topics
			X	Drinking and driving motor vehicles[b]
				Mental Health
			X	Depression/anxiety awareness[c]
X	X	X	X	Coping skills/stress reduction[c]
				Sleep?

[a] There is "*good*" evidence to support the recommendation and it should be included in a periodic health examination

[b] There is "*fair*" evidence to support the recommendation and it should be included in a periodic health examination

[c] There is *insufficient* **"direct"** evidence that counseling on these topics leads to a specific change of behavior; but there **"is"** evidence linking these topics to health conditions/or diseases

Source: Adapted from www.guidelines.gov

TABLE 11.25
Evidence for Evaluation and Treatment Guidelines [81]

BMI at each health care encounter for children and youth age 2–20 yr (**Level I**)
BMI ≥ 85th percentile: rule out hypertension (HTN), dyslipidemia, and diabetes (DM2) (**Level I**)
A BMI ≥ 95th percentile: rule out exogenous obesity and complications (**Level I**)
Early intervention begins with children greater than or equal to 2 yr (**Level I**)
The family must be ready for change; probe for readiness to change (**Level IIa**)
Educate the family on related medical complications (e.g., HTN, dyslipidemia, DM2) (**Level I**)
Educate the family on psychosocial complications (e.g., depression, self-esteem) (**Level I**)
Involve the entire family and/or all caregivers in the plan (**Level I**)
The family should be in agreement with the interventions (**Level I**)
Emphasize long-term permanent changes, not rapid weight loss or short-term diet and exercise programs; seek small, gradual, but lifelong changes (**Level I**)
Support family activities that provide everyone with exercise (**Level I**)
Low fat, low cholesterol, reduced sugar diet per age weight and nutritional requirements (**Level I**)
Encourage planned meals (e.g., eating breakfast); discourage skipping meals (**Level I**)
Discourage eating while watching television (**Level I**)
Avoid the use of food as a reward or punishment (**Level I**)
Stock refrigerator with healthy food and drink choices (**Level I**)
Encourage 30 to 60 min of moderate physical activity most days of the week (**Level I**)
Promote a variety exercise to prevent boredom or overtraining (**Level I**)
Maintain an open and accepting relationship to all family members involved (**Level I**)
May utilize a multidisciplinary approach for comprehensive management (**Level I**)
Consider cultural norms and socioeconomic status (**Level I**)

Source: Adapted from *Preventive counseling and education*. http://www.guideline.gov. Accessed November 17, 2005

management using a training curriculum and a referral model that includes specialists, multidisciplinary weight management clinics, and community-based nutrition and fitness programs. In addition to developing a model for care and training clinicians to care for underserved populations, there is an acute need for community-based nutrition and fitness programs resources and guides, increase in access to dietician and psychologists, increase in reimbursement of care, and practical tools for assessment and monitoring. As suggested previously by the American Heart Association, the development of a chronic care model for obesity is long overdue.

Chapter or CME Reviewers

Shaheen Lakhani, PsyD
Margaret Marino, PhD
Stephen Luippold, ARPN
Cheryl Jesuit, MS, RD
Vivien Morris, RD, MPH
Caroline Apovian, MD
Douglas Hoffman, MD
Suleiman Mustafa-Kutana, MD
Sharon O'Brien, MD
Shirley Huang, MD

BMC Department of Pediatrics
Barry Zuckerman, MD
Howard Bauchner, MD
Robert Vinci, MD
Cynthia Rodriguez, MA

BMC Office of Development
Norman Stein
Meredith Benedict
Larry Hanawalt
Douglas Ferguson

Research
Kayoung Rhee, MD
Allison Brown, MD
Vijay Srinivasen, MD
Traynor Canny
Rishi Shukla, MA

CME Instructors

Caroline Apovian, MD
T. Desmond Brown, MD
Gerald Cox, MD, PhD
Suleiman Mustafa-Kutana, MD
Sharon O'Brien, MD
Rishi Shukla, BA
Claudio Morera, MD
Kara Gross, MD
Shirley Huang, MD
Inger Hustrulid, RD, LDN
Natalie Egan, MS, RD
Cheryl Jesuit, MS, RD
Harry Pino, PhD
Catherine Logan, MSPT
Gita Rao, BA
Julie Vanier, BA
Meredith Harris, PhD
Shaheen Lakhani, PsyD
Marlene Schwartz, PhD
Margaret Marino, PhD
Diane Willis, PhD
Martha Perry, MD
Kay Rhee, MD

HealthNet Partners
Codman Square Health Center
Dorchester House Multi-Service Center
Mattapan Community Health Center
Whittier Street Health Center
South Boston Community Health Center
East Boston Neighborhood Health Center
Greater Roslindale Medical and Dental Center
Upham's Corner Health Center
South End Community Health Center

11.7 ACKNOWLEDGMENTS

This clinical guide for pediatric ambulatory weight management is the result of a collaboration between the BMC Divisions of Pediatric Nutrition, General Pediatrics, and Community Pediatrics, Boston HealthNet, the Massachusetts chapter of the American Academy of Pediatrics, the NewBalance Foundation, the Physician Specialist Award from the American Society for Nutrition, and the Joel and Barbara Alpert Endowment for the Children of the City. Funding was provided in part by the NewBalance Foundation and the Joel and Barbara Alpert Endowment for the Children of the City.

We would like to specially thank the following pediatricians for their commitment: Leslie Scherl (East Boston Neighborhood Health Center), Morris Borten (South End Community Health Center), Jean Kelley and Giuseppina Romano-Clarke (Dorchester House Multi-Service Center), Alexandria Lespinasse (Mattapan Community Health Center), Paul Gustafson (Geiger Gibson), Carol Cancro (Whittier Street Health Center), Edward Levy and Tanya Sullivan (Upham's Corner Health Center), Janet Protiva (Greater Roslindale Medical Center), and Nisha Thakrar (South Boston Health Center).

REFERENCES

1. Summerbell CD, Ashton V, Campbell KJ, Edmunds L, Kelly S, Waters E, Interventions for treating obesity in children. *Cochrane Database Syst Rev* 2003 and 2004; (3):CD001872.
2. Glenny A, O'Mearas S, Melville A, Sheldion TA, Wilson C. The treatment and prevention of obesity: a systematic review of the literature. *Int J Obes Metab Disord* 1997; 21:715–737.
3. Summerbell CD, Waters E, Edmunds LD, Kelly S, Brown T, Campbell KJ. Interventions for preventing obesity in children. *Cochrane Database Syst Rev* 2005; 20;(3):CD001871.
4. American Academy of Pediatrics, Committee on Nutrition. Prevention of Pediatric Overweight and Obesity (policy statement). *Pediatrics* 2003; 112:424–430. http://aappolicy.aappublications.org. Accessed November 11, 2005.
5. Whitaker, RC, Wright, JA, Pepe, MS, Seidel, KD, Dietz, WH. Predicting obesity in young adulthood from childhood and parental obesity. *New Engl J Med* 1997; 337:869–873.
6. Must A, Jacques PF, Dallal GE, Bajema CJ, Dietz WH. Long-term morbidity and mortality of overweight adolescents: a follow-up of the Harvard Growth Study 1922 to 1935. *New Engl J Med* 1992; 327:1350–1355.
7. Vanhala M, Vanhala P, Kumpusalo E, Halonen P, Takala J. Relation between obesity from childhood to adulthood and the metabolic syndrome: population based study. *BMJ* 1998; 317:319–320.
8. Kumanyika S. Obesity, health disparities, and prevention paradigms: hard questions and hard choices. Preventing Chronic Disease. Public Health research, practice, and policy. 2(4). 2005. www.cdc.gov/pcd/issues/2005/oct/05_0025.htm. Accessed November 14, 2005.
9. Strauss RS, Pollack HA. Epidemic increase in childhood overweight, 1986–1998. *JAMA* 2001; 286:2845–2848.

10. U.S. Census Bureau. Projected Population of the United States, by Race and Hispanic Origin: 2000 to 2050 (Table 1a.) http://www.census.gov/ipc/www/usinterimproj/ Accessed September 2004.
11. Haas JS, Lee LB, Kaplan CP, Sonneborn D, Phillips KA, Liang S-Y. The association of race, socioeconomic status, and health insurance status with the prevalence of overweight among children and adolescents. *Am J Public Health* 2003; 93:2 105–2110.
12. Tershakovec AM, Kuppler K. Ethnicity, insurance type, and follow-up in a pediatric weight management program. *Obes Res.* 2003; 11(1):17–20.
13. Rhee KE, De Lago CW, Arscott-Mills T, Mehta SD, Davis RK. Factors associated with parental readiness to make changes for overweight children. *Pediatrics* 2005; 116(1):e94–e101.
14. Kolagotla L, Adams W. Ambulatory management of childhood obesity. *Obes Res* 2004; 12(2):275–283.
15. O'Brien SH, Holubkov R, Reis EC. Identification, evaluation, and management of obesity in an academic primary care center. *Pediatrics* 2004; 114(2):e154–e159.
16. Story, MT, Neumark-Stzainer, DR, Sherwood, NE, Holt K, Sofka D, Trowbridge FL, Barlow SE.. Management of child and adolescent obesity: attitudes, barriers, skills, and training needs among health care professionals *Pediatrics* 2002; 110: 210–214.
17. Reisinger KS, Bires JA. Anticipatory guidance in pediatric practice. *Pediatrics* 1980; 66(6):889–892.
18. Lyznicki JM, Young DC, Riggs JA, Davis RM; Council on Scientific Affairs, American Medical Association. Obesity: assessment and management in primary care. *Am Fam Physician* 2001; 63(11):2185–2196.
19. Davis DA, Thomson MA, Oxman AD, Haynes B. Changing physician performance: a systematic review of the effect of continuing medical education strategies. *JAMA* 1995; 274(9):700–705.
20. Dietz WH, Robinson TN. Use of the body mass index (BMI) as a measure of overweight in children and adolescents. *J Pediatr* 1998; 132(2):191–193.
21. Li S, Chen W, Srinivasan SR, Bond MG, Tang R, Urbina EM, Berenson GS. Childhood cardiovascular risk factors and carotid vascular changes in adulthood: the Bogalusa Heart Study. *JAMA* 2003; 290(17):2271–2276. Erratum in *JAMA* 2003 Dec 10; 290(22):2943.
22. Koplan JP, Liverman CT, Kraak VA, Eds. Committee on Prevention of Obesity in Children and Youth. *Preventing Childhood Obesity: Health in the Balance.* Institute of Medicine. The National Academy Press. 2004.
23. Weight-for-length and BMI growth charts. www.cdc.gov/growthcharts/. Accessed November 14, 2005
24. Ogden CL, Carroll MD, Curtin LR, McDowell NA, Tabok CJ, Flegol KM. Prevalence of overweight and obesity in the United States, 1999–2004. *JAMA* 2006 Apr 5;295(13): 1549–1555.
25. Hendricks K.M. Weaning: pathophysiology, practice and policy. In: Walker W, Watkins J, Duggan C, Eds. *Nutrition in Pediatrics: Basic Science and Clinical Applications*, 3rd ed. B.C. Decker; 2003; 531–561.
26. Kivitie-Kallio S, Norio R. Cohen syndrome: essential features, natural history, and heterogeneity. *Am J Med Genet* 2001; 102(2):125–135.
27. Beales PL, Elcioglu N, Woolf AS, Parker D, Flinter FA. New criteria for improved diagnosis of Bardet-Biedl syndrome: results of a population survey. *J Med Genet* 1999; 36(6):437–446.

28. de Sanctis C, Lala R, Matarazzo P, Balsamo A, Bergamaschi R, Cappa M, Cisternino M, de Sanctis V, Lucci M, Franzese A, Ghizzoni L, Pasquino AM, Segni M, Rigon F, Saggese G, Bertelloni S, Buzi F. McCune-Albright syndrome: a longitudinal clinical study of 32 patients. *J Pediatr Endocrinol Metab* 1999; 12(6):817–826.
29. Barlow SE, Dietz WH. Obesity evaluation and treatment: Expert Committee recommendations. The Maternal and Child Health Bureau, Health Resources and Services Administration and the Department of Health and Human Services. *Pediatrics* 1998; 102(3):E29.
30. Lenders C, Hoppin A. Management and Treatment of Obesity. In: Walker W, Watkins J, Duggan C, Eds. *Nutrition in Pediatrics: Basic Science and Clinical Applications*, 3rd ed. B.C. Decker; 2003; 917–934.
31. Rosenbaum M. Obesity in children. In: Caro JF, Ed. Obesity. Endotext.com. 2002. www.endotext.org. Accessed November 11, 2005.
32. Fishman L, Lenders C, Fortunato C, Noonan C, Nurko S. Increased prevalence of constipation and fecal soiling in a population of obese children. *J Pediatr* 2004; 145(2):253–254.
33. Nead KG, Halterman JS, Kaczorowski JM, Auinger P, Weitzman M. Overweight children and adolescents: a risk group for iron deficiency. *Pediatrics* 2004; 114(1):104–108.
34. Lenders C, Lee K, Kapoor B, Jonas M. Abnormal alanine aminotransferase in a pediatric obesity program: prevalence and risk factors. *Ped Res* 2000; 47(4):44.
35. American Psychiatric Association: *Diagnostic and Statistical Manual of Mental Disease*. DSMIV-TR. 4th ed. American Psychiatric Association, Washington, DC, 2000.
36. Bodin AM. Teasing and Bullying Survey: Clinical Version, 2004. Visit www.familyandmarriage.com to contact author for instrument and permission to use.
37. Kovacs M. Children's Depression Inventory. Multi-Health Systems. New York, 1982
38. Achenbach TM. *Integrative Guide to the 1991 CBCL/4-18, YSR, and TRF Profiles.* Burlington: University of Vermont, Department of Psychology, 1991.
39. Maloney MJ, McGuire JB, Daniels SR. Reliability testing of a children's version of the Eating Attitude Test. *J Am Acad Child Adol Psych* 1988; 27:541–543.
40. Cooper Z, Fairburn C. The Eating Disorders Examination: a semi-structured interview for the assessment of the specific psychopathology of eating disorders. *Int J Eating Disord* 1987; 6:1–8.
41. Johnson WG, Grieve F, Adams CD, Sandy J. Measuring binge eating in adolescents: adolescent and parent versions of the questionnaire of eating and weight patterns. *Int J Eating Disord* 1999; 26:301–314.
42. Vila G, Zipper E, Dabbas M, Bertrand C, Robert JJ, Ricour C, Mouren-Simeoni M., Mental disorders in obese children and adolescents. *Psychosom Med* 2004; 66: 387–394.
43. Report of the Expert Committee on the Diagnosis and Classification of Diabetes Mellitus. *Diabetes Care* 1997; 20:1183–1197.
44. American Diabetes Association. Type 2 diabetes in children and adolescents. *Diabetes Care* 2000; 23(3):381–389.
45. American Diabetes Association. Standards of medical care in diabetes. *Diabetes Care* 2005; 28:S4–S36.
46. Fagot-Campagna A, Saaddine JB, Engelgau MM. Is testing children for type 2 diabetes a lost battle? *Diabetes Care* 2000; 23(9):1442–1443.
47. American Academy of Pediatrics. National Cholesterol Education Program, Report of the Expert Panel on Blood Cholesterol Levels in Children and Adolescents. *Pediatrics* 1992; 89:525–584.

48. Fletcher B, Bezzak, Ades, P et al. Managing abnormal blood lipids: a collaborative approach. *Circulation* 2005, 112(20): 3184–3209.
49. Kavey RE, Daniels SR, Lauer RL, Atkins DL, Hayman LL, Taubert K. American Heart Association. American Heart Association guidelines for primary prevention of atherosclerotic cardiovascular disease beginning in childhood. *Circulation* 2003, 107:1562–1566.
50. National High Blood Pressure Education Program Working Group on High Blood Pressure in Children and Adolescents. The fourth report on the diagnosis, evaluation, and treatment of high blood pressure in children and adolescents. *Pediatrics* 2004; 114:555–576.
51. Strauss R. Childhood obesity. *Curr Probl Pediatr.* 1999; 29(1):1–29.
52. Daniels SR, Arnett DK, Eckel RH, Gidding SS, Hayman LL, Kumanyika S, Robinson TN, Scott BJ, St Jeor S, Williams CL. Overweight in children and adolescents: pathophysiology, consequences, prevention, and treatment. *Circulation* 2005; 111(15):1999–2012.
53. Winter W., Schatz W. Pediatric Lipid Disorders in Clinical Practice. Emedicine. January 1, 2005 http://www.emedicine.com/ped/topic2787.htm. Accessed November 11, 2005.
54. American Academy of Pediatrics. Clinical Guideline: diagnosis and management of childhood obstructive sleep apnea syndrome. *Pediatrics* 2002; 109:704–712.
55. Foster GD, McGuckin BG. Estimating resting energy expenditure in obesity. *Obes Res* 2001; 9S5:367S–372S; discussion 373S–374S.
56. Gidding SS, Dennison BA, Birch LL, Daniels SR, Gilman MW, Lichtenstein AH, Rattay KT, Steinberger J, Stettler N, Van Horn L. American Heart Association. American Academy of Pediatrics. Dietary recommendations for children and adolescents: a guide for practitioners: consensus statement from the AHA. *Circulation* 2005; 112(13):2061-75. Summarized in www.guidelines.gov and endorsed by the American Academy of Pediatrics. *Pediatrics* 2006; 117: 544–559.
57. American Academy of Pediatrics: Policy statement. Breastfeeding and the use of human milk. *Pediatrics* 2005; 115(2):496–506. http://aappolicy.aappublications.org. Accessed November 11, 2005.
58. Maillet JO, Young EA. Nutrition education for healthcare professionals: position of the ADA. *J Am Diet Assoc* 1998; 98:343–346.
59. Figueroa-Colon R, von Almen TK, Franklin FA, Schuftan C, Suskind RM. Comparison of two hypocaloric diets in obese children. *Am J Dis Child* 1993; 147:160–166.
60. Wadden TA, Foster GD, Sarwer DB, Anderson DA, Gladis M, Sanderson RS, Letchak RV, Berkowitz RI, Phelan S. Dieting and the development of eating disorders in obese women: results of a randomized controlled trial. *Am J Clin Nutr* 2004; 80(3):560–568.
61. Van Loan MD, Wang MC, Bachrach LK, Crawford PB. Effect of drive to thinness during adolescence on adult bone mass. Abstract presentation. 22nd Annual Meeting of the American Society for Bone and Mineral Research, Toronto, Canada, 2001.
62. Harvey EL, Glenny A-M, Kirk SFL, Summerbell CD. Improving health professionals' management and the organisation of care for overweight and obese people. *Cochrane Database Syst Rev.* 1, John Wiley and Sons: Chichester, UK, 2004.
63. Epstein LH, Valoski A, Wing RR, McCurley J. Ten-year follow-up of behavioral, family-based treatment for obese children. *JAMA* 1990; 264:2519–2523.
64. Golan M, Weizman A, Apter A, et al. Parents as the exclusive agents of change in the treatment of childhood obesity. *Am J Clin Nutr* 1998; 67:1130–1135.
65. Brownell KD, Kelman JH, Stunkard AJ. Treatment of obese children with and without their mothers: changes in weight and blood pressure. *Pediatrics* 1983; 71:515–523.

66. Robinson TN. Reducing children's television viewing to prevent obesity: a randomized controlled trial. *JAMA* 1999; 282:1561–1567.
67. Gortmaker SL, Must A, Sobol AM, Peterson K, Colditz GA, Dietz WH. Television viewing as a cause of increasing obesity among children in the United States, 1986–1990. *Arch Pediatr Adolesc Med* 1996; 150(4):356–362.
68. Kids & Media @ the New Millennium: A Kaiser Family Foundation Report Key Data (1999). http://www.kff.org/entmedia/1535-pressreleasefinal-doc.cfm. Accessed September, 2004.
69. Dennison BA, Erb TA, Jenkins PL. Television viewing and television in bedroom associated with overweight risk among low-income preschool children. *Pediatrics* 2002; 109(6):1028–1035.
70. Epstein LH, Valoski A, Wing RR, McCurley J. Ten-year follow-up of behavioral, family-based treatment for childhood obesity. *Health Psychol* 1994; 3:373–383.
71. Strong WB, Malina RM, Blimkie CJ, Daniels SR, Dishman RK, Gutin B, Hergenroeder AC, Must A, Nixon PA, Pivarnik JM, Rowland T, Trost S, Trudeau F. Evidence based physical activity for school-age youth. *J Pediatr* 2005; 146(6):732–737.
72. Epstein LH, Myers MD, Raynor HA, Saelens BE. Treatment of pediatric obesity. *Pediatrics* 1998; 101(3):554–570.
73. Figueroa-Colon R, von Almen TK, Franklin FA, Schuftan C, Suskind RM. Comparison of two hypocaloric diets in obese children. *Am J Dis Child* 1993; 147(2):160–166.
74. James J, Thomas P, Cavan D, Kerr D. Preventing childhood obesity by reducing consumption of carbonated drinks: cluster randomized controlled trial. *BMJ* 2004; 328(7450):1237.
75. Munoz KA, Krebs-Smith SM, Ballard-Barbash R, Cleveland LE. Food intakes of US children and adolescents compared with recommendations. *Pediatrics* 1997; 100(3):323–329.
76. Morland K, Wing S, Diez Roux A. The contextual effect of the local food environment on residents' diets: the atherosclerosis risk in communities study. *Am J Public Health* 2002; 92(11):1761–1767.
77. Sloane DC, Diamant AL, Lewis LB, Yancey AK, Flynn G, Nascimento LM, McCarthy WJ, Guinyard JJ, Cousineau MR; REACH Coalition of the African American Building a Legacy of Health Project. Improving the nutritional resource environment for healthy living through community-based participatory research. *J Gen Intern Med* 2003; 18(7):568–575.
78. American Dietetic Association. Position of the American Dietetic Association: Dietary Guidance for healthy children ages 2-11 years. *J Am Diet Assoc* 2004; 104:660–677.
79. Apovian CM, Baker C, Ludwig DS, Hoppin AG, Hsu G, Lenders C, Pratt JS, Forse RA, O'brien A, Tarnoff M. Best practice guidelines in pediatric/adolescent weight loss surgery. *Obes Res* 2005; 13(2):274–282.
80. *Preventive counseling and education.* Bloomington (MN): Institute for Clinical Systems Improvement (ICSI); 2004. http://www.guideline.gov/summary/summary.aspx?doc_id=5365&nbr=3668. Accessed November 17, 2005.
81. University of Texas at Austin, School of Nursing, Family Nurse Practitioner Program. Evaluation and treatment of childhood obesity. Austin (TX): University of Texas at Austin, School of Nursing; 2004. http://www.guideline.gov/summary/ summary.aspx?ss=15&doc_id=5431&nbr=3725. Accessed November, 17 2005.

12 Behavioral Health Considerations for the Management of Pediatric Obesity in Primary Care

Shaheen U. Lakhani, Margaret Marino, Timothy M. Rivinus, and Stephen Luippold

CONTENTS

12.1 INTRODUCTION

Obesity continues to rise at an alarming rate among youth, worldwide, with no immediate signs of slowing down [1]. As gatekeepers of both physical and mental health, primary care clinicians increasingly are expected to assume a greater role as a valuable informational and counseling resource on weight management for children and adolescents. They are accessible to youth and their families, as well as most familiar with their medical and physical history. During the last decade, expert committees and providers have been developing guidelines for primary care clinicians in the medical and dietary assessment, treatment, and overall management of pediatric obesity. However, most clinicians will agree that the most widespread of sequelae of pediatric obesity is psychosocial [2] and ultimately treatment and management is about behavior change [3]. Primary care clinicians continue to feel less proficient in behavioral management strategies, parent guidance/intervention, and addressing family dynamics impacting weight-control treatment [4]. In general, both expertise and time constraints appear to influence the quality and outcome of care [5]. Therefore, the overarching goal of this chapter is to increase the level of competence and comfort of primary care clinicians to independently screen for behavioral health concerns (psychiatric, psychosocial, readiness to change) related to the management of pediatric obesity, as well as to apply counseling strategies in the primary care setting. Behavioral health considerations for the primary care clinician, presented in this chapter, are derived from a combination of research findings, expert consensus recommendations, and the authors' clinical experience. Therefore it is left to clinicians to use their own clinical judgment when using information provided in this chapter.

12.2 BEHAVIORAL ASSESSMENT

Weight management ultimately is about behavior change. For the primary care clinician, the goal of conducting a brief behavioral assessment is to deliver the diagnosis of obesity in a sensitive way, to assess patient and family readiness to change, and to screen for psychiatric, family, and other environmental conditions that may interfere with treatment effectiveness. The reader is referred to Figure 12.1 for an assessment algorithm.

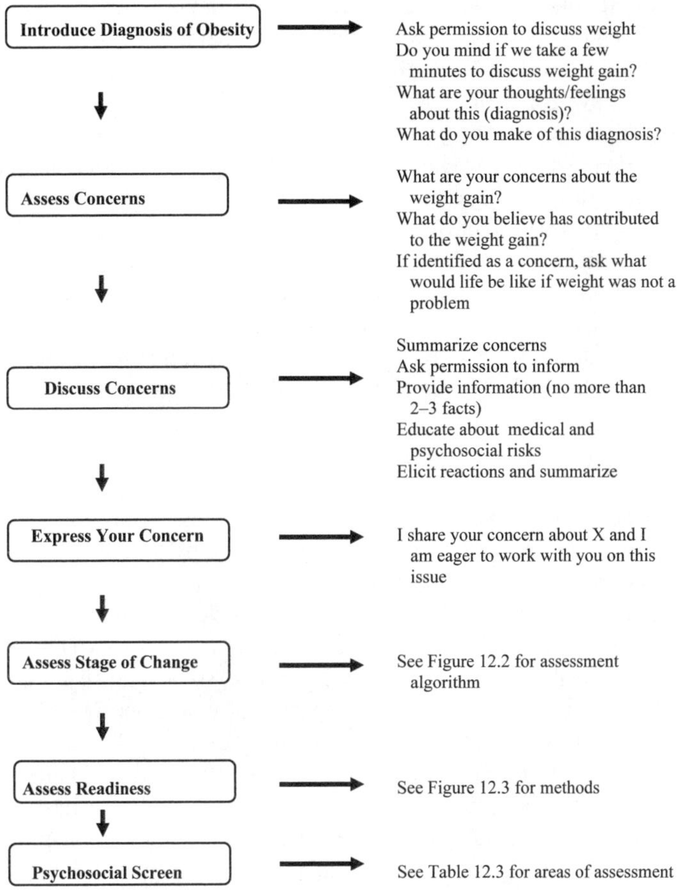

FIGURE 12.1 Primary care behavioral assessment algorithm for pediatric weight management (ages 2–20).

12.3 DELIVERING THE DIAGNOSIS

Negative health beliefs of illness and health care can significantly impact treatment. Given societal stigma surrounding obesity, obesity may well just be considered the next taboo to confront in doctor–patient–family communication following sexuality/fertility and death/dying. Primary care clinicians therefore are encouraged to pay attention to the child–parent response to the diagnosis of obesity. Emotional response by the older child or adolescent may include feelings of betrayal (i.e., parents or health clinicians did not intervene earlier in life), anger, embarrassment, sadness, denial, worry (about own health risks or parental response) and, in some circumstances, relief/hope (i.e., someone is willing to talk about it and help).

As Satter [6] describes well, feeding a child is about the connection between parent and child, trust and control, providing and neglect, and acceptance and rejection. Therefore, it should not be that surprising to the primary care clinician that the diagnosis of child obesity has the potential to evoke a powerful parental response. The diagnosis can be perceived by the parent as a personal criticism or attack by the clinician [42] on parenting ability (i.e., I cannot control my child's eating or I do not know how to nurture/feed my child, therefore, I am a bad parent) or for the overweight parent may trigger current beliefs, feelings, or memories associated with his/her own weight problem. Parental response may include feelings of disbelief, anger, guilt/shame, embarrassment, denial and hope or relief. The clinician who takes the time (however brief) to investigate the emotional and cognitive response to the diagnosis of obesity will find that the patient/family will possibly be more willing to consider a more open, mutual discussion of the problem — it is an effective rapport-building strategy. It is recommended that primary care clinicians consider the involvement of mental health professionals if the patient/family response is causing significant distress.

12.4 LANGUAGE AND DEMEANOR

Outcome of a consultation often is affected by the clinician's consulting behavior [7]. Language and demeanor that convey respect and empathy toward the patient/family may build rapport quickly. Language such as "fat," "lazy," "massive," or "huge" are not appropriate for clinicians to use. Terms such as "overweight" or "weight concern/issue" are more acceptable. Avoidance of using the word "weight" altogether, however, may send the message that weight gain is something to be ashamed of. Although there is no empirical data showing that the use of terms such as "obese," "overweight," or "weight gain" cause an eating disorder, care should be taken when discussing weight with patients who present with a highly distorted body image.

The use of a narrative counseling style [8] to introduce the diagnosis of obesity allows the primary care clinician to create enough distance between the problem (obesity), child (i.e., the child is not viewed as the problem), and parent (i.e., parent is not solely blamed) to facilitate the expansion of responsibility, choice, and family agency to change during the course of treatment. This gap created between obesity and the child, in particular, also may help alleviate feelings of self-blame, as obesity often is viewed by others as a sign of lack of willpower and control [9]. We have found this counseling style to be particularly effective for shifting attitudes about obesity/weight gain with adolescents. The reader is referred to Table 12.1 for examples of using a

TABLE 12.1
Examples of Using a Narrative Approach to Discuss Weight

How has weight impacted your (*your child's*) life?
In what situation are you (*is your child*) stronger than your (their) weight?
In what situation is the weight problem stronger than you (*your*) child?
If I were watching you earlier as a parent to your child, what do you think I would have seen that would have helped me to understand how your child became overweight?
If weight was not a problem, what would life be like for you (*your child*) right now?
What would life be like for the family?

narrative approach. Clinicians themselves, even health professionals who specialize in obesity, demonstrate weight bias [44–49]. Therefore, clinicians should consider examining their own beliefs about their weight, body image, and parenting adequacy (if parents), as these beliefs may inadvertently shape attitude toward the overweight child and/or their caregiver, which can have both positive and negative effects.

12.5 ASSESSING PATIENT/FAMILY READINESS TO CHANGE

Although educating the patient/family on the medical etiology of obesity may be the first step to helping recognize obesity as a health problem, alone it may not be sufficient for helping make positive and permanent changes in beliefs, attitudes, and behaviors that may impact weight gain [9]. In fact, most families already know what they should be doing (e.g. increase physical activity, reduce caloric intake) [10]. Therefore, it is essential for clinicians to also focus their attention on elements of behavior change theory with their patients and families.

There have been considerable advances in behavior change theory during the last 20 years; however, a significant gap continues to exist between clinicians' familiarity with these models and their ability to apply them in practice [11]. Of these models, the transtheoretical model [12,13], more commonly known as the stages of change model (SOCM), holds promise for helping patients increase their motivation or readiness to change (RTC) behaviors impacting weight gain when coupled with Motivational Interviewing (MI) [14]. SOCM proposes that the process of change is the same regardless of the target behavior [12]. Furthermore, optimal interventions (see Section 12.11) are those that match the individual stage of change [12]. Table 12.2 provides a summary of definitions and prescriptive guidelines for SOCM.

Two RTC concepts, (1) importance of change for a person (elicits health beliefs and expectations of outcome) and (2) confidence about doing what is necessary to succeed (self-efficacy) are key elements for the assessment of RTC [7]. Although SOCM/RTC approach looks promising for the area of weight control, research for applicability in children and adolescents is limited [11]. Therefore, clinicians are advised to use these ideas with parents of children/younger adolescents or with older adolescents alone only as a framework to understand behavior and for determining appropriate counseling strategies [11]. The reader is referred to Figure 12.2 and Figure 12.3 for SOCM and RTC assessment methods.

12.6 PSYCHOSOCIAL SCREENING

The psychological, social, and emotional stability of each child, adolescent, and his or her family can affect their ability to control weight successfully [3]. Therefore, clinicians need to be able to identify who would benefit further from behavioral health services prior to or during weight control treatment. Screening for psychiatric conditions and assessing individual and family psychosocial functioning helps the primary care clinician determine which patient is at risk or more vulnerable to psychological, social, and environmental problems that may aggravate the weight gain or negatively affect the course of weight control treatment. Although there are

TABLE 12.2
Definitions and Prescriptive Guidelines for Stages of Change Model

Stage	Definition	Practitioner's Role
Precontemplation	No intention to change behavior in the foreseeable future æ unaware or underaware of their problems	Nurturing parent
Contemplation	Aware that a problem exists	Socratic teacher Seriously thinking about making a change Have not yet made a commitment to take action
Preparation	Intend to take action in the next month	Experienced coach Have unsuccessfully taken action in the past year — report small behavioral changes but have not yet reached a criterion for effective action
Action	Modify behavior and/or environment to overcome problem	Consultant Have successfully altered the target behavior to an acceptable criterion for a period of 1 day – 6 months
Maintenance	Work to prevent relapse and consolidate gains attained during action	Consultant Extends from 6 months to an indeterminate period past the initial action

Prescriptive Guidelines for Use of Stages of Change Model in Counseling

Assess stage of change
Be aware of treating all patients as though they are in action
Assist patient/family in moving one stage at a time
Recognize patient/family in action stage more likely to achieve better and quicker outcomes
Facilitate thinking about a problem to doing things to overcome the problem
Anticipate recycling through stages of change before achievement of long-term maintenance æ include relapse-prevention strategies in treatment
Conceptualize change mechanisms as processes, not as specific techniques
Do the right things (processes) as the right time (stages) — avoid mismatching stages and processes

Source: Extracts (c.260 words) from pp.230–235 "Stages of Change: prescriptive guidelines for behavioral medicine and psychotherapy" by James O. Prochaska, C.C. DiClemente, and J.C. Norcross to construct Table 12.2: Definitions and prescriptive guidelines for stages of change model and Figure 12.2: Stages of change assessment from *Psychologists Desk Reference* edited by Gerald P. Koocher et al. (1998). By permission of Oxford University Press, Inc.

Do you think behavior X is a problem for you now?

If **YES:** contemplation, preparation, or action stage
If **NO:** precontemplation or maintenance

When do you intend to change X?

someday or not soon...................contemplation
in the next month........................preparation
right now...................................action

FIGURE 12.2 Stages of change assessment algorithm. (Adapted from Extracts (c.260 words) from pp.230–235, Stages of change: prescriptive guidelines for behavioral medicine and psychotherapy by James O. Prochaska, C.C. DiClemente. and J.C. Norcross to construct Table 12.2: Definitions and prescriptive guidelines for stages of change model and Figure 12.2: Stages of change assessment from *Psychologists Desk Reference*, Gerald P. Koocher et al., Eds. (1998). By permission of Oxford University Press, Inc.

no studies that compare different methods for psychiatric screening or assessment of obese children, clinicians may use a combination of screening mechanisms that includes interviews, routine chart reviews, multidisciplinary rounds, and use of well-validated instruments used in normal as well as psychiatric populations. Table 12.3a and 12.3b provide suggested topic areas to consider when conducting a psychosocial

Method 1: Use open-ended questions†

Examples: Teens/parents can differ a lot in how ready they are to change their behavior X.
What about you?
How ready are you to change?

Method 2: Use scaling questions†

How important is it for you to change in general? change behavior "X"?
On a scale of 1 to 10, what number would you give yourself where 1 means not at all important and 10 means absolutely important?
Why are you at X and not Y? Y should be a lower number.
What would need to happen for you to raise your score a couple of points?

Repeat this query replacing "important" with "confident."

Method 3 Use a readiness ruler‡

How ready are you to change behavior X? Please show me where you are on this ruler?

NOT READY AT ALL		UNSURE		TOTALLY READY

FIGURE 12.3 Readiness to change assessment methods. †Reprinted from *Health Behavior Change: A Guide for Practitioners*, Rollnick, S., Mason, P., and Butler, C., p 68, 1999, with permission from Elsevier. ‡A readiness ruler. Adapted from Stott et al., *Family Practice* 12(4), 413–418, 1995. Figure 2, by permission of Oxford University Press, Inc.

TABLE 12.3A
Psychosocial Screening – Psychiatric Conditions

Area of Inquiry	Sample Questions
Depression	Have you been more sad or irritable lately? Assess for suicidal ideation.
Anxiety	Inquire about current/past exposure to stressful life events, losses, exposure to violence, witnessing violence, abuse and neglect — note age, distress response and coping strategies.
Psychosis	Do you hear/see things that other people don't hear/see?
Eating disorder	See Tables 12.7 and 12.8 for classification distinctions and sample screening questions.
Substance use/abuse	Ask about use of alcohol, drugs, caffeine, herbal supplements, diet pills, and steroids.
Behavioral problems	Any difficulty with concentrating? Paying attention?
Sleep problems	Is it easy/hard to fall or stay asleep, wake up? Do you fall asleep with the TV on?
Psychiatric treatment history	Current/past patient/family psychotherapy and psychopharmacological treatment history

TABLE 12.3B
Psychosocial Screening — Impact of Weight

Area of Inquiry	Sample Questions
Emotional	Does weight ever make you feel X? (sad, angry, worried, guilty, scared, low self-esteem) — probe response.
Avoidance	Does weight ever make you stop doing activities you have an interest in or like doing? Inquire about physical as well as social activities — note that these can be one of the same for some children and adolescents.
Weight teasing	See Tables 12.4 and 12.6 for questions and definitions of teasing.
Early maturation	Do others treat you older than you are? Can you give me an example?
Relationships	Does weight ever make your relationship with parents, siblings, friends worse or better? How many close friends do you have? Do you date? Is it easy or hard to make friends? To keep friends? Quickly assess family structure and functioning using a genogram.
Academic Performance	What school do you go to? What grade are you in? Is this year better, worse, or the same as last year? How? Have you missed any school? How much? Why? Do you get any special help during or after school for X? Do you have any concerns about your child's learning?
Activity	What sit-down activities do you like to do outside of school? (TV, phone, homework, computer time)

TABLE 12.3B (Continued)
Psychosocial Screening — Impact of Weight

Area of Inquiry	Sample Questions
	What physical activities do you participate in? How much time do you spend doing these activities on school days? Weekends? Are you alone or with someone when doing these activities? Do you have a television in your bedroom? Do you eat your snacks/meals while watching TV? Alone? With someone?
Interests and personal strengths	What do you want to be when you grow up? What do you like to do when you are on your own? With friends? With family? If someone was to tell me something they admire about you, what would he or she say?

screening for the overweight/obese patient (ages 2–20). This may be completed over a couple of visits alongside a medical or dietary assessment and/or revisited at a later time if there are new or continued concerns. The primary care clinician who is constrained by time or has limited access to behavioral health services should at least screen for mood and eating disorders as well as assess family functioning.

12.6.1 Weight Teasing and Peer Rejection

When screening for psychiatric conditions, the primary care clinician will need to disentangle the psychiatric problems from the physical. In an obese pediatric population, this may be complicated as the relationship between obesity and psychopathology is still not clearly understood [15]. Some studies show that obese children seeking clinical treatment have increased levels of depression, anxiety, somatoform, and eating disorders [15]. However, there is no clear indication of higher rates of psychiatric comorbidity in the general population of obese children, especially when factors for maternal psychopathology or body dissatisfaction are controlled for [15]. In general, there is no empirical evidence to suggest a direct relationship between obesity and psychopathology in children or adolescents. Friedman and Brownell [16] attribute this to a generation of studies that failed to establish a risk factor model and to examine the temporal relationship between obesity and psychopathology.

Studies on the prevalence and impact of weight-teasing in obese youth as well as our own clinical observations suggests that subgroups of obese children and adolescents who are distressed by incidents of weight teasing or peer rejection often present with psychological factors such as lower self-esteem, depressive symptoms, anxiety, body dissatisfaction, or suicidal ideation and attempts [17,18]. These children are subjected to societal views that discriminate on the basis that their obesity is a reflection of poor character [9] and, thereby, tend to receive fewer friendship nominations compared to normal-weight youth [19]. It is our clinical observation that children who are distressed by weight teasing and peer rejection are at risk for further avoidance of physical and social activities of interest (due to physical limitations, poor social skills, or body dissatisfaction related to obesity). Overweight children tend to internalize social messages that weight is within their personal control and subsequently blame themselves for the negative social experiences that they confront [19]. Studies also show that obese youth are vulnerable to both becoming a victim or perpertrator of bullying and that methods of teasing/bullying maybe gender and age specific [50,51]. Therefore, it is imperative for the primary care clinician to assess (see Table 12.4) for the impact of weight teasing/peer rejection as part of psychosocial screening.

Primary care clinicians can educate parents about the psychosocial impact of weight-teasing and the risk for psychiatric conditions. By asking the patient about weight teasing, clinicians model for parents what questions to ask their child about teasing. Parents need to learn what coping strategies (see Table 12.5) to teach their child, as well as how to advocate for them. Too often, parents instruct their weight-teased children to simply "ignore" or "walk away" when confronted with weight teasing. This may be an appropriate instruction for actual or perceived dangerous situations. However, in other situations that are not physically harmful, this kind of advice has the potential to lower self-esteem as it does not allow the child to feel in control of the situation and may lead to the internalization of negative emotion and self-blame.

TABLE 12.4
Suggested Questions for Clinician and Parent Assessment of Weight-Teasing of Obese Child/Adolescent

Who is the teaser? (friend, teacher, parent, sibling, cousin?)
What is child/adolescent being teased about?
What does the teasing/bullying look like? (taunting, hitting, withdrawal of friendships?)
Where is the teasing happening? (home, bus, classroom?)
Is the child being bullied? Is the child physically safe?
How long has it been happening?
Who has the child/adolescent notified about this?
What does it make him/her feel like?
How does the child/adolescent respond to situation? what are their coping strategies?
Is the parent aware of situation? If so, how has parent responded to situation?
Repeat back to the child what was told in order to understand the experience carefully
What is his/her sense of self-worth/self esteem?
What assistance does the child or parent need to handle the situation? (behavioral health counseling, parental or provider advocacy with school, government)
Does child believe that weight loss will cease weight-teasing and/or he/she would have more friends?

Source: Adapted from Freedman, J.S. *Easing the Teasing: Helping Your Child Cope with Name-Calling, Ridicule and Verbal Bullying*. Chicago: Contemporary Books, 2002.

TABLE 12.5
Parent–Child Guidance for Weight-Teasing Intervention

Start your own anti-teasing campaign at home
- Examine own behavior for teasing child and well as others at home
- Educate family members about potential harm towards child that arises from weight-teasing
- Educate family members about the differences between joking (acceptable) and teasing (not acceptable) (See Table 12.6)

Choose a quiet, private space (no siblings) to inquire about weight teasing with your child.
Discuss weight-teasing when your child is experiencing a positive mood
Monitor for changes in child's mood
Help child develop coping strategies — role play some of these strategies
Teach child to self-talk (i.e., Whose opinion counts here?)
Plan ahead (identify time and place of teasing, safe places, teaser and helpers)
Role play just say "so?" and walk away
Ignore, walk away and join other children or pretend to be interested in something else happening elsewhere (good for younger kids)
Ask for help
Seek behavioral health counseling
Advocate for a bullying/teasing program at your child's school/class

Source: Adapted from Freedman, J.S. *Easing the Teasing: Helping Your Child Cope with Name-Calling, Ridicule and Verbal Bullying*. Chicago: Contemporary Books, 2002.

Primary care clinicians may encourage parents of obese children and adolescents to examine their own weight-teasing behavior toward their child as parents often describe their joking as either being meaningless or being helpful (i.e., "calling him fat will make him do something about his weight"). Use of such language will be perceived by the child as hurtful. Making distinctions between joking, teasing, and bullying (see Table 12.6) with a parent may help parents to assess what language is harmful to their child. Parents need to respect their child and show acceptance of their size. Primary care clinicians are strongly encouraged to involve mental health

TABLE 12.6
Weight-Teasing Definitions

Joking	X and Y are both smiling
Teasing	X feels hurt, Y engages in name-calling, put-downs, ridicule, annoying gestures. Forms of teasing for adolescents are more relational (i.e., spreading rumors and lies, withdrawal of friendship).
Bullying	X feels threatened and unsafe, Y repeatedly teases, torments, taunts. Common forms in children are acts of kicking, stealing and hitting. Physical aggression and threatening verbal taunting may occur among adolescents.

Source: Adapted from Freedman, J.S. *Easing the Teasing: Helping Your Child Cope with Name-Calling, Ridicule and Verbal Bullying*. Chicago: Contemporary Books, 2002.

clinicians for further assessment and counseling if a child's distress is significantly interfering with daily functioning.

12.6.2 Early Maturation

Although no peer-reviewed empirical studies have examined the psychosocial impact of early physical maturation in obese children, from our own clinical experience and that of others [2] strongly suggests that this subgroup of obese children is often socially marginalized as a result of their physical appearance and may develop psychological symptoms of low self-esteem, depression, or anxiety. It is not uncommon for adults at home or at school to mistake the overweight child for being older than their chronological age. Often these children appear taller than their nonoverweight peers [2] and/or physically and sexually mature. Expectations set by adults both at home and at school or by age-related peers may be developmentally inappropriate. Children who feel they are unable to fulfill such expectations are at risk for experiencing feelings of failure and inadequacy [2]. Perceived inadequacy may further lower self-esteem, aggravate negative body image, and result in social marginalization, or rejection [2]. Expectations set by peers or sometimes by parents (i.e., wearing a bra, dressing older, having sexual knowledge, dating or having sex), which are beyond the child's developmental limitations, may potentially pressure youth to engage in high-risk behaviors such as alcohol and substance abuse [2]. Although epidemiological data about the incidence and prevalence of substance abuse in the obese adolescent population are not yet available, the psychological factors associated with social marginalization have implications for engaging in substance abuse as well as other high-risk health behaviors [15,17,18]. Therefore, clinicians are strongly encouraged to consider screening for the psychosocial impact on obese children who show physical signs of early maturation.

12.7 EATING PROBLEMS

Screening for eating problems is critical, as it could be a significant contributing factor to weight gain. Eating problems exist on a continuum. Problems can range from a simple lack of information about nutrition and physical activity, to failure to respond to satiety cues, to complex behavioral patterns that help to cope with deep emotional need and unresolved pain. There are many terms for the disorders of eating and weight. Clinician and patient tend to use terms interchangeably (e.g. confusing compulsive eating with binge eating). This confusion can interfere with an accurate assessment. It is important for the primary care clinician to have a basic understanding of the different eating disturbance classifications (see Table 12.7). The main purpose of primary care clinicians screening for eating problems is to determine if weight control counseling is an appropriate intervention at the time. Patients presenting with symptoms of an eating disorder should be referred for further assessment and treatment to a mental health clinician with expertise in pediatric eating disorders and obesity.

Obese children may be overeating as a consequence of lack of information on the one hand or, on the other hand, deprivation, neglect, or familial psychopathology. It is

TABLE 12.7
Summary of Eating Problems

Problem	Classification
Overeating	Symptom
Compulsive eating	Symptom
Binge eating disorder	Proposed DSM-IV-TR psychiatric disorder
Bulimia nervosa	DSM-IV-TR Psychiatric disorder
Anorexia nervosa	DSM-IV-TR Psychiatric disorder
Eating disorder NOS	DSM-IV-TR Psychiatric disorder
Night eating	Syndrome

up to the primary care clinician to discern where the problem lies. As part of a routine screening for obesity in children and adolescents, it is important that the clinician keep in mind the many factors that can impact eating problems. Overeating can be an issue unto itself — a discreet problem. But it may potentially co-occur with dysregulation in other areas of functioning, such as physiological (e.g., sleep awakenings, urinary incontinence, encopresis), behavioral (i.e., following the rules at home/school, attention and impulsivity problems), social (i.e., difficulties with friendships and relationships with family), and emotional. Overeating can also be a consequence of difficulties the parents have with setting limits in many areas of the child's life, not just with food.

When screening for eating problems (see Table 12.8 for suggested questions), another important area to investigate is the provision of practical and emotional

TABLE 12.8
Suggested Questions for Screening for Eating Problems in Obese Children/Adolescents

Tell me what happens with food?
Have you ever been on a diet? Why? Who started it? (yourself, parent? grandparent?)
Do you ever binge?
  What does a binge mean for you?
  When was the last time it happened?
  What started it?
  What stops it?
  Have you ever tried to do anything to get rid of the food you have eaten? What? Do you use laxatives? Overexercise? (Key symptoms of a binge are: amount of food consumed and perceived loss of control)
What meals do you have during the day?
  Walk me through your day of meals and snacks. For young children ask the parent to do this
  If skipping meals or snacks ask why? (to lose weight, not hungry, no time, food security?)
  Have you ever restricted your food intake?
How much time do you think about food and weight?
How do you feel about the way you look?
To parent: Have you ever found food missing, wrappers, bag, sauce lying around? Does your child sneak food?

support to the child by caregivers at home. Clinicians need to discern if overeating is a consequence of the lack of caregiver supervision, involvement, or availability. Not only does this create the opportunity for unsupervised eating, but it also creates the potential for unmet emotional needs that may potentially be fulfilled with food.

For example, a primary care clinician might ask how long children are left home alone without an adult present. Lissau and Sorensen [20] found that neglected children are nine times more likely than others to become obese. In the most extreme situation, there has been a link between child abuse and eating problems. Felitti et al. [21] reported that adults seeking treatment for obesity demonstrated a fourfold increase in the prevalence of childhood sexual abuse, as well as a twofold increase in nonsexual abuse, compared to a control population. These factors are very critical when decisions are made about what the next step should be and what other services to enlist to address the problem. Clearly, if safety or protective issues exist, they become the primary target of intervention. If larger behavioral issues exist alongside the overeating, clinicians are encouraged to involve licensed mental health clinicians for the most positive outcome.

Primary care clinicians who address the problem of pediatric obesity should routinely inquire about disordered eating behaviors, such as binge eating, food restriction, and use of diet pills/herbal supplements, laxative, and diuretics. There would be several reasons that this is critical. Eating problems in this culture exist on a continuum throughout someone's lifetime. Some researchers have concluded that there is an increased risk for eating disorders among an obese population [22–25]. The interventions for eating disorders are very different than those that are applied in the treatment of obesity. This is especially true for children and adolescents. Applying the same model of intervention for someone who is obese, but who also has an eating disorder, will result in several things: 1) poor outcome relative to weight loss, 2) a worsening of the symptoms of their eating disorder, and 3) a sense of failure that the patient and their family feels from yet another attempt to intervene with the problem, which only lowers their sense of hope to address the problem in the future. Like children suffering from depression, children with eating disorders require psychological treatment and frequent primary care follow-up rather than referral to a tertiary weight control program.

12.7.1 Binge Eating Disorder

Within the population of overweight children, the primary diagnostic distinction relative to eating disorders would be between binge eating disorder and the medical condition of obesity. Not all children who overeat are binge eaters. Binge eating is an eating disorder that has the following symptoms: bingeing on large quantity of food in a discreet time period; an experience of loss of control — the sense that the person cannot stop eating — as well as feeling significant negative feelings after the binge — shame/guilt/disgust. People with binge eating disorder are very concerned about their body image and often express great dissatisfaction with their size and shape, even as children. Parental observation or report from others of child sneaking food, finding hidden food wrappers or taking food from peers at school are signals that the eating problem might be more than overeating. A child who is overeating, but not binging, will not experience the same sense of loss of control and body dissatisfaction.

12.7.2 "Compulsive Eating"

"Compulsive eating" is a popular term that is often used by families. It is important for clinicians to carefully inquire what is meant when families use that term. Typically, it implies an emotional component to overeating; eating without regard to physical hunger. It is distinguished from binge eating in a number of ways; the quantity of food that is consumed is much less and there is not the same experience of loss of control and shame afterwards. Also critically different is the lack of body shame and self-hatred.

12.7.3 Bulimia Nervosa

Another critical distinction is between the medical conditions of obesity and bulimia. Bulimia is an eating disorder that involves binge eating, as well as some method to get rid of the food, via purging or intense overexercising. It is similar to binge eating in that it involves binge eating as well as intense body dissatisfaction. But it is different in that there are compensatory weight loss behaviors — purging via vomiting or use of laxatives or diuretics or overexercising to the point of obsession, without regard to physical pain, injury, or illness. Bulimia can be found among normal weight as well as an overweight population.

12.7.4 Anorexia Nervosa

Anorexia nervosa is also an eating disorder that affects children, but more often adolescents. It involves the refusal to maintain a safe body weight, intense fear of getting fat, and food restriction and, sometimes, purging. Anorexia would obviously not be ruled out at the time of evaluation of an overweight child or adolescent. However, it is worth discussion for several reasons. It would be critical information to know where anorexia fits, relative to their current difficulties. For example, was their weight gain the result of severe food restriction at some point in their life. It is also important to ask if they have family members who are anorexic.

12.7.5 Eating Disorder NOS

Eating disorder not otherwise specified (ED NOS) is a classification for people who have many key features of an eating disorder, but do not meet all of the criteria for either bulimia or anorexia. The lack of meeting full criteria should not be confused with the lack of concern or seriousness of this disorder. The symptoms can be quite severe, even though they do not meet full criteria. Someone who is binging and vomiting, but not often enough to meet criteria, is clearly at risk both from a medical and psychiatric perspective and also for having their eating disorder become more severe if left untreated.

12.7.6 Night Eating Syndrome

Night eating syndrome (NES) is believed to consist of four core symptoms: morning anorexia, evening hyperphagia, nocturnal awakenings, and eating during waking episodes [26]. Preliminary data suggest that eating patterns of persons with NES may be distinct from those seen in other eating or sleep disorders; however, more research is needed. Unfortunately, to the best of our knowledge, there are no published studies examining this syndrome in the obese pediatric population.

Lastly, while the identified patient is being evaluated, it is important for the primary care clinician to ask about family history of an eating disorder. Parents are powerful role models for their children. If they have an eating disorder, the impact on the home is very profound. Parents, mothers in particular, shop, cook, and feed their families. If their eating pattern is dysregulated as a result of their own eating disorder, the impact on the family relative to normalized eating patterns will be large. There is likely to be an overfocus on weight, shape, and physical appearance, and perhaps the use or abuse of exercise as a coping method. In addition, parents who themselves have eating disorders will clearly have greater difficulty complying with suggested behavioral interventions.

12.8 FAMILY FUNCTIONING

For children and younger adolescents, family functioning is key to determining if the patient (even if motivated) will be able to carry out treatment recommendations, as parents, often, are the agents of change. For the psychosocial screening, clinicians can quickly assess this by drawing a simple genogram that documents how family structure and functioning impacts the child's weight gain. Clinicians may also choose to gather this information when screening for eating problems, as discussed earlier. Table 12.9 provides a summary of areas to screen for regarding family functioning. If constrained by time, the primary care clinician may consider focusing on assessing the level of parental involvement, supervision, availability, and ability to set limits, provide routine, and identify current psychosocial stressors and coping strategies.

12.9 PSYCHOTROPIC MEDICATION AND WEIGHT CHANGES

Parents of overweight children who are treated with medication to control psychiatric symptoms may note weight gain to the start of medication. Medication-related weight gain is one of the most common secondary causes of obesity. Primary care and mental health clinicians alike struggle with the management of this problem. Weight gain is also one of the most troublesome side effects of prescription psychotropic medication. It is difficult enough to accept, much less require, medication treatment for a psychiatric disorder. But when, as part of the personal cost of that treatment, a person's weight becomes difficult to control, that cost may be seen as too high by a patient and result in medication noncompliance. For example, if weight gain should result from the medication treatment of a mood disorder such as depression, unwanted weight gain clearly runs counter to the antidepressant treatment objectives. This is a dilemma for patients of both sexes, but, particularly, for adolescent girls. Therefore, a thorough discussion of this dilemma at the onset of medication prescription and a close working relationship between pediatrician and psychopharmacologist regarding the management of side effects are essential.

TABLE 12.9
Suggested Areas to Screen for Family Functioning

Family history for obesity and other associated medical problems (i.e., diabetes)
Intactness of family
Are patients meals supervised and/or prepared at more than one home?
Are joint custody parents supportive of patient weight control?
Which adults in child's life "share the fridge"?
Any history of family deaths associated with obesity?
Impact of patient weight gain on family relationships (i.e., distancing, alliances, sabotaging family members, weight teasing)
Level of parental involvement and supervision (i.e., how available are parents, work schedules, etc.)
Parenting styles [41]
- Authoritarian = high degree of control and without or low warmth
- Authoritative = rational degree of control with warmth ideal
- Permissive = low degree of control with warmth
- Rejecting–neglecting = low degree of control and little warmth

Feeding styles
- Emotional (use food to cope with emotional distress)
- Pressure (insist that child eats, i.e., usually for historical, cultural, or pride reasons)
- Convenience (use food to cope with environmental stressor)
- Excessive control (restrict foods often, note least preferred style for weight management)
- Instrumental (use food to reward or punish behaviors)
- Healthy control (encourages and respects child to self-regulate; note: most preferred style for weight management)

Current/past environmental barriers to family weight control attempts (i.e., food security, unsafe neighborhood, lack of insurance, transportation, legal)

Primary prevention of weight gain is of course the best approach and should be actively pursued early in medication treatment. Concomitant treatment with a nutritionist and an exercise program commitment is the best recommendation. If such a plan is not possible at the beginning of treatment, it should be initiated and recommended during treatment. It is sometimes possible, as the psychiatric illness improves, to switch to a less offending medication, so that the weight gain tendencies are often reversed. Vigilance for comorbid substance abuse or dependence with psychiatric disorder is prudent. Alcohol and cannabis are associated with weight gain, and the abused stimulants (cocaine, methamphetamine) with weight loss and with treatment resistance.

It is sometimes difficult to disentangle the obesity of the primary psychiatric problem from its medication treatment. Table 12.10 ranks the currently used groups of prescribed psychotropic medications associated with weight gain (and, sometimes, weight loss).

12.9.1 Antidepressants

Weight gain with the newer antidepressants such as the serotonin and serotonin–norepinephrine reuptake inhibitors (SSRIs and SNRIs) is possible but far less frequent

TABLE 12.10
Rank of Psychotropic Medication by Weight Gain

Generic Name	Brand Name	Weight Gain Risk
Antidepressants		
TCA		
Amitriptilyne	Elavil	High
Imipramine	Tofranil	High
SSRI		
Paroxetine	Paxil	Moderate
Sertraline	Zoloft	Low
Fluoxetine	Prozac	Low
Escitalopram	Lexapro	Low
Fluvoxamine	Luvox	Low
Others		
Mirtazapine	Remeron	High
Venlafaxine	Effexor	Low
Buproprion	Wellbutrin	May cause weight loss
Antipsychotics		
First generation		
Fluphenazine	Prolixin	Moderate
Haloperidol	Haldol	Low
Molindone	Moban	May cause weight loss
Second generation		
Clozapine	Clozaril	Very high
Olanzapine	Zyprexa	Very high
Risperidone	Risperdal	High
Quintiapine	Seroquel	High
Aripiprazole	Abilify	Low
Ziprasidone	Geodon	Low
Mood stabilizers		
Lithium	Lithobid	High
Valproate	Depakote	High
Carbamazepine[a]	Tegretol	Moderate
Oxcarbazepine[a]	Trileptal	Moderate
Lamotrigine	Lamictal	Low
Topiramate[a]	Topamax	May cause weight loss

[a] Not FDA approved for mood disorders.

than with the older antidepressants, particularly the tricyclics (TCA), which are used far less often than in the past.

12.9.2 Antipsychotic Medications

The antipsychotic medications are common causes of weight gain. It is hypothesized that hypothalamic stimulation of the appetite centers may be part of the cause.

Furthermore, most antipsychotics cause a "metabolic" syndrome in which an individual's "set point" (the variable that affects calories burned in relation to intake) is altered, resulting in weight gain relative to previous nutritional and metabolic experience. Most of the older antipsychotic medications cause weight gain. Of the second generation of antipsychotics, olanzapine (Zyprexa) and clozapine (Clozaril) are the most common offenders. The triglycerides and low-density lipoproteins (LDLs) become elevated, associated with a relative insulin resistance and type II diabetes-proneness. Therefore, baseline and regular measurements of these laboratory parameters are recommended. Also, before starting an antipsychotic medication, all patients must be weighed and their BMI periodically monitored throughout treatment.

12.9.3 Mood-Stabilizing Medications

Mood stabilizers are used for the cyclic mood disorders: bipolar and cyclothymic disorder. Of these lithium, valproate (Depakote, Depakane), and carbamazepine (Tegretol, Carbatrol) are most likely to cause weight gain.

12.9.4 "Weight-Neutral" Medications and Weight Loss

No discussion of weight issues and psychoactive medications would be complete without mentioning that for a minority of people taking the medications mentioned above, weight gain does not usually occur, i.e., which are relatively "weight neutral." There are even some medications: molidone in the first generation antipsychotic group, atomoxetine (Strattera) (a medication used for the treatment of attention deficit disorder) and topirmate (Topomax) in the mood stabilizer group, which have been occasionally associated with moderate weight loss. Topiramate, for example, is sometimes strategically used by the psychopharmacologist to counter or avoid weight gain from other psychiatric medications.

12.9.5 Stimulant Medications

Some relative suppression of appetite is associated with stimulant medication (methylphenidate, dextro- or mixed amphetamine salts). Rarely is the appetite suppression so severe as to require that the stimulant be switched or stopped. However, stimulants should never be used to promote weight loss. Tolerance to the relative weight loss propensity of the stimulant medications develops quickly, and abuse and dependence are the frequent results.

In general, it is good practice for the primary care clinician to understand the obese patient's weight gain trajectory prior to the use of psychotropic medication as well as thereafter.

12.10 TREATMENT CONSIDERATION FOR THE PSYCHIATRIC PATIENT

There is no evidence-based guideline to determine who starts treatment for obesity on the basis of a presenting psychiatric disorder. In practice, clinical group treatment programs tend to refer patients with serious psychiatric conditions, patients with

TABLE 12.11
Suggested Behavioral Factors to Consider for Delaying Weight-Control Treatment

Actively suicidal, homicidal, psychotic, manic
Severe depression or anxiety response (i.e., ASD, PTSD)
History of multiple suicide attempts during last 3 years
Engaging in high-risk behaviors within last 6 months (e.g., fire setting, running away)
Concern or evidence of alcohol or drug abuse
Concern or evidence of an eating disorder
Serious preoccupation with body image, i.e., patient believes only weight loss will alleviate or eliminate psychosocial problems
Repeated lack of adherence with medical and/or psychiatric regimens in the short-term
Patient or parent not concerned about obesity
Hostile interpersonal relationship between patient and parent
Concern or evidence about sexual or physical abuse, neglect, or other serious maltreatment conditions

poor social skills, patient preference for individual treatment, or the patient/family who are not ready to change. Refer to Table 12.11 for suggested behavioral factors to consider when deciding whether a patient should start treatment. Primary care clinicians considering the delay of starting weight control counseling due to behavioral factors should continue to monitor patients with frequent routine care follow-up visits and work closely with patients' mental health clinicians.

12.11 COUNSELING CONSIDERATIONS

There is growing acceptance that behavioral and family counseling plays a significant role in evidence-based multicomponent treatments for pediatric weight management. Of most promise are counseling strategies that focus on readiness to change (i.e., MI), behavior modification, and improving parenting skills. Primary care clinicians are encouraged to structure their sessions (see Figure 12.4) so that key elements of effective behavior change counseling strategies (i.e., setting an agenda) are included in routine follow-up visits.

12.11.1 Motivational Interviewing (MI)

The success of modern medicine has been to transform acute illness into chronic conditions. The management of chronic illnesses, however, has proven to be complicated as it depends on the patient/family being able to make changes in health behavior, which will lead to more desirable health outcomes in the long term. The challenge to primary care clinicians often is that behavior change is a slow, gradual process. In a health care climate that is highly constrained by time and encourages a consultation style of direct persuasion, most clinicians would agree that the concept of "process" and "patient-centeredness," in reality, have a limited role in medical consultation. Lower-intensity, time-limited counseling

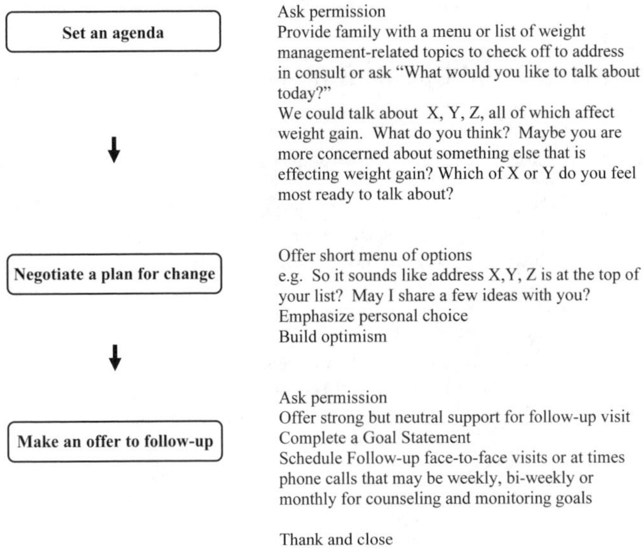

FIGURE 12.4 Suggested follow-up session structure for behavioral counseling. (Adapted from Rollnick, S., Mason, P., and Butler, C. *Health Behavior Change: A Guide for Practitioners*. Edinburgh: Church Livingston, 44, 1999.)

strategies such as phone counseling or web-based self-help/self-monitoring programs may be more desirable to the primary care clinician; however, more research is needed to assess benefits/costs and long-term efficacy [27] in pediatric weight management.

MI is gaining acceptance in the medical field as an alternative counseling style to the traditional one, direct persuasion (i.e., advice giving), which often results in argumentative or passive communication patterns between the clinician and patient when discussing health behavior change. For further discussion of MI please refer to Chapter 3 on MI counseling in this book as well as *Health Behavior Change: A Guide for Practitioners* [7].

Although studies on the applicability of MI with a pediatric population are limited, clinicians may consider using MI to increase readiness in parents of children/young adolescents or with older adolescents alone, who present with either no apparent or obvious ambivalence (precontemplation) or are highly ambivalent (contemplation) about behavior change. Primary care clinicians need to be aware that a majority of families will be in precontemplation or contemplation. Prochaska and colleagues [12] estimate that approximately 10 to 15% of adults referred to programs that involve changing health behavior (i.e., smoking cessation, addictions) are prepared for action, approximately 30 to 40% are in contemplation, and 50 to 60% are in precontemplation. Therefore, the goal of the primary care clinician is to create movement toward a workable ambivalence (preparation) where the patient/family feels confident enough to work on small, doable goals set by both clinician and parent/adolescent. See Table 12.12 for suggested strategies and questions

TABLE 12.12
Suggested Strategies and Questions for Patient/Parent in Early Stages of Change

Stage of Change	Goals	Strategy*	Questions
Precontemplation	Recognize there is a problem Personalize risks	Raise knowledge about problem and negative effects Raise knowledge nature of their behavior Arouse emotion regarding problem Recognize how current behavior conflicts with personal goals and behavior and effects on others and environment Weighing the pros and cons of staying the same or making a change	What would have to happen for you to know overweight is a problem? What would be the warning signs? Has anyone ever expressed concern about the weight? If so, who? What are they? Have you ever tried to change in the past? What are the positives/negatives of staying the same?
Contemplation	Raise self-confidence Be ready to make a commitment	Examine reasons for current behavior Recognize how current behavior conflicts with personal goals and behavior and effects on others and environment Identify barriers to change, coping strategies Make changes in social environment that encourages behavior change	Why do you want to change now? What are the reasons for not changing? What are the barriers that keep you from changing? What would help you (how could I help you) at this time? What/who helped in past? What do you think you need to know about changing?
Preparation	Initiate change Develop a plan	Increase self-confidence to change Avoid/alter cues for behavior problem Substitute healthy behaviors for unhealthy ones Enlist social support	

* Adapted from Velasquez, M.M., Maurer, G.G., Crouch, C., and DiClemente, C.C. *Group Treatment for Substance Abuse: A Stages-of-Change Manual*. New York: The Guilford Press, 8–9, 2001.

to help move the patient/family through earlier stages of change. These strategies may also be used to work with the patient/family who has slipped or relapsed from maintenance to precontemplation or contemplation. Those families who are in preparation are most appropriate for referral to general nutrition services, exercise professionals, and tertiary weight management centers as they primarily offer action-orientated counseling and programming. Lastly, another key MI strategy that may be helpful to the clinician working with families is the setting of an agenda. This will help the primary care clinician to prioritize behaviors to work on, as weight management involves targeting multiple behaviors [7].

12.11.2 Parent Training and Behavior Modification

Obesity is a function of its environment. Families represent a significant environmental influence that affects the development and maintenance of positive health habits and appear to have a powerful influence on weight control treatment effectiveness [28]. Studies show that the influence of parents or primary caregivers plays a key role key in pediatric weight control [29,30]. Golan and colleagues [31,32] go further to suggest that parents alone serve as exclusive agents of change and that their own behavior more than the child's should be targeted in pediatric weight management. Parents of children or young adolescents may be considered by the clinician as the sole recipient of counseling; however, adolescents benefit from their own counseling as well. One program has shown that weight control outcomes improve when adolescents and parents receive their own training, which respects the adolescent's need to become more independent [33].

When parents are ready to make lifestyle modifications, they can learn to support the child or adolescent with behavior modification strategies such as monitoring behaviors, realistic goal setting, contracting, and problem solving. Other behavioral strategies found effective in helping families make changes include controlling cues in the environment (stimulus control), stress management, and rewarding successful changes or efforts to change behavior (not weight loss). For guiding principles and examples of effective weight control strategies with pediatric families, the reader is referred to Dietz and Robinson [34].

Parent training primarily focuses on improving parenting skills. Parents are educated and coached by the primary care clinician to change problem behaviors that may be affecting weight gain, using concepts of learning theory and behavior modification, such as those just mentioned above. Before a parent is asked to engage in interventions that require the ability to plan ahead, supervise, organize, set limits, routine, and structure, reward successful behavior, or model desirable behavior, primary care clinicians need to assess parent competency in these areas and family functioning. Tables 12.13a and b provide suggested questions to consider for assessment, as well as clinician counseling strategies for when provider and parent get "stuck" communicating. Another method of gathering this information quickly is to review a patient/family typical day with both parent and child. Parental modeling of dietary practices is a powerful determinant of children's eating behaviors [35,36] and should be encouraged. Therefore for obvious reason, clinicians are cautioned to ask parents with poor target behaviors to model behavior. Yet, a willingness by parents to change their own health habits affecting weight gain, as well as to consider making changes in parenting style (i.e., firm but respectful and accepting), is a positive sign for patient/family readiness to participate in weight control treatment. Primary care clinicians can take on the role of educator and coach to help parents improve quality of communication and level of involvement with their child (see Table 12.14 for a summary of behavioral parent guidance tips). In addition, clinicians may be helpful in providing guidance on the division of responsibilities for feeding (see Table 12.15). Parents with restrictive or passive parenting styles that are interfering with responsibilities for feeding may benefit from referrals to a parenting

TABLE 12.13A
Suggested Questions and Counseling Probes to Consider in the Assessment of Parenting Skills and Family Dynamics

What are parent's concerns regarding their child's weight gain/obesity? (future health risk, stigmatization)
What does parent attribute weight gain to? (genetic, hormonal, environmental factors)
What are parent's feelings/attitudes towards child's weight gain? (surprised, guilty, embarrassment)
What are parent's current feelings about/towards child in general? (acceptance, proud, frustrated with)
What is parent's feeding style? (convenience, emotional, balanced, etc)
What level of supervision does parent provide to child? (over meals/snacks, homework, etc)
How available is parent to child? (work schedules, who provides care when parent away)
How involved is parent in child's life? (how much do they know about their child's life/functioning)
What is the parent's parenting style? (authoritarian, authoritative, passive)
Is there evidence of abuse/neglect by parent?
What are perceived barriers to starting treatment? (transportation, child care, child motivation)
Is parent experiencing any current distress? What are the precipitating stressors?
What are parent's thoughts about being referred to a weight management program? (if this is an available resource)
What matters to you about your child's weight?
What is your child's routine for the day and night? Who is involved in their care? What adults eat with your child?

TABLE 12.13B
Troubleshooting "Stuck" Conversations: Unpacking the Meaning

IF:

Parent/adolescent stuck in the behavior change process.
You realize you have been doing all the talking for a while.
You hear something that sounds important to you and you are not sure it is important to the client.
You find yourself arguing with parent/adolescent.
You are puzzled and realize you may be proceeding with a mistaken understanding of what parent/adolescent wants.
You here a generic word/phrase such as "I want to feel better" or "That doesn't work." (Do you know exactly what "that "refers to?)

THEN:

Slow down the consultation.
Be curious about what the parent's/adolescents priority concerns are and accept as true for the parent/adolescent.
Ask some questions to unpack what parent/adolescent is trying to say:
"I'm wondering. Would it be helpful to explore what this is all about for you?"
"What matters to you about...?"
"What does ... mean to you?"
"What are the best and worst parts? Would it help to talk more about that part?"
"What matters most about it?"
"Are there parts of this that mean more to you than others?"
"Is this what matters the most to you or is there something else we are missing?"

Source: Adapted from Kellogg M. Unpacking Meaning. In *Counseling Tips for Nutrition Therapists:* Practice *Workbook,* Vol.1, Kg Press 2006. Permission granted by author.

TABLE 12.14
Suggested Tips for Parents

Praise positive behaviors and efforts
Problem-solve with child about alleviating boredom — limit sedentary behaviors
Model positive health habits for the whole family
Do not criticize own self-worth or body appearance in front of child
Do not use food to reward/punish desirable/undesirable behavior
Do not reward children for eating all food especially when they are not hungry
Create an environment where primarily healthy foods are available
Avoid endorsing stereotypes of obesity (i.e., he's lazy, lacks discipline)
Expose family members to a variety of healthy foods
Ensure family eats together at least one meal a week
Create a family space to eat free of distractions (i.e., no TV, radio, phones or reading materials)
Ensure family plays together at least once a week
Plan ahead — maintain a household routine/schedule
Avoid hiding unhealthy foods — just don't buy them instead
Be consistent, available and responsible for your child/adolescent

group, parent educator, or family therapist, as well as being provided with a resource list that includes information on parent support hotlines, books, and website references that provide parenting education.

12.11.3 Cultural/Socioeconomic Considerations

Although a complete discussion of cultural, socioeconomic, legal/ethical issues in the context of obesity and weight management is beyond the scope of this chapter, the primary care clinician is strongly encouraged to consider the possibility that these issues may significantly impact the patient/family's readiness to change as well as

TABLE 12.15
Parent/Child Feeding Responsibilities for the Overweight Child

Parent is responsible for:
What, when, where and how much
- To teach the child "how much" until child can self-regulate
- To set limits (firm but warm) and not restrict
- To respect child/adolescent

Children and Adolescents are responsible for:
To learn and apply signs of hunger/thirst and fullness to self-regulate
For adolescents to understand and live up to parental expectations and own obligations around healthy consumption

Source: Adapted from Satter, E. *Your Child's Weight: Helping without Harming, Birth through Adolescence*. Madison: Kelcy Press, 2005.

treatment effectiveness. Culture/ethnicity may shape health beliefs about weight gain. For example, some cultures may value a more full-bodied appearance, which may be seen as a sign of good health. A family with this value, therefore, may not perceive obesity to be a problem. Clinicians are encouraged to avoid "correcting" the belief and instead educate on some of the physiological concerns and risks associated with the obesity, which have little to do with appearance.

Some cultural norms may value limited questioning of clinicians (i.e., sign of disrespect) or expect clinicians to do most of the talking during a consult (i.e., a sign of expertise). The clinician who considers using MI counseling may, therefore, need to modify key elements of the approach (i.e., limiting the handing over of some of the decision-making responsibility to the family or not push or expect the patient/family to do the talking) and focus on building self-efficacy to change behavior, instead. With respect to motivation, clinicians are also cautioned of mistaking minimal eye contact and limited questioning by the family as a sign of poor motivation. Socioeconomic issues such as food security (see Chapter 13 for community perspective), health insurance, and impact of immigration (i.e., changes in diet, access to physical activity, status, etc.) should also be considered.

12.11.4 Counseling Setting

Often, primary care clinicians struggle with the question of whether children, adolescents, and their parents should be seen together or apart during counseling sessions. Clinicians often struggle with this issue when having to deliver bad news or to discuss sensitive health topics such as obesity and weight management. As a rule of thumb, parents of infants, toddlers, and preschoolers should be the main recipients of counseling since they provide most of the child's food selections as well as being most responsible for providing structure for most of the day [6]. For school-aged children up to age 10, parents are still considered to be the primary recipient of counseling; however, clinicians should strive occasionally to meet one-on-one with the child in order to monitor psychosocial functioning, to confirm accuracy of parent report regarding interventions, to praise accomplishments that were part of the plan [6]. For children aged 10 to 12, clinicians are encouraged to meet with child and parent together, as children have more autonomy over food selection and joint counseling provides an opportunity to understand rules of feeding responsibilities [6]. Clearly, adolescents and parents typically benefit from having separate sessions, as the division of responsibilities is different where the parent plays a more supportive role. Clinicians at anytime are encouraged to hold separate sessions for parent and child if there are serious psychosocial concerns that require further screening or signs of a deteriorating parent–child relationship.

Lastly, the physical surroundings of the counseling setting are as important to consider as the use of appropriate language. Primary care clinicians are encouraged to consider creating a physical environment for the obese patient and their family that feels supportive, private, and safe (see Table 12.16 for suggestions).

TABLE 12.16
Practice-Setting Recommendations

Equip examination rooms and waiting areas with larger furniture (e.g., chairs and tables) and medical equipment (e.g., scales and blood pressure cuffs).
Obtain measurements as well as counsel patients/families in a private room — not in corridors or waiting areas.
Provide the option to remain clothed when measuring or examining the patient.
Stock waiting area with print and/or electronic materials that encourage self-assessment and build knowledge around health habits. Ensure that materials do not further stigmatize patient/family.

12.12 ADOLESCENT WEIGHT LOSS SURGERY (WLS)

Given more recent considerations by the medical community in treating adolescent morbid obesity with surgical options, the authors have decided to provide some discussion on this topic as the issue may be raised by parent or adolescent during a primary care consultation. For morbidly obese adults, WLS has been found to be an effective yet controversial treatment option with well-defined risks. However, for the morbidly obese adolescent patient, research is limited. There are no national guidelines for pediatric weight loss surgery; however, recently, an expert panel in the state of Massachusetts issued an executive report [37] that provides expert recommendations for use of WLS — for best practice guidelines on adolescent WLS refer to Apovian and colleagues [38]. Although there is no consensus among health professionals on whether or not psychiatric comorbidities are contraindications to surgery, individual institutions have developed their own guidelines for preoperative behavioral health evaluation and counseling in order to reduce anticipatory anxiety regarding surgery, as well as to improve postoperative behavior change and compliance, respectively [39].

Primary care clinicians are encouraged to consider the psychological maturity and environmental stability (see Table 12.17) of their patients in addition to BMI and physiological maturity eligibility factors when considering a WLS referral. Unless emancipated, the adolescent patient is still legally bound to the decision-making rights of the parent or legal guardian and does not have independent control over their living environment. Therefore, clinicians need to set higher standards than it would for an adult being considered for WLS. The primary care clinician may want to consider involving a child/adolescent mental health clinician who is preferably familiar with obesity and WLS. As a rule of thumb, however, WLS for the adolescent patient should be considered as a last resort treatment option.

12.13 CONCLUSION

Behavioral family-based treatment is now considered to be a key element of multicomponent treatments recommended for pediatric weight management. Primary care clinicians, therefore, will be expected to be involved in helping families

TABLE 12.17
Psychological Factors to Consider for Adolescent WLS Referral

Psychological maturity
Able to provided informed assent without coercion
Able to comply with medical regimens in the short term
Able to demonstrate compliance with lifestyle changes in the short-term
Able to demonstrate an awareness of potential psychological distress if family does not provide adequate instrumental and emotional support
Able to realize that surgery itself does not guarantee weight loss
Environment stability
Parental acceptance and respect of child
Parental social support (involved in care, practically and emotionally available)
Absence of current maltreatment conditions (abuse or neglect)
Plan for addressing practical barriers such as insurance, transportation
School support (academic/vocational)
Parental/family functioning relatively stable with appropriate supports in place
Absence of active drug and alcohol abuse in parent or child

prioritize competing concerns to weight control management; to increase family-efficacy for modification of health habits; to help families control for environmental factors that may be contributing to weight gain; to reinforce positive changes made; and to monitor patient/family psychosocial functioning, which may require further assessment and treatment by qualified mental health professionals [34]. Although these tasks may at times seem to go beyond one's scope of practice, the primary care clinician can increase their proficiency by freely modifying behavioral considerations presented in this chapter in response to primary care setting pressures. Given the multicomponent treatment demands primary care clinicians often need to coordinate in pediatric weight management, it is recommended that clinicians consider the involvement of their mental health colleagues to help with assessment, education, and family-based behavioral counseling in order to reduce some of the patient care burden.

REFERENCES

1. Ogden, C.L., Carroll, M.D., Curtin, L.R., McDowell, M.A., Tabak, C.J., Flegal, K.M. Prevalence of overweight and obesity in the United States, 1999–2004, *JAMA* 295(13), 1549–1555, 2006.
2. Dietz, W.H., Health consequences of obesity in youth: childhood predictors of adult disease, *Pediatrics* 101(suppl), 518–525, 1998.
3. Jonides, L., Buschbacher, V., and Barlow, S.E., Management of child and adolescent obesity: psychological, emotional, and behavioral assessment, *Pediatrics* 110(1), 215–221, 2002.
4. Story, M.T., Neumark-Stzainer, D.R., Sherwood, N.E., Holt, K., Sofka, D., Trowbridge, F.L., and Barlow, S.E., Management of child and adolescent obesity: attitudes, barriers, skills, and training needs among health care professionals, *Pediatrics* 110(1), 210–214, 2002.

5. Barlow, S.E., Trowbridge, F.L., Klish, W.J., and Dietz, W.H., Treatment of child and adolescent obesity: reports from pediatricians, pediatric nurse practitioners, and registered dieticians, *Pediatrics* 110, 229–235, 2002.
6. Satter, E., *Your Child's Weight: Helping without Harming, Birth through Adolescence* Kelcy Press, Madison, WI, 2005.
7. Rollnick, S., Mason, P., and Butler, C., *Health Behavior Change: A Guide for Practitioners*, Church Livingstone, Edinburgh, 1999.
8. White, M. and Epston, D., *Narrative Means to Therapeutic Ends*, W.W. Norton, New York, 1990.
9. Schwartz, M.B. and Puhl, R., Childhood obesity: a societal problem to solve, *Obes Rev* 4, 57–71, 2003.
10. Epstein, L.H., Roemmich, J.N., and Raynor, H.A., Behavioral therapy in the treatment of pediatric obesity, *Ped Clin North Am* 48, 981–993, 2001.
11. Mullen, M.S. and Shield, J., *Childhood and Adolescent Overweight: The Health Professional's Guide to Identification, Treatment and Prevention,* American Dietician Association, 2004.
12. Prochaska, J.O., DiClemente, C.C., and Norcross, J.C., Stages of change: prescriptive guidelines for behavioral medicine and psychotherapy, in *Psychologists' Desk Reference*, Koocher, G.P., Norcross, J.C., and Hill, S.S., III, Oxford University Press, New York, 1998.
13. Prochaska, J.Q. and DiClemente, C.C., Stages and processes of self-change in smoking: toward an integrative model of change, *J Consult Clin Psychol* 5, 390–395, 1983.
14. Miller, W.R. and Rollnick, S., *Motivational Interviewing: Preparing People to Change Addictive Behavior,* The Guilford Press, New York, 1991.
15. Zametkin, A.J., Zoon, C.R., Klein, H.W., and Munson, S., Psychiatric aspects of child and adolescent obesity: a review of the past 10 years, *J Am Acad Child Adolesc Psychiatry* 43(2), 134–150, 2004.
16. Friedman, M.A. and Brownell, K.D., Psychological correlates of obesity: moving to the next research generation, *Psychol Bull* 117, 3–20, 1995.
17. Jackson, T.D., Grilo, C.M., and Masheb, R.M., Teasing history, onset of obesity, current eating disorder psychopathology, body dissatisfaction, and psychological functioning in binge eating disorder, *Obes Res* 8, 451–458, 2000.
18. Eisenberg, M.E., Neumark-Sztainer, D., and Story, M., Associations of weight-based teasing and emotional well-being among adolescents, *Arch Pediatr Adolesc Med* 157, 733–738, 2003.
19. Strauss, R.S. and Pollack, H.A., Social marginalization of overweight children, *Arch Pediatr Adolesc Med* 157, 746–752, 2003.
20. Lissau, I. and Sorensen, T., Parental neglect during childhood and increased risk of obesity in young adulthood, *Lancet* 343, 324–327, 1994.
21. Felitti, V.J., Anda, R.F., Nordenberg, D., Williamson, D.F., Spitz, A.M., Edwards, V., Koss, M.P., and Marks, J.S., Relationship of childhood abuse and household dysfunction to many of the leading causes of death in adults: the adverse childhood experiences (ACE) study, *Am J Prev Med* 14, 245–258, 1998.
22. Neumark-Sztainer, D., Story, M., Falkner, N.H., Beuhring, T., and Resnick, M.D., Sociodemographic and personal characteristics of adolescents engaged in weight loss and weight/muscle gain behaviors: who is doing what?, *Prev Med* 28, 4–50, 1999.
23. Berkowitz, R., Stunkard, A.J., and Stallings, V.A., Binge eating disorder in obese adolescent girls, *Ann NY Acad Sci* 699, 200–206, 1993.

24. Britz, B., Siegfried, W., Ziegler, A., Lamertz, C., Herpertz-Dahlmann, B.M., Remschmidt, H., Wittchen, H.U., and Hebebrand, J., Rates of psychiatric disorders in a clinical study group of adolescents with extreme obesity and in obese adolescents ascertained via a population based study, *Int J Obes Relat Metab Disord* 24, 1707–1714, 2000.
25. Neumark-Sztainer, D., Story, M., French, S., Hannan, P.J., Resnick, M.D., and Blum, R.W., Psychosocial concerns and health-compromising behaviors among overweight and nonoverweight adolescents, *Obes Res* 5, 237–249, 1997.
26. Stunkard, A.J. and Allison, K.C., Two forms of disordered eating in obesity: binge eating and night eating, *Int J Obes Relat Metab Disord* 27(1), 1–12, 2003.
27. U.S. Preventive Services Task Force, Behavioral counseling in primary care to promote a healthy diet: recommendations and rationale, *Am J Prev Med* 24(1), 93–100, 2003.
28. White, M.A., Martin, P.D., Newton, R.L., Walden, H.M., York-Crowe, E.E., Gordon, S.T., Ryan, D.H., and Williamson, D.A., Mediators of weight loss in a family-based intervention presented over the internet, *Obes Res* 12(7), 1050–1059, 2004.
29. Epstein, L.H., McKenzie, S.J., Valoski, A., Klein, K.R., and Wing, R.R., Effects of mastery criteria and contingent reinforcement for family-based child weight control, *Addict Behav* 19, 135–145, 1994.
30. Epstein, L.H., Valoski, A., Wing, R.R., and McCurely, J., Ten-year follow-up of behavioral family-based treatment for obese children, *JAMA* 264, 2519–2523, 1990.
31. Golan, M. and Crow, S., Targeting parents exclusively in the treatment of childhood obesity: long-term results, *Obes Res* 12(2), 357–361, 2004.
32. Golan, M., Weizman, A., Apter, A., and Fainaru, M., Parents as exclusive agents of change in the treatment of childhood obesity, *Am J Clin Nutr* 67, 1130–1135, 1998.
33. Brownell, K.D., Kelman, J.H., and Stunkard, A.J., Treatment of obese children with and without their mothers: changes in weight and blood pressure, *Pediatrics* 71, 515–523, 1983.
34. Dietz, W.H. and Robinson, T.N., Overweight children and adolescents, *N Engl J Med* 352 (20), 2100–2109, 2005.
35. Golan, M., Fainaru, M., and Weizman, A., Familial approach to the treatment of childhood obesity: a conceptual model, *J Nutr Educ* 33(2), 102, 2001.
36. Wrotniak, B.H., Epstein, L.H., Paluch, R.A., and Roemmich, J.N., The relationship between parent and child self-reported adherence and weight loss, *Obes Res* 13(6), 1089–1096, 2005.
37. Betsy Lehman Center for Patient Safety and Medical Error Reduction, expert panel on weight loss surgery, Massachusetts Department of Public Health, 2004.
38. Apovian, C.M., Baker, C., Ludwig, D.S., Hoppin, A.G., Hsu, G., Lenders, C., Pratt, J.S.A., Forse, A., O'Brien, A., and Tarnoff, M., Best practice guidelines in pediatric/adolescent weight loss surgery, *Obes Res* 13, 274–282, 2005.
39. Sogg, S. and Mori, D.L., The Boston interview for gastric bypass: determining the psychological suitability of surgical candidates, *Obes Surg* 14(3), 370–380(11), 2004.
40. Freedman, J.S., *Easing the Teasing: Helping Your Child Cope with Name-Calling, Ridicule and Verbal Bullying,* Contemporary Books, Chicago, 2002.
41. Baumrind, D., Parenting styles and adolescent development, In *Encyclopedia of Adolescence*, Lerner, R.M., Petersen, A.C., and Brooks-Gunn, J. Garland, New York, 1991.
42. Edmunds, L.D. Parents' perceptions of health professionals' responses when seeking help for their overweight children. *Fam Pract* 22, 287–292, 2005.
43. Puhl, R. and Brownell, K.D. Bias, discrimination, and obesity. *Obes Res* 9, 788–805, 2001.

44. Brownell, K.D., Puhl, R., Schwartz, M.B., and Rudd, L. (Eds.). *Weight Bias: Nature, Consequences, and Remedies,* Guilford Publications, Guilford Press, 2005.
45. Latner, J.D. and Stunkard, A.J. Getting worse: the stigmatization of obese children. *Obes Res* 11, 452–456, 2003.
46. Schwartz, M,B., O'Neal, H., Brownell, K.D., Blair, S., and Billington, C. Weight bias among health professionals specializing in obesity. *Obes Res* 11, 1033–1039, 2003.
47. Maroney, D. and Golub, S. Nurses' attitudes toward obese persons and certain ethnic groups. *Percept Motor Skills* 75, 387–391, 1992.
48. Klein D., Najman, J., Kohrman, AF., and Munro, C. Patient characteristics that elicit negative responses from family physicians. *J Family Practice* 14, 881–888, 1982.
49. Price, J.H., Desmond, S.M., Krol, R.A., Synder, F.F., and O'Connell, J.K. Family practice physicians' beliefs, attitudes, and practices regarding obesity. *Am J Prevent Med,* 339–345, 1987.
50. Janssen, I., Craig, W.M., Boyce, W.F., and Picket, W. Associations between overweight and obesity with bullying behaviors in school-aged children. *Pediatrics* 113, 1187–1194, 2004.
51. Griffiths, L.J., Wolke, D., Page, A.S., and Horwood, J.P. Obesity and bullying: different effects for boys and girls. *Arch Dis Childhood* 91, 121–125, 2006.

13 The Community as a Resource to Support Positive Nutrition and Physical Activity Behaviors in Youth

Vivien Morris and Gita Rao

CONTENTS

13.1 INTRODUCTION

Combatting the obesity epidemic among children requires a holistic approach to prevention and treatment. Clinical office-based responsibilities to patients and their families are described in great detail in other chapters of this text. Once patients leave clinical settings, they need additional support to implement strategies and maintain behaviors that promote healthy diets and adequate physical activity in the face of environments that work against them. Understanding the environment in which the patient and family lives is critical to the long-term success of weight management. The rationale for including community-based initiatives in the arsenal of tools available to clinicians to prevent and treat obesity is outlined and illustrations using promising and successful programs provided.

13.2 THE SOCIAL ECOLOGICAL MODEL

Overweight and obesity are public health problems, and as such must be addressed at multiple levels simultaneously and in an integrated way. Environmental risk factors as diverse as family dynamics, food insecurity, lack of safe places for physical activity, limited support for physical education in the schools, and lack of consistent access to healthful food choices all speak to the need for an approach that is multifaceted. The socioecological model provides a useful framework for approaching childhood overweight and obesity.[1] This model includes five levels of influence. The individual child is at the center of this model, surrounded by family, friends, and peers who provide support and identity. The next level includes institutions and organizations. Key institutions and organizations for children are school and afterschool programs, as well as social and religious organizations. These institutions and organizations have their own rules, policies, and environments that affect nutrition and physical activity behaviors. The community level includes social networks, norms, and practices among organizations. Media influences, the food supply, health care, and built environment can also be placed here. The final level is the public policy and is often the target of advocacy for changes in policies, regulations, and laws at the local, state, and federal government levels. Each of these levels will be discussed in this chapter in the context of providing a supportive and healthy environment for children aiming to reach and maintain a healthy weight (Figure 13.1).

13.2.1 Individual Support

Obese children have their own food likes and dislikes as well as varied interests in physical activity. Family access to food and physical activity resources also vary. Getting to know these and making recommendations in line with individual preferences and resource availability increases the likelihood of successful interventions.

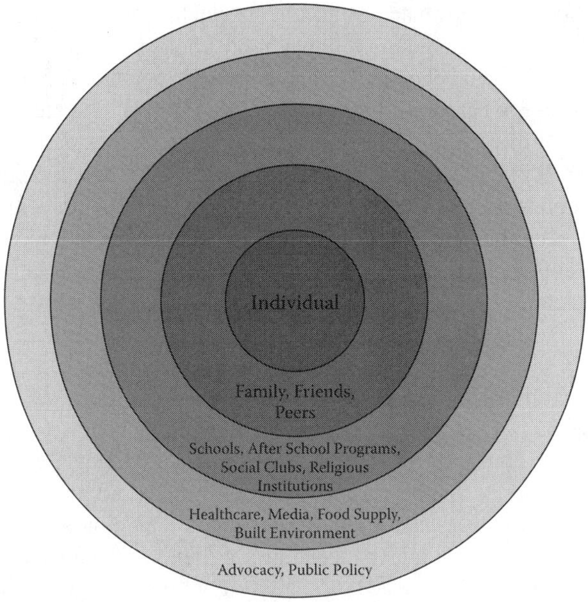

FIGURE 13.1 The social ecological model as a framework for approaching childhood overweight and obesity.

Individualized health support for obese children may take place in the primary care clinician office, in specialty clinics or in specialized community-based programs. Primary care clinicians are often the first health resource sought by overweight children and adolescents or their families. Counseling sessions with a multidisciplinary team that includes doctors, nurses, dietitians, clinical psychologists, social workers, and exercise specialists are able to focus on the special needs of the obese child. Detailed descriptions of appropriate clinical care are described within other chapters of this book. Outside of the clinic session, individuals may be referred to community-based programs that support their efforts to engage in safe physical activity and make nutrition behavior changes. Young people who have had negative experiences with physical activity, those who lack basic physical activity skills, or those who need a specialized supportive environment to begin necessary lifelong behavior changes may benefit from a program designed for overweight youth. Several examples of group programs designed to support weight management in youth are described in this chapter.

13.2.2 Family, Friends, and Peers

13.2.2.1 Families

Families play a critical role in providing environments that support young children to develop lifelong healthy eating and physical activity behaviors. The family role in determining what and how first foods are offered sets the stage for lifelong eating habits.

One of the earliest decisions made by parents is whether to breast feed or bottle feed their infant. This decision and subsequent food choices lay the basis for lifelong nutritional health. Clinical behavioral interventions for treatment of childhood obesity have found that family-based programs have long-term (10 yr) effectiveness.[2] Parents exert more control over eating behavior in early years (3–5 yr old)[3] and less control in later years (8–9 yr old).[4] Characteristics that affect both food intake and physical activity of children in the family setting include age and gender, ethnicity, social norms, socioeconomic class, family composition, and the knowledge attitudes and behaviors of both the parents and the children.[5] Cultural traditions also play a significant role. Parents should determine what foods are offered to children and when they are offered; children should be supported to decide how much they will consume. Role modeling healthy eating behaviors at mealtime through family meals offers an important opportunity to support children in adopting good health habits.[6] Laboratory studies found that parental child-feeding practices impact child-eating behaviors and subsequent overweight in some families.[7] However, a contrasting study found that parental control over children's intake in middle-class Caucasian families did not generalize to 8- to 9-yr-olds in families with diverse socioeconomic and ethnic backgrounds.[4]

Parents play an important role in mediating children's sedentary and activity behaviors. Television viewing is a sedentary activity commonly engaged in by children. Parents setting limits on the amount of television children are allowed to watch and not placing a television in children's bedrooms have significant impacts on the use of screen media by youth.[8] Parents may both encourage independent play by children and engage in active play alongside their children. Although the Centers for Disease Control Task Force on Community Preventive Services did not find sufficient evidence that family-based social support programs on physical activity changed behaviors of family members in their review of 11 qualifying studies,[9] encouraging parents to plan family physical activity opportunities remains a reasonable recommendation. The role of the family in influencing child behavior is addressed in depth in another chapter (see Chapter 12). An expert committee of the Institutes of Medicine summarized the recommendation for parents and families: Engage in and promote healthful dietary intake and active lifestyles (e.g., increased physical activity, reduced television and other screen time, and more healthful dietary behaviors) (Table 13.1).[10]

A collaborative effort between the National Institutes of Health's National Heart, Lung and Blood Institute (NHLBI), National Institute of Diabetes and Digestive and Kidney Diseases (NIDDK), National Institute of Child Health and Human Development (NICHD), and National Cancer Institute (NCI) developed the We Can! (Ways to Enhance Children's Activity and Nutrition) project. We Can! is a national public education and childhood obesity prevention program that focuses on supporting the

TABLE 13.1
Institute of Medicine Recommendation for Parents and Families for the Prevention of Childhood Obesity

Engage in and promote more healthful dietary intake and active lifestyles (e.g., increased physical activity, reduced television and other screen time, and more healthful dietary behaviors)[10]

capacity of parents of youth ages 8–13 to provide healthy home environments.[11] Targeted behaviors include improved nutritional choices, increased physical activity, and reduced screen time. Local experience by the Boston Organization of Nutritionists and Dietitians of Color in implementing the We Can! Curriculum with African-American, Afro-Caribbean, and Latino parents has been very positive. The group attributes its success to having a sound curriculum delivered in a supportive environment by culturally attuned health educators.[12]

13.2.2.2 Friends and Peers

Social worth, emotional growth, and well-being are derived from spending time with peers. In addition to home-based socializing, schools, clubs, enrichment programs, physical activity programs, and sports provide opportunities for youth to interact with friends and peers. Many programs utilize group health education activities in social environments that capitalize on the building of friendship networks and peer support. No large clinical trials have studied the efficacy of utilizing peer leaders as health educators to support weight management in children. Peer-based strategies have been used successfully in youth-focused violence prevention, smoking prevention, and alcohol and drug use prevention programs.[13–15] The Teens Eating for Energy and Nutrition in Schools (TEENS) study, a school-based nutrition intervention for young adolescents designed to increase fruit and vegetable intake and lower fat intake, found that peer-led nutrition education approaches are feasible and highly acceptable among students and peer leaders.[16] Similarly, the Trying Alternative Cafeteria Options in Schools (TACOS) project used student-led promotional activities to encourage healthier food choices among secondary school students.[17] Youth-led health promotion activities provide opportunities for youth to become involved and empowered. Additionally, some programs have been able to capitalize on older youth's ability to relate to the special interests and concerns of younger children.[18] FANtastic Girls, a model program for weight management utilizing teen peer leaders, is discussed in the section of this chapter, that focuses on afterschool programs.[19]

Children also spend time daily communicating with their peers, often through electronic media like telephones and the Internet. This utilization of media may encourage sedentary behavior, as youth may be sitting or lounging for long periods of time. The Kaiser Family Foundation study of more than 2000 third through twelfth graders found that youths spend nearly 6.5 hr/d (6 hr and 21 min) with media. 53 min/d are spent talking on the telephone and 62 min/d using a computer.[20] Instant messaging has become one of the most popular computer and cellular phone activities. The Kaiser Family Foundation study describes bedrooms as multimedia centers for youth. Children are often utilizing multiple media outlets at once. The study found that youth have changed how they use media as well as which media they use. Sixty-four percent of youth have downloaded music from the Internet; 48% have streamed a radio station through the Internet; 66% use instant messaging; 39% have a cell phone, 34% say they have a digital video recorder in their homes; 32% have created a personal Web site or Web page; 18% have an MP3 player; and 13% have a handheld device that connects to the Internet. While some of these media options have the potential to provide encouragement for physical activity (e.g., listening to music while exercising or dancing), in the bedroom they are often used while being relatively sedentary.

13.2.3 Schools and Afterschool Programs as Community Resources to Promote Healthy Eating and Increased Physical Activity

13.2.3.1 Schools

Schools are a key venue for supporting the development of healthy lifestyles among youth and families, reaching almost all children and adolescents in the nation. A child's schooling may begin as early as age three. Since children may spend over half their awake hours in school, schools provide key opportunities to promote healthy behaviors.[21] School contact with parents also provides opportunities to influence family-health behaviors.[22] Areas of intervention in schools that may support healthy weights in children include: comprehensive school health, modifications in school lunch and school breakfast programs, improved access to healthy a la carte foods in schools, improved access to quality physical education programs, increased opportunities for physical activity outside of physical education classes, and supports for decreased television viewing (Table 13.2).

13.2.3.2 Health Education

Health education classes, once a cornerstone of healthy education programs in schools, have been cut in many states due to budgetary constraints. Advocacy for restoration of funds for these programs and general health services for school-based programs continues. Health education is one of the eight components of a coordinated school health approach, which also includes health services, a healthy school environment, health promotion for staff, counseling, nutrition services, and physical education.[23] This approach emphasizes improvement in quality in each component as well as integration of components for unified and reinforced health messages. Nutrition education is one element of health education. Nutrition education is further enhanced when it is combined with support for positive health behavior change in the coordinated school health model. Action for Healthy Kids (AFHK), a collaboration of more than 40 national organizations and government agencies representing the education, health, fitness, and nutrition fields, as well as 51 state teams developed an action plan to assist America's schools fight the epidemic of overweight. Change in health education is a key component of AFHK's action plan. The AFHK health education goal is: "to provide students in pre-kindergarten through

TABLE 13.2
Common Goals of School-Based Interventions Promoting Nutrition and Physical Activity

Plan and implement comprehensive school health
Improve access to healthy foods (a la carte and school meals programs)
Increase physical activity and quality physical education
Reduce television viewing

grade 12 with behavior-focused nutrition education integrated into the curriculum that is interactive and teaches the skills they need to adopt healthy eating habits."[24] The Centers for Disease Control and Prevention has described eight action steps for implementing quality health education courses of study, which include education to promote physical activity and healthy eating.[25]

13.2.3.3 School Nutrition Programs

The National School Lunch (NSL) and School Breakfast (SB) programs are meal programs administered locally by schools and school authorities, at the state level by state education agencies, and federally by the Food and Nutrition Service of the U.S. Department of Agriculture. In 2005, 29.6 million children participated in the NSL program, and 9.37 million children participated in the SB program.[26] More than one-half of youths in the U.S. eat one of their three major meals in school, and 1 in 10 children and adolescents eats two of three main meals in school.[27] Free and reduced priced meals must be provided to children who meet income eligibility requirements. Federal school food standards require that no more than 30% of calories come from fat and less than 10% from saturated fat. Lunches must provide 33% of the Recommended Dietary Allowances (RDA) of protein, Vitamin A, Vitamin C, iron, calcium, and calories, while lunch must provide 25% of these RDAs as well as 25% of calories. Evaluation of the diets of children who participate in NSL and SB programs found that students who participate in these programs have a higher mean intake of food energy, seven vitamins and minerals, total fat, saturated fat, fiber, and sodium than do students who do not participate in either of these programs.[28] Providing consistency in food quality and taste appeal serves to encourage youth to seek out and consume healthy foods offered in schools.

Foods of minimal nutritional value, such as soda, chewing gum, and some candies, are not allowed to be sold in the cafeteria during school meals in schools participating in the NSL and SB programs. Compliance with this regulation is not consistently enforced, and many unhealthful foods have escaped that label and are free to compete directly with school meals. Also, foods of minimal nutritional value may be sold outside of the cafeteria. School-vending machines, a la carte food sales, and foods sold at special school events have become the focuses of these discussions. Local, state, and federal level efforts are underway to limit the sale of competitive foods of low nutritional value in schools. Local schools and school boards have at times been reluctant to remove these foods from schools, because of the significant revenue they provide for school functioning. While mindful of the revenues provided to schools through a la carte and vending machine sales, advocates for improved nutrition in schools have joined with local school boards and state legislators to promulgate regulations to limit access to unhealthy foods in schools. Work to remove unhealthy food options from schools complements efforts to encourage increased student selection of healthy food choices, including fruits and vegetables and foods low in total fat and saturated fat. Several evaluated programs have been effective in increasing fruit and vegetable intake[29–32] and in decreasing the fat content of school meals.[33,34] Thus clinicians should be mindful of the benefits of encouraging the participation of their young patients in school-feeding programs while advocating for systemic improvements in the school-feeding environment (Table 13.3).

TABLE 13.3
Strategies for School-Based Promotion of Healthy Eating

Changes in food service and the food environments
- Changing food availability
  - Provide appealing, low-fat, low-sodium foods in vending machines and at school meetings and events
  - Introduce salad bars into cafeteria
- Altering the food environment
  - Placing healthier foods in the most prominent positions
  - Eliminating advertisements in schools promoting high-fat and high-sugar foods
- Changing food preparation methods
  - Discontinuing frying
- Altering prices on competitive foods/healthy food

Promotional activities (cafeteria or school-wide)
- Healthy Media campaigns — school newspapers and Website development
- Free samples of lower-fat foods distributed with taste test
- Poster contest for advertisements of healthier foods

Classroom curricula on nutrition education and behavioral skills
- Peer-led nutrition education
- Multidisciplinary curriculum with nutrition messages integrated into major subject areas that comply with state curriculum frameworks

Parental involvement
- Newsletters sent home on changes in food service at school
- Family nights promoting nutrition activities

Source: Adapted from[10].

13.2.3.4 Physical Education and Physical Activity

Along with efforts to promote healthier eating environments and behaviors among students, school-based health promotion has aimed to increase the amount of time that students spend engaged in physical activity students receive. The National Association for Sport and Physical Education recommends that all children engage in moderate to vigorous physical activity for at least 60 min each day.[35] Given that children spend half of their day in school, the Institute of Medicine recommends that children engage in 30 minutes of moderate-to-vigorous physical activity during the school day.[21] The Robert Wood Johnson Foundation "Healthy Schools for Healthy Kids" report recommends that schools provide 30 min of physical education for every child, every day in every grade.[36] Unfortunately, given budgetary and academic pressures, only 8% of elementary schools, 6.4% of middle/junior high schools, and 5.8% of senior high schools in the nation provide daily physical education (PE) or its equivalent for the entire school for all grades.[37] According to the Youth Risk Behavior Survey, only 28% of high school students reported attending PE class daily in 2003 as opposed to 42% in 1991.[37]

Age, ethnic, and sex differences also exist in physical activity levels. Researchers have noted a decline in physical activity among adolescent black girls and white girls compared to boys, with more pronounced decreases in activity by black girls. By age 16 or 17, 56% of black girls and 31% of white girls reported no habitual leisure-time activity.[38] These concerning facts warrant interventions that promote physical activity, including a high-quality physical education program, in schools. A high-quality physical education program is characterized by: its emphasis on knowledge and skills for a lifetime of physical activity; meets the needs of all students; keeps students active for most of physical education class time; teaches self-management as well as movement skills, and is an enjoyable experience for students.[39] Two nationally recognized physical education programs found to improve both the quantity and the quality of physical activity among school students are the Sports, Play, and Active Recreation for Kids (SPARK) and the Child and Adolescent Trial for Cardiovascular Health (CATCH) programs. One SPARK intervention found that the amount of moderate to vigorous physical activity by students was significantly increased when physical education specialists taught the sessions (40 min), compared to those sessions taught by teachers (33 min) or the control classes (18 min).[40] Modifications in physical education programming in elementary schools were also a key component of the CATCH program. An evaluation of the CATCH program found that students at the CATCH schools reported more moderate to vigorous activity and more vigorous activity than control schools.[41]

Increasing physical activity through regular activities of daily living provides passive opportunities for physical activity across the life cycle. Walking and biking to school provide regular, predictable, and important opportunities for physical activity. There has been a significant decline in the percentage of walking trips for children aged 5 to 15 from 1977 to 2001, dropping from 20.2% of school trips in 1977 to 12.5% of school trips in 2001.[42] For adolescents, the percentage of walking trips dropped even more significantly from 20.9% in 1977 to 13.6% in 1990 to 10.9% in 2001. According to the Centers for Disease Control (CDC), if an additional one-quarter of children were to walk to school, total active travel time could increase by 50% nationwide (Table 13.4).[43]

13.2.3.5 Employing the Strategies: CATCH Study

An example of a large-scale school-based intervention that utilizes multifaceted strategies to improve child health is the CATCH program. Piloted in schools, the CATCH

TABLE 13.4
Strategies for School-Based Promotion of Physical Activity

Provide physical education instruction
Establish and/or enforce requirements for mandatory daily physical education in schools
Change PE curricula
Utilize curricula that engage all students, regardless of athletic ability, in moderate to vigorous activity
Provide age appropriate and culturally sensitive instruction in physical education
Expand physical activity opportunities
Expand afterschool physical activity programs for all students
Provide daily recess periods for elementary school students, featuring time for unstructured but supervised active play
Promote walking and bicycling to school

Source: Adapted from[10].

intervention was designed to decrease cardiovascular risk factors in children through integrated classroom curriculum, parent education, physical education curriculum, and school food service modification. Results from the study found that CATCH intervention schools had significantly lower consumption of fat and saturated fat and higher levels of self-reported physical activity compared to comparison schools. At a schoolwide level, intervention schools showed a significantly greater proportion of time spent in moderate to vigorous physical activity in physical education classes, and cafeterias offered school meals that were significantly lower in fat and saturated fat when compared with comparison schools. With a multifaceted approach, the CATCH intervention has shown that schools have the ability to influence students' dietary intake and physical activity through both student-level education and schoolwide environmental change.[34]

13.2.3.6 The Afterschool Program: A Resource for Promoting Nutrition and Physical Activity

Given reductions in physical education during the school day, it is increasingly important to engage students in physical activity during afterschool hours. Afterschool programs can be a venue for conveying important messages regarding nutrition and physical activity via hands-on activities and curricula. For many youth, the afterschool hours consist of sedentary behaviors and excessive snacking. In contrast, youth who participate in structured afterschool programming may engage in a variety of activities that promote healthy lifestyles, academic achievement, and social development. These programs are an opportunity for influential adults and peers to role-model healthy eating and physical activities for youth. Free from school curriculum constraints, afterschool programs have a unique quality that encourages youth to learn new skills and information through innovative and engaging practices (Table 13.5).[44]

There is a strong need for such engaging afterschool programs for families in the U.S. While 6.5 million K-12 children (11%) participate in afterschool programs, an additional 15 million families report their child would participate, if a quality program were available in their community.[45] The need for afterschool programs for school-age children is especially apparent among low-income families where both parents or a single parent is working.[44] Only 14% of children ages 5 to 12 with employed mothers attend afterschool programs, while an additional 15% are involved in alternative enrichment activities or lessons.[46] It is estimated that 18% of children ages 5 and 14 regularly spend afterschool hours without the supervision of an adult.[47] For these children, afterschool programs are a missed opportunity for education, social development, enrichment activities, and health promotion.

TABLE 13.5
Health Promotion in Afterschool Programs

Educate youth on importance of nutrition and physical activity via creative curriculums
Reduce sedentary behaviors and excessive snacking among youth
Facilitate role-modeling of healthy eating and physical activities for youth

TABLE 13.6
Afterschool Providers

Private Organizations (ex: YMCA, Boys and Girls Clubs)
Municipal (Community Centers)
Schools
Local Nonprofits
Churches
Community Health Centers

Afterschool providers include a broad variety of organizations and government divisions. Of the 94 cities sampled in the 2003 U.S. Conference of Mayor's on Afterschool Programs, 89% of cities offered afterschool programs in schools, 63% in community centers, 57% in other public or private facilities, and 31% in childcare centers. Eight of the 94 cities had church-based programs. In 72% of the cities, afterschool programs were operated by the city government.[48] Of cities surveyed, 84% contained afterschool programs in which snacks were served to participants (Table 13.6).

Afterschool programs greatly vary in content of activities, size and type of facilities, class size, staff training, and child-to-staff ratios.[46] According to the Harvard Family Research Project, of the 27 afterschool programs surveyed from their 2003 database, only approximately 50% offered structured sports or recreation while nearly all offered academic support for youth.[49] With rising academic pressures on students, the priority of many afterschool programs may be to provide academic support rather than alternative enrichment activities. As with schools, afterschool programs may face challenges in incorporating organized physical activity into their structure. Accordingly, the afterschool time remains an underutilized resource for supporting youth in nutrition education and physical activity.

Various strategies can be employed to incorporate nutrition education and physical activity into existing afterschool programs. Recognizing that youth lacking experience in sports may shy away from larger afterschool programs, communities must strive to offer smaller, mentor-based programs promoting healthy lifestyles among youths who face additional social or physical barriers to participation. A community's afterschool programs should offer a range of physical activities such that youth with minimal sports skills, not just competitive athletes, are empowered to participate (Table 13.7).

TABLE 13.7
Strategies for Promoting Healthy Lifestyles in Afterschool Programs

Encourage established afterschool providers to incorporate structured physical activity and nutrition education into their program structure
Develop afterschool programs that specialize in culturally appropriate nutrition and physical activity promotion for youth populations disproportionately affected by overweight
Launch afterschool programs that specifically support overweight youth in developing the skills necessary to be physically active and eat healthily

13.2.3.6.1 Strategy 1: Encourage Established Afterschool Providers to Incorporate Structured Physical Activity and Nutrition Education into Their Program Structure

Afterschool programs that are currently serving youth can build or strengthen components of their curriculum dedicated to promoting healthy lifestyles among youth. While the majority of youth participating in these programs may not be overweight, all youth can benefit from creative physical and nutrition activities. This strategy employs a large-scale, broad prevention effort to guide youth in developing and sustaining healthy habits that can ultimately prevent the onset of overweight and associated chronic diseases. The goal is not to overshadow the fundamental objectives of these existing afterschool programs; an academic-enrichment program should continue to focus on boosting academic performance in youth. Rather, the goal is to complement the established academic enrichment with health promotion that will enable the youth to better reach their academic goals.[44] In addition to incorporating health-based activities, afterschool programs that offer snacks to participants are in a key position to provide youth with appealing, healthy alternatives to the usual high-fat, salt, and sugar snacks consumed by youth. The attitude of afterschool program staff toward the health-promoting activities and snacks is crucial to the success of these components. Staff who actively participate in the nutrition and physical activities as well as try new healthy snacks offered will serve as influential role models for youth.

The process of incorporating new activities into a long-standing programs infrastructure may appear daunting for afterschool program administrators and staff. Use of existing standards and training tools recently developed can aid programs with this process by providing target goals as well as content and curriculums for nutrition and physical activities. Several organizations have developed a series of resources to assist other programs in developing and implementing health-based activities. California Adolescent Nutrition and Fitness (CANfit) is one organization that provides training and technical assistance to youth-serving organizations on culturally appropriate nutrition and physical activity education. Since 1993, CANfit has awarded grants to community organizations that have implemented a variety of nutrition and physical activity programs specifically focusing on low-income, multiethnic youth. They have developed the CANfit Super Manual, a comprehensive guide created to enable youth service providers to effectively incorporate nutrition and physical activity into their programming. This manual contains nutrition and fitness research and curricula.[50] The Nutrition and Fitness for Life Program at the Boston Medical Center is in the process of piloting its "Healthy Me" curriculum with several afterschool providers in the Boston area. The "Healthy Me" resource consists of a series of nutrition and physical activities along with a self-assessment tool to encourage afterschool providers to evaluate their program environment and brainstorm changes to promote activity and healthy eating in their communities.[51]

One national afterschool provider, the Boys and Girls Clubs of America, has developed a new component to more strongly promote physical activity and nutrition titled "Triple Play" (Table 13.8).[52]

TABLE 13.8
Boys and Girls Clubs: "Triple Play"

Triple Play is an initiative of the Boys and Girls Clubs designed to improve participants' knowledge of healthy habits, good nutrition, and physical fitness; increase the amount of physical activity; and foster positive social development. Program components include daily physical challenges, sports clubs, sports leadership camps, healthy habits nutrition curriculum, games, and social recreation.

Source: Boys and Girls Clubs, 2006.

13.2.3.6.2 Strategy 2: Develop Afterschool Programs That Specialize in Culturally Appropriate Nutrition and Physical Activity Promotion for Youth Populations Disproportionately Affected by Overweight

As previously discussed, pediatric overweight disproportionately affects minorities in the U.S. Between 1999 and 2002, 21% of non-Hispanic black and 23% of Mexican-American adolescents ages 12–19 were overweight compared with 14% non-Hispanic white adolescents.[53] These statistics warrant the development of afterschool programs focusing on prevention of overweight in youth populations most at risk. Prevention efforts for these youth should be rooted in communities with large populations of disproportionately affected minorities. To most effectively role-model healthy behaviors, afterschool program staff should reflect the culture of the community served and should reside locally. In addition, programs should engage the broader community in promoting health as much as possible. For example, an afterschool program may showcase the nutrition and physical activities they have learned via a community health fair or family day. Two examples of afterschool program models promoting healthy eating and increased physical activity among minority youth include the Mission Girls Program and the Girls Health Enrichment Multi-Site Study (GEMS) "Girlfriends for Keeps" program (Tables 13.9 and 13.10).[50,54]

TABLE 13.9
The Mission Girls Program

The Mission Girls Program educates low-income Latina girls about nutrition, fitness, and body image, utilizing the Latina-specific ritual of Quincinera. Activities include culturally appropriate weekly healthy cooking classes; physical activities including Latin dancing, sports, fitness games, hiking, swimming, and yoga. Girls also completed a peer education project in which they were trained to lead classes on healthy lifestyles in San Francisco middle schools[50]

Source: CANfit program.

TABLE 13.10
GEMS: "Girlfriends for Keeps"

The Girls Health Enrichment Multisite Studies (GEMS) included a pilot community-based obesity prevention afterschool program for African-American girls aged 8–10 yr. The 12-week program focused on increasing physical activity and healthy eating. Family education events were held to foster parent involvement. This afterschool model for obesity prevention was well-received, as evidenced by strong attendance rates and high reported satisfaction levels among participants.[54]

13.2.3.6.3 Strategy 3: Launch Afterschool Programs That Specifically Support Overweight Youth in Developing the Skills Necessary to Be Physically Active and Eat Healthily

While all youth face barriers to attending afterschool programs (transportation, safety, and cost), youth who are overweight may face additional social and physical barriers to participating in afterschool programs with structured or, even more so, unstructured sports and recreation. Although overweight youth may benefit from afterschool physical activity, a variety of barriers may hinder their participation. Low-income families may face greater obstacles affording program fees for their children. In addition, overweight children with disabilities may require specialized transportation that is not available or affordable. A history of social isolation or teasing may deter overweight youth from participating in afterschool group-based activities. Therefore, overweight youth may require additional support through smaller afterschool programs that integrate physical activity and health education in a safe, comfortable setting. An example of a pilot community-based afterschool program specifically supporting overweight girls is the FANtastic Girls Program developed by the Nutrition and Fitness for Life Program at the Boston Medical Center (Table 13.11).

While the afterschool hours present a key opportunity to promote healthy eating and increased physical activity, communities face common challenges in incorporating additional activities into existing program infrastructures and launching new programs that broaden the population of youth served (Table 13.12).

Ideally, all afterschool programs would have easy access to both recreational spaces, such as youth-friendly swimming pools and gyms, and safe cooking facilities.

TABLE 13.11
FANtastic Girls (Fitness and Nutrition) Program

The FANtastic Girls Program is an afterschool program developed to support overweight girls in achieving and maintaining healthy weights through increased physical activity and healthy eating. The 12-wk program consists of peer-led nutrition education and noncompetitive physical activities, recreational trips, and family nutrition nights. The program serves as a launching point, providing each participant with information on affordable, appealing afterschool programs in their neighborhoods upon the last session.[19]

TABLE 13.12
Challenges to Health Promotion in Afterschool Programs

Limited facilities
High turnover of staff
Low participant attendance

Yet, in reality, afterschool programs may be faced with inadequate classrooms and no access to larger rooms or physical recreational facilities. Afterschool programs with such hurdles may either seek out physical activity and nutrition curriculums specifically designed for afterschool programs with only classroom space, such as Healthy Me,[51] or may advocate for access to local recreational facilities. For example, an afterschool provider may try to partner with a local school to keep the school's gyms open during afterschool hours for organized programming. The benefits of expanding school facilities to afterschool programs include a heightened sense of community and reduction in youth crime. As schools in the U.S. are now being built or modified, communities may have the opportunity to better design schools that can accommodate afterschool programming.[21]

Another challenge posed to afterschool programs expanding their curriculums for health promotion is the high staff turnover rate. Every year, afterschool programs lose two of every six program staff members to turnover, thus creating constant pressure to hire and train new staff.[55] The retention of program staff is crucial to maintain high-quality programs and to expand the services and components of any afterschool program. The California School-Age Consortium is currently addressing the issue of staff turnover through its "Partners to Advance Training and Hiring of Workers in Afterschool Youth Services" (PATHWAYS) program. The PATHWAYS program recruits local qualified individuals for jobs in local afterschool programs while simultaneously providing them with the training and skills they need to succeed. Young adults are recruited from local job placement services, screened for likely success as afterschool workers, enrolled in preparation classes at a local community college, recruited by local partnering afterschool providers in need of staff, and enrolled in career development programs at a community college that will lead to a degree or certification in education or related fields.[56] By investing in the professional development of their staff, afterschool program providers can better retain talented staff members, and thus more easily expand the quality and depth of their program curricula to incorporate health promotion.

All afterschool programs face challenges in attendance and retention of participants, especially among older youth. While a variety of factors may contribute to poor attendance — cost, transportation, and neighborhood safety — enhancing program appeal to youth will only improve the family's motivation to enable their children to attend the program. Some youth may have taken health and physical education in school and may already have negative attitudes toward these health topics. It is crucial that the afterschool program present physical activity and nutrition education in hands-on, creative ways that differ from more traditional school-based curricula. One strategy for increasing the appeal of nutrition education in afterschool programs is the use of peer leaders to implement the health-promoting activities. Peer-led health interventions make a positive impact on young people's skills, confidence, and sense of efficacy.[56] Evaluation of the FANtastic Girls Program found that employing peer leaders as health educators may increase the acceptability and receptivity of an afterschool program focusing on promotion of healthy eating and physical activity among overweight minority girls.[19] Peer leader programs can give youth a sense of empowerment and influence over program activities, thus inspiring a higher degree of investment among older adolescents. In addition, the mentoring peer leaders provide to younger children may give the additional personal support younger children need to remain engaged in an afterschool program.

13.2.3.7 Health Care Providers: Advocating for Afterschool Programs

Health care providers can play a key role in enabling afterschool programs to effectively promote healthy eating and increased physical activity in their communities by encouraging youth attendance. A team of health care providers can become familiar with the local afterschool providers, accessing information regarding local YMCAs, Boys and Girls Clubs, and municipal community centers via the Internet. Clinics may ask for student volunteers to survey the area for existing afterschool programs, visit sites, and generate more in-depth lists of neighborhood afterschool programs. By discussing afterschool opportunities with families, health care providers are supporting local afterschool programs in broadening the youth populations they serve (Table 13.13).

13.2.4 Community-Based Religious Organizations

Families find support for raising healthy children in many community-based organizations. Families often find support and guidance on health issues in religious institutions. Low-income and minority communities often rely heavily on faith communities to provide social supports and needed services. In addition to religious and ethical instruction, these institutions often provide important family supports including afterschool care, food pantries, and health education. Health promotion organizations have increasingly looked outside of traditional health-focused community organizations to find partners for health education, behavior change, and advocacy. Partnerships have been built with religious institutions in order to better reach the public and to utilize the influence of religious leaders to support

TABLE 13.13
Health Care Providers Advocating for Afterschool Programs

Inquire about how patients spend their afterschool hours
Discuss the benefits of afterschool programs with patients and families
Gain familiarity with local afterschool program providers
Educate patients on afterschool opportunities in their neighborhood

health-behavior change. Where there is a commonality of interest and mutual understanding, these projects have a higher likelihood of success. Working with religious institutions to promote adolescent and youth health is an often untapped resource. Although not directly youth focused, the North Carolina Black Churches United for Better Health Project provides an example of a community-based health intervention aimed at increasing fruit and vegetable consumption for cancer and chronic disease prevention.[57] This project was supported by the National Cancer Institute. This multicomponent intervention within 24 black churches from five rural counties in eastern North Carolina included a variety of activities including garden and fruit tree planning, individualized health communications with members, congregation-wide educational materials, cooking and food-preserving classes, recipe tasting and cookbook development, and serving fruits and vegetables at church functions. The project demonstrated significant improvements in fruit and vegetable consumption and associated psychosocial measures, which were maintained during a 2-yr period. Another program, Healthy Body/Healthy Spirit utilized motivational interviewing and culturally tailored self-help nutrition and physical activity interventions in African-American church settings.[58] Motivational interviewing (see Chapter 3) is an individual-centered technique for enhancing a person's motivation for change by helping him or her to explore and resolve their ambivalence about change.[59] The cultural interventions included culture-based approaches to increase physical activity and increase fruit and vegetable consumption. Religious institutions often routinely offer special programming for youth, including social clubs, liturgical dance classes, sports teams, community service activities, and child-care, school, and afterschool programs that provide opportunities to support healthy lifestyles for youth.

13.2.5 Media and Advertising

A Kaiser Family Foundation study found that the total amount of recreational media content young people are exposed to each day has increased by more than an hour over the past 5 yr, with most of the increase coming from video games and computers.[20] While the actual number of hours devoted to media use has remained constant at just under 6.5 hr/d, the use of multiple media outlets at once, or multitasking, means more media exposure. Electronic media use exceeds the amount of time children spending doing anything else besides sleeping. Studies have found that children who watch more than 4 hr of television per day had significantly greater body mass index (BMI), compared with those watching fewer than 2 hr/d.[60] Having a television located in the bedroom has been reported to be a strong predictor of childhood overweight.[61] In response to these and other concerns, the American Academy of Pediatrics recommends the limitation of television and video time to a maximum of 2 hr/d.[62]

13.2.5.1 Advertising

Commercial advertising of food and beverages is a high-stakes industry, with more than $11 billion in industry expenditures in 2004, including $5 billion for television advertising.[63] Marketing vehicles include television, product placement, character licensing, special events, and in-school activities, among others. Children and youth are a special target for marketing and advertising. Marketing to children begins early in life, with a goal of developing early product loyalty. Yet before age 8 and up to age 11, children may not be able to discriminate commercial from noncommercial content or to attribute persuasive intent in advertising. Because many of the foods and beverages advertised are high in calories and low in nutrients, there is concern that marketing practices are adversely impacting the health of children and youth. The Institute of Medicine expert panel on food marketing to children and youth concluded that there is strong evidence that television advertising affects the preferences, purchase requests, and short-term consumption of foods and beverages of children ages 2–11 yr.[63] Additionally, strong evidence was found of a statistical association between television advertising of food and beverages on adiposity in children aged 2–11 yr and teens aged 12–18 yr.[63] Low-income and minority communities are especially vulnerable to marketing of unhealthy food items.[64] High rates of television viewing among ethnic minority children (black youth spends 4 hr/d; Hispanic youth 3.38 hr/d) compared to white youth (Caucasian youth spends 2.75 hr/d) leads to more advertising exposure.[20] Marketing sectors also receive differing content messages. A study of food marketing messages targeting the African-American market versus the general market found more food commercials appeared during African-American programs than general market programs, and more of these food commercials were for high fat foods.[65,66] Health care providers have important roles to play in helping children and families resist the pressures placed to consume excess amounts of food and make unhealthy food choices. Additionally, advocacy is needed to encourage government and industry to make far-reaching changes in practices and policies that adversely affect children's health (Table 13.14).

13.2.6 The Built Environment

The built environment has a profound impact on health. Heart disease, diabetes, obesity, asthma, and depression are diseases that can be moderated by the design of the human environment.[67] Following the needs of the automobile, urban sprawl has become ubi-quitous in planning. Larger, older cities face tough choices to invest in public

TABLE 13.14
Conclusions of the IOM Expert Panel on Food Marketing to Children and Youth

Food and beverage marketing influences the diets and health of children and youth
Marketing practices geared to children and youth contribute to an environment that puts their health at risk
Food and beverage companies, restaurants, and marketers have underutilized potential to devote creativity and resources to develop and promote food, beverages, and meals that support healthful diets for children and youth
Achieving healthful diets for children and youth will require sustained, multisectoral, and integrated efforts that include industry leadership and initiative
Public policy programs and incentives do not currently have the support or authority to address many of the current and emerging marketing practices that influence the diets of children and youth[63]

transportation and walkable/bikeable neighborhoods rather than widening expressways. Environmental design may make it easier or more difficult for youth to walk and bike to school or work. National transportation surveys have found a 50% decrease in walking and bicycling to school among children aged 5 to 15 from 1977 to 2001.[68] From 1995 to 2001, there was a modest increase of 4.6% in trips made to school by walking. Safe routes to school programs aim to accelerate this trend of increased walking to school.[69] These programs may require infrastructure supports like improved sidewalks, street-crossing supports, designated bicycle lanes, and improved public safety, all of which improve overall neighborhood quality and may support children and families to be more active beyond the school day. Planning and zoning decisions also have an impact on children's physical activity patterns. Planning decisions that place retail establishments in walkable proximity to population centers and discourage use of cars for shopping support increased physical activity. Locating parks, green spaces, and newly constructed schools in walkable distances to large numbers of youth rather than in locations that require car or bus transportation increase the likelihood of youth accessing these resources through walking. Zoning codes may need to be changed to encourage multiuse land development patterns, which make it possible to work, shop, and go to school within walking distance of people's homes.[68] In new construction, elevators may be prominently located while stairs are hidden, promoting passive travel between floors. Recommendations for action from the National Center for Environmental Health of the Centers for Disease Control and Prevention for the public health sector to create a healthier environment are described (Table 13.15).[67]

13.2.7 Community Food Resources

The relationship between access to food resources and weight status is a complex one. Both underweight and overweight may be related to food insecurity. Food-insecure households may not have access to adequate nutritious food for a healthy diet. This may be because they lack sufficient financial resources or because reliable sources of affordable healthy food are not available. In 2004, 13.5 million American households were food insecure.[71] Rates of food insecurity are highest among low-income families, although families above the official poverty line may also be food insecure. Food-insecure houseolds with incomes below the official poverty line numbered 36.8% in 2004.[70]

TABLE 13.15
Recommendations for Action: National Center for Environmental Health of the CDC

Support research to determine the impact that changes in the built environment can have on public health, such as the addition of green space, sidewalks, and bike paths, and the reduction in impervious surfaces
Participate in local planning processes such as comprehensive planning meetings, zoning hearings, and urban planning workshops
Work with planners and other land-use professionals to provide them with the strong public health arguments they need to support "smart-growth" designs and initiatives[67]

Overall, households with children reported food insecurity at about double the rate for households without children (17.6% vs. 8.9%). Since 1999, there has been a steady increase in the number of food-insecure households in the U.S.

Among women, a positive association between food insecurity and overweight has been found.[71,72] The relationship between food insecurity and overweight status remains somewhat ambiguous in children and adolescents. In a 1994 pediatric case study, Dietz hypothesized that episodic food shortages may cause increased body fat.[73] A recent study of kindergarten children found that low income but not food insecurity was a predictor of overweight status in children. In this study, there was no difference between the weight status of children from food-secure and food-insecure households.[74] Researchers have suggested that in households with food insecurity, young children may be selectively protected.[75] This explanation was confirmed, utilizing nationally representative data on food intake.[76]

Studies of purchasing patterns of low-income families have shown that food-insecure families purchase a limited variety of cheap, energy-dense foods high in fat, and added sweeteners and poor in nutritional quality. Additionally, these households reduce their consumption of fresh fruits and vegetables, whole grains, low-fat dairy, fish, and vegetable protein. A contributor to these purchasing practices may be that these energy-dense diets are more affordable than are healthier diets based on lean meats, fish, fresh vegetables, and fruit.[76] Families participating in the food stamp program receive a supportive service that lessens the impact of poverty on food insecurity. Clinicians should facilitate the enrollment of eligible families into nutrition programs like food stamps and WIC, and serve as advocates to ensure maximal access by families that would benefit from these services. However, food stamp participation may not be sufficient to meet the costs of purchasing a healthy diet.[77]

In young children, a dose–response relationship has been seen between fair/poor health status and severity of food insecurity.[78] Thus health practitioners must concern themselves with efforts to ensure adequate access to healthy foods to pediatric patients.

Increasing the availability and affordability of healthy foods for food-insecure families are important areas of environmental change. Some ways to increase access to healthy foods at the community level include improving access to government food programs, decreasing food prices through special price supports, assisting stores, and markets in making produce more available, establishing farmers' markets, and increasing the number of community gardens.

13.2.8 Advocacy

The American Academy of Pediatrics Policy Statement on Prevention of Pediatric Overweight and Obesity states "as leaders in their communities, pediatricians can be effective advocates for health- and fitness-promoting programs and policies."[63] Areas of advocacy may include but are not limited to:

- Working with local communities and schools to support needed counseling and school health services, increased access to quality physical education programs, and changes in school food policies to assure access to healthy foods
- Support for needed funding for research to test prevention strategies and develop effective treatment approaches

Legislation to improve food security and access to healthful foods in homes, schools, and communities
Legislation to support walkable and bikeable communities

Clinician scholars play a pivotal role in providing background research to support advocacy efforts. One example of such background research is the "Real Cost of a Healthy Diet" study conducted at Boston Medical Center.[77] By sampling food costs across neighborhoods and among differing-sized stores, researchers were able to show that a family of four receiving the maximum Food Stamp allotment would be unable to purchase either the foods comprising the U.S. Department of Agriculture Thrifty Food Plan meal pattern (with a monthly deficit of $27) or a healthier diet based on the American Heart Association dietary recommendations (with a monthly deficit of $148). This information was then used to advocate for improved access to affordable and healthy foods at the local and national level.

Advocacy efforts can include, among others, letter writing, news editorials, and public testimony. They can be local, regional, national, or international in scope. Advocacy can be done as an individual, as a singular professional association, or as part of larger coalitions. There is a place for all forms of advocacy in a well-coordinated effort. Local medical and public health associations are an important resource available to clinicians as they develop an advocacy agenda related to overweight in children. The Massachusetts Public Health Association has developed a tool kit available online to assist community organizations and individuals, including clinicians, in advocating for positive changes to promote good nutrition in schools.[79] This resource can be found at the Website http://www.mphaweb.org. Many important policies and practices need to be changed at the national and even international levels to make the broad impact needed to curb the epidemic of childhood obesity. Working within national organizations and collaboratively across national and international organizations will give health care providers opportunities to join with others to create health-promoting environments and care systems.

13.3 CONCLUSION

The scope of work needed to turn the tide on childhood obesity at the community level is very broad. Clinicians are needed to support children and families at every level of the socioecological model. Pediatric clinicians help the individual child and family implement health-promoting behavior changes as part of the clinical scope of practice. Clinicians may help families establish new practices, policies, and traditions such as family walks and limitations on television viewing. Support for individual and family health behavior change often takes place in the health practitioner's office. The pediatric clinician has an equally large role to play in helping families access food, nutrition, and physical activity resources in their community. Where those resources are less than optimal, the clinician may serve as a change agent to help improve the quality of these resources. School and afterschool programs, community social and religious institutions, and media outlets and policy change efforts at the local, state, and national level are all areas that benefit from direct involvement by pediatric clinicians interested in the well-being of their overweight and obese patients.

REFERENCES

1. McElray, K.R. et al. An ecological perspective on health promotion programs. *Health Ed Quarterly* 15,351–377, 1988.
2. Epstein, L.H. et al. Ten-year outcomes of behavioral family-based treatment for childhood obesity. *Health Psych* 13,373, 1994.
3. Birch, L. and Fisher, J. Development of eating behaviors among children and adolescents. *J Peds* 101,539, 1998.
4. Robinson, T.N. et al. Is parental control over children's eating associated with childhood obesity? Results from a population-based sample of third graders. *Obes Res* 9,306, 2001.
5. Dietz, W.H. and Gortmaker, S.L. Preventing obesity in children and adolescents. *Annu Rev Public Health* 22,337, 2001.
6. Gillman, M.W. et al. Family dinner and diet quality among older children and adolescents. *Arch Fam Med* 9,235, 2000.
7. Birch, L.L. and Davison, K.K. Family environmental factors influencing the developing behavioral controls of food intake and childhood overweight. *Pediatr Clin North Am* 48,893, 2001.
8. Wiecha, J.L. et al. Household television access: associations with screen time, reading, and homework among youth. *Amb Pediatr* 1,244, 2001.
9. Task Force on Community Preventive Services. Recommendations to increase physical activity in communities. *Am J Prev Med* 22,67S, 2002.
10. Koplan, J.P., Liverman, C.T., and Kraak, V.I. (eds.) *Preventing Childhood Obesity: Health in the Balance.* Chapter 8: Home. Institute of Medicine. The National Academies Press, Washington, DC, 2005.
11. We Can! (Ways to Enhance Children's Activity and Nutrition) project. Accessed: www.nhlbi.nih.gov/health/public/heart/obesity/wecan/.
12. Morris, V. et al. Cultural approach to utilizing the National Institutes of Health's *WE CAN!* (Ways to Enhance Children's Activity& Nutrition) Parent Education Curriculum. Accepted for poster session. American Public Health Association 134th Annual Meeting and Exposition, Boston, MA, November 2006.
13. Carroll, G.B., Hebert, D.M., and Foy, J.M. Youth action strategies in violence prevention. *J Adolesc Health* 25(1),7–13, 1999.
14. Gibson, P.G., Shah, S., and Mamoon, A.H. Peer-led asthma education for adolescents: impact evaluation. *J Adolesc Health* 22,66–72, 1998.
15. Holden, D.J. et al. Conceptualizing youth empowerment within tobacco control. *Health Educ Behav* 31,548, 2004.
16. Story, M. et al. Peer-led, school-based nutrition education for young adolescents: feasibility and process evaluation of the TEENS study. *J Sch Health* 72,121, 2002.
17. French, S.A. et al. An environmental intervention to promote lower-fat food choices in secondary schools: outcomes of the TACOS study. *Am J Pub Health* 94,1507, 2004.
18. Fisher, L.A. et al. Peer-led alcohol education program: a pharmacy student-led program for seventh graders. *J Am Pharm Assoc* 40,82, 2000.
19. Rao, G. et al. FANtastic Girls: a community intervention to reduce overweight among adolescents in Boston. *J Urban Health. Supplement* 82(2), 2005.
20. Robertss, D.F., Foehr, U.G., and Rideout, V. Generation M: Media in the Lives of 8-18 Year-Olds. A Kaiser Family Foundation Study. March 2005. Accessed: http:// www.kff.org/entmedia/upload/Generation-M-Media-in-the-Lives-of-8-18-Year-Olds-Report.pdf.

21. Koplan, J.P., Liverman, C.T., and Kraak, V.I. (eds.) *Preventing Childhood Obesity: Health in the Balance.* Chapter 7: Schools. Institute of Medicine. National Academies Press, Washington, DC, 2005.
22. Haskins, R., Paxson, C., and Donahue, E. Fighting obesity in the public schools. Policy brief. *Future Child.* Spring 2006. Accessed: http://www.futureofchildren.org/.
23. Wechsler, H. et al. The role of schools in preventing childhood obesity. *State Ed Standard* 5,5, 2004.
24. Moag-Stahlberg, A. Creating and evaluating school-based initiatives to improve nutrition and physical activity. *State Ed Standard* 5,43, 2004.
25. Centers for Disease Control and Prevention. Ten Strategies for Promoting Physical Activity, Healthy Eating, and a Tobacco-Free Lifestyle Through School Health Programs. 2003. Accessed: http://www.cdc.gov/healthyyouth/putlications/pdf/ten_strategies.pdf.
26. National School Lunch Program. Participation Summary. Data as of February 27, 2006. Accessed: http://www.fns.usda.gov/pd/slsummar.htm.
27. Dwyer, J. The school nutrition dietary assessment study. *AJCN* 61,173S, 1995.
28. U.S. Department of Agriculture, Food and Nutrition Service, Office of Analysis, Nutrition and Evaluation, Children's Diets in the Mid-1990s. Dietary Intake and Its Relationship with School Meal Participation, CN-01-CD1, by Phil Gleason and Carol Suitor. Project Officer, Ed Herzog, Alexandria, VA: 2001. Accessed: http://www.fns.usda.gov/oane/MENU/Published/CNP/FILES/ChilDiet.pdf.
29. Stables, G.J. et al. Small school-based effectiveness trials increase vegetable and fruit consumption among youth. *J Am Diet Assoc* 105,252, 2005.
30. Story, M et al. Peer-led, school-based nutrition education for young adolescents: feasibility and process evaluation of the TEENS study. *J Sch Health* 72,121, 2002.
31. Gortmaker, S.L. et al. Impact of a school-based interdisciplinary intervention on diet and physical activity among urban primary school children: eat well and keep moving. *Arch Pediatr Adolesc Med* 153,975, 1999.
32. Gortmaker, S.L. et al. Reducing obesity via a school-based interdisciplinary intervention among youth: planet health. *Arch Pediatr Adolesc Med* 153,409, 1999.
33. Snyder, P. et al. The pathways study: a model for lowering the fat in school meals. *Am J Clin Nutr* 69,810S, 1999.
34. Hoelscher, D.M. et al. School-based health education programs can be maintained over time: results from the CATCH institutionalization study. *Prev Med* 38,594, 2004.
35. National Association for Sport and Physical Education. Physical Activity for Children: A Statement of Guidelines for Children Ages 5-12, 2nd edition. Accessed: http://aahperd.org/naspe/template.cfm?template=ns_children.html.
36. The Robert Wood Johnson Foundation: Healthy Schools for Healthy Kids. Accessed http://www.rwj.org.
37. Grunbaum, J.A. et al. Youth risk behavior surveillance — United States, 2003. *Morb Mortal Wkly Rep* 533,3536, 2004.
38. Kim, S.Y.S. et al. Decline in physical activity in black girls and white girls during adolescence. *N Engl J Med* 347,709, 2002.
39. Wechsler, H. et al. The role of schools in preventing childhood obesity. *State Ed Standard* 5,5, 2004.
40. Sallis, J.F. et al. The effects of a 2-year physical education program (SPARK) on physical activity and fitness in elementary school students. Sports, Play and Active Recreation for Kids. *Am J Public Health* 87,1328, 1997.
41. McKenzie, T.L. et al. School physical education: effect of the Child and Adolescent Trial for Cardiovascular Health. *Prev Med* 25,423, 1996. Accessed: http://www.cdc.gov/healthyyouth/putlications/pdf/ten_strategies.pdf.

42. Bureau of Transportation Statistics. National Household Travel Survey (Internet). Washington, D.C.: U.S. Department of Transportation, 2003.
43. Centers for Disease Control and Prevention. Preventing Chronic Disease: Public Health Research, Practice and Policy. 2,2005 Accessed: www.cdc.gov/pcd/issues/2005/apr/04_0039.htm.
44. California Adolescent Nutrition and Fitness Program. *Promoting Health and Preventing Obesity in After School Programs: Critical Issues to Consider.* Appendix A: CANFIT Guidelines for After School Program Content. 1,2004.
45. The Afterschool Alliance. Working Families and America: Special Report from America after 3 pm. A household survey on afterschool in America. 2004. Accessed: http://www.afterschoolalliance.org/press_archives/Working_Families_Rpt.pdf
46. Vandell, D.L. and Shumow, L. After-school child care programs. *Future Child* 9, 26, 1999.
47. Smith, K. Who's Minding the Kids? Child Care Arrangement. *Current Population Reports.* United States Census Bureau. October, 2000. Accessed: http://www.census.gov/prod/2000pubs/p70-70.pdf.
48. The United States Conference of Mayors. Afterschool Programs in Cities across the United States. 2003. Accessed: http://www.usmayors.org/USCM/uscm_projects_services/education/afterschoolreport03.pdf.
49. A Review of Activity Implementation in Out-of-Time Programs. Harvard Family Research Project. 2,2003. Accessed: http://www.gse.harvard.edu/hfrp/content/projects/afterschool/resources/snapshot2.pdf.
50. California Adolescent Nutrition and Fitness Program. Mission and Components. Accessed: http://www.canfit.org.
51. Morris, V. et al. Healthy Me: A nutrition and physical activity curriculum for after school programs, Nutrition and Fitness for Life Program, Boston Medical Center, unpublished.
52. Boys and Girls Clubs of America. Triple Play: A Game Plan for Mind, Body, and Soul. Sports, Fitness, and Recreation. 2006. Accessed: http://www.bgca.org/programs/sportfitness.asp.
53. Centers for Disease Control and Prevention. National Center for Health Statistics: Prevalence of Overweight among Children and Adolescents: United States, 1999-202. Accessed: http://www.cdc.gov/nchs/products/pubs/pubd/hestats/overwght99.htm.
54. Story, M. et al. An afterschool obesity prevention program for African-American girls: The Minnesota GEMS pilot study. *Ethn Dis* 13,S1, 2003.
55. California School Age Consortium. The High Stakes of Afterschool Program Staff Turnover. Accessed: http://calsac.org/files_cms/PATHWAYS%20complete.pdf.
56. Turner, G. Peer support and young people's health. *J Adolesc* 22,567, 1999.
57. Campbell, M. et al. Fruit and vegetable consumption and prevention of cancer: The Black Churches United for Better Health project. *Am J Pub Health* 89,1390, 1999.
58. Resnicow K. et al. Healthy Body/Healthy Spirit: a church-based nutrition and physical activity intervention. *Health Ed Res* 17,562, 2002.
59. Rollnick, S. and Miller, W.R. What is motivational interviewing? *Behav Cognitize Psychother* 23,325, 1995.
60. Anderson, R.E. et al. Relationship of physical activity and television watching with body weight and level of fatness among children: results from the Third National Health and Nutrition Examination Survey. *JAMA* 79,938, 1998.
61. Dennison, B.A., Erb, T.A., and Jenkins, P.L. Television viewing and television in bedroom associated with overweight risk among low-income preschool children. *J Pediatr* 109,1028, 2002.
62. American Academy of Pediatrics. AAP Policy Statement. *J Pediatr* 112,424, 2003.

63. McGinnis, J.M., Gootman, J.A., and Kraak, V.I. (eds.) *Food Marketing to Children and Youth: Threat or Opportunity*: IOM, National Academies Press, Washington, DC 2006. Accessed: www.nap.edu/books/0309097134/html.
64. Kumanyika, S. and Grier, S. Targeting interventions for ethnic minority and low-income populations. *Future Child* 16,187,2006. Accessed: http://www.futureofchildren.org.
65. Tirodkar, M.A. and Jain, A. Food messages on African American television shows. *Am J Pub Health* 93,439, 2003.
66. Henderson, V.R. and Kelly, B. Food advertising in the age of obesity: content analysis of food advertising on general market and African American television. *J Nutr Educ Behav* 37,191, 2005.
67. Jackson, R.J. and Kochtitzky, C. Creating a Healthy Environment: The Impact of the Built Environment on Public Health, *Sprawl Watch Clearinghouse Monograph Series*, 2004. Accessed: http://www.sprawlwatch.org.
68. Strum, R. Childhood obesity—what we can learn from existing data on societal trends, part 2. *Prev Chronic Dis* (serial online) 2,1, 2005. Accessed: http://www.cdc.gov/pcd/issues/2005/apr/04_0039.htm.
69. Ham, S.A., Macera, C.A. and Lindley, C. Trends in walking for transportation in the United States, 1995 and 2001. *Prev Chronic Dis* (serial online) 2005 Oct (date cited). Available from: http://www.cdc.gov/pcd/issues/2005/oct/05_0138.htm.
70. Nord, M., Andrews, M., and Carson, S. Household food security in the United States, 2004, *Economic Research Service Report No. 11*, Washington, DC, October 2005. Accessed: www.ers.usda.gov/publications/err11.
71. Olson, C.M. Nutrition and health outcomes associated with food insecurity and hunger. *J Nutr* 129,521S, 1999.
72. Townsend, M.S. et al. Food insecurity is positively related to overweight in women. *J Nutr* 131,1738, 2001.
73. Dietz, W.H. Does hunger cause obesity? *J Pediatr* 95,766, 1995.
74. Rose, D. Economic determinants and dietary consequences of food insecurity in the United States. *J Nutr* 129,517S, 1999.
75. Radimer, K.L. et al. Understanding hunger and developing indicators to assess it in women and children. *J Nutr Educ* 24,36S, 1992.
76. Drewnowski, A. and Specter, S.E. Poverty and obesity: the role of energy density and energy costs. *Am J Clin Nutr* 79,6, 2004.
77. Neault, N. et al. The Real Cost of a Healthy Diet: Healthful Foods Are Out of Reach for Low-Income Families in Boston, Massachusetts. Report published by the Boston Medical Center Department of Pediatrics. Aug 2005. Available at: http://doc2.bumc.bu.edu/csnappublic/HealthyDiet_Aug2005.pdf).
78. Cook, J.T. et al. Food insecurity is associated with adverse health outcomes among human infants and toddlers. *J Nutr* 134,1432, 2004.
79. Massachusetts Public Health Association. Community action to change school food policy: an organizing kit. 2005. Accessed: http://www.mphaweb.org/home_food_policy_kit.pdf.

Index

A

B

C

D

E

N

O

P

Q

R

S